Emergency Surgery and Critical Care

Emergency Surgery and Critical Care

Editor: Gideon Allen

AMERICAN
MEDICAL PUBLISHERS
www.americanmedicalpublishers.com

AMERICAN
MEDICAL PUBLISHERS
www.americanmedicalpublishers.com

Cataloging-in-Publication Data

Emergency surgery and critical care / edited by Gideon Allen.
p. cm.
Includes bibliographical references and index.
ISBN 978-1-63927-488-8
1. Surgical emergencies. 2. Critical care medicine. 3. Medical emergencies. 4. Surgery.
5. Emergency medical services. 6. Intensive care units. I. Allen, Gideon.
RD93 .E44 2022
617. 026--dc23

American Medical Publishers,
41 Flatbush Avenue,
1st Floor, New York,
NY 11217, USA

ISBN 978-1-63927-488-8 (Hardback)

Contents

Preface

This book has been a concerted effort by a group of academicians, researchers and scientists, who have contributed their research works for the realization of the book. This book has materialized in the wake of emerging advancements and innovations in this field. Therefore, the need of the hour was to compile all the required researches and disseminate the knowledge to a broad spectrum of people comprising of students, researchers and specialists of the field.

A surgical emergency refers to a medical emergency which requires an immediate surgical intervention in order to save life and resolve the clinical issue. Emergency surgeries can be required in case of acute trauma, cardiothoracic emergencies, gynecological complications and acute gastrointestinal, neurological/ophthalmic and vascular conditions. This may include the treatment of acute airway obstruction, acute appendicitis, gastrointestinal perforation, acute mesenteric ischemia, retinal detachment, bleeding ectopic pregnancy, etc. Critical care is a dedicated branch of medicine aimed at the provision of medical care to patients with life-threatening conditions through life support and intensive monitoring. Mechanical ventilation, hemofiltration, total parenteral nutrition, etc. as well as frequent nursing assessments and nursing care are provided to critically ill patients. This book traces the progress of emergency surgery and critical care and highlights some of their key practices. It unfolds the innovative aspects of emergency surgery which will be crucial for the progress of the field in the future. It is meant for students who are looking for an elaborate reference text in these fields.

At the end of the preface, I would like to thank the authors for their brilliant chapters and the publisher for guiding us all-through the making of the book till its final stage. Also, I would like to thank my family for providing the support and encouragement throughout my academic career and research projects.

Editor

1

Primary omental torsion (POT): a review of literature and case report

Jacopo Andreuccetti*, Cecilia Ceribelli, Ottavia Manto, Massimo Chiaretti, Paolo Negro, Domenico Tuscano

Abstract

Eitel first described omental torsion in 1899, since then, fewer than 250 cases have been reported. Although omental torsion is rarely diagnosed preoperatively, knowledge of this pathology is important to the surgeon because it mimics the common causes of acute surgical abdomen. For this reason, in the absence of diagnosed preexisting abdominal pathology, including cysts, tumors, foci of intra-abdominal inflammation, postsurgical wounds or scarring, and hernial sacs, omental torsion still can represent a surprise. Explorative laparotomy represents the diagnostic and definitive therapeutic procedure. Presently laparoscopy is the first choice procedure.

Introduction

Omental Torsion (OT) is a condition in which a pedicle of the omental apron twists on its longer axis to such an extent that its vascularity is compromised. Eitel [1] in 1899 first reported a case of omental torsion unassociated with a hernia. Since that time many reports have appeared in the literature, notably that by Morris [2] in which 164 authentic cases of torsion of the omentum were gathered from 1905 to 1930. OT may be Primary Omental Torsion (POT) because a mobile, thicken segment of omentum rotates around a proximal fixed point in the absence of any associated or secondary intra-abdominal pathology. Morris [3] reported that, while POT may occur at any age, it most frequently occurs between 30 and 50 years (83 cases, 52.5%), the males are more commonly affected than females (ratio of 2:1), and that the Secondary Omental Torsion (SOT) is mostly associated with predisposing pathology (50.3%). Morris [2], Adam [3] and Barcia & Nelson [4] emphasized the fact that the hernias were of the right inguinal variety, were scrotal type, of long duration, easily reducible, and that they almost invariably contained omentum. In this condition, patients suffering from recurring abdominal pain may have temporary twists of the omentum. The "omental ball" and the omental fibrotic thickenings occasionally found, result from these recurring attacks of incomplete OT. The chronic changes occasionally found in the omentum in acute (complete) OT [5], seem to substantiate the occurrence of the recurring type of OT. A certain number of OT are caused by inflammatory foci within the abdominal cavity, which produce an inflammation by contiguity in the neighbouring omentum. This may be true in cases of mild or subsiding appendicitis or cholecystitis in which the original focus subsides, but the changes induced in the omentum persist. In conclusion POT is unipolar when the proximal omentum remains fixed and the other tongues are free. SOT is bipolar due to a fixation of the omental tongue both proximally to the colon and distally, subsequently to adhesions for pathological conditions.

Case Report

S. C., a retired man, aged 83, was admitted to our Hospital because of an intra-abdominal pain started a few days before in the absence of fever, vomiting or nausea. The patient felt a dull pain in right side of the abdomen for one day, he did not sleep during the subsequent night, then he was visited at home by his Practitioner who treated the patient pharmacologically. In the same day, when the abdominal pain became steady and dull, the patient was brought to First Aid Service of our University General Hospital. The Patient was affected by glaucoma, hypertension had a pace maker and had received right saphenectomy and right eye cataract interventions ten years before. At physical examination the abdomen appeared bloated, tenderly, with slow peristalsis, last evacuation the day before. There was moderate rigidity of the upper right side of the abdomen, with tenderness in the right and in the lower quadrants. At the admittance laboratory findings showed white blood

* Correspondence: jacopo.andreuccetti@gmail.com
Department of General Surgery and Organ Transplantation, "Sapienza" Università di Roma, Umberto I Policlinico di Roma, Rome, Italy

cells count 7,640/mmc with 81.6% polymorphonuclear cells, increasing at the next days evaluations (91.6% polymorphonuclear cells), alfa-1 seroproteins 10.8 g/dl and glycaemia 173 mg/dl. As this disease may mimic other surgical emergencies, extensive imaging studies were performed.

- Ultrasonography (US), which gave negative result,
- Computerized Tomography (CT) (Figure 1, 2) scan which showed an inhomogeneous, irregular edge profile mass of 38 × 30 × 25 cm of great omental appearance, localized at the right side, moreover, concentric distribution of fibrous and fatty folds converging radially toward the torsion with oedema of the fat tissue was evidenced.

The operation was performed on the third day after admittance, in improved metabolic conditions. After a healthy appendix was found, we did inspect the cecum for a perforated diverticulum, the terminal ileum was then examined for Meckel diverticulum and regional enteritis, the pelvic organs were inspected and palpated, gallbladder and duodenum were observed, mesentery was evaluated for mesenteric lymphadenitis, no peritoneal pedicle torsion was found inside the umbilicus. Then we did observe the "omental ball" of 18 × 13 × 6 cm in size, which was suspended by a pedicle twisted on its axis four times (Figure 3) and was easily resected. Our patient had an uneventful recovery and was discharged two days after. **Histology Findings**: omental pedicle of 18 × 13 × 6 cm in size, with lobed and cyanotic look. Evidence of hemorrhagic infarction and focal fat necrosis areas at the section. **Microscopic**: Omental tissue characterized by acute extensive hemorrhagic infarction and fat necrosis, with polymorph nuclear cells infiltration of vein vessels and focal necrosis areas.

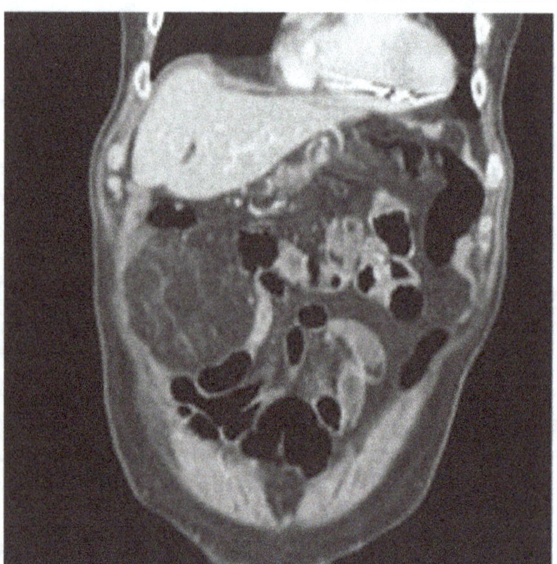

Figure 1 Computerized tomography (CT) scan shows a characteristic fat pattern. The vascular pedicle extends caudally and enters a large well-circumscribed heterogeneous fatty mass in the right lower quadrant and increased fat density.

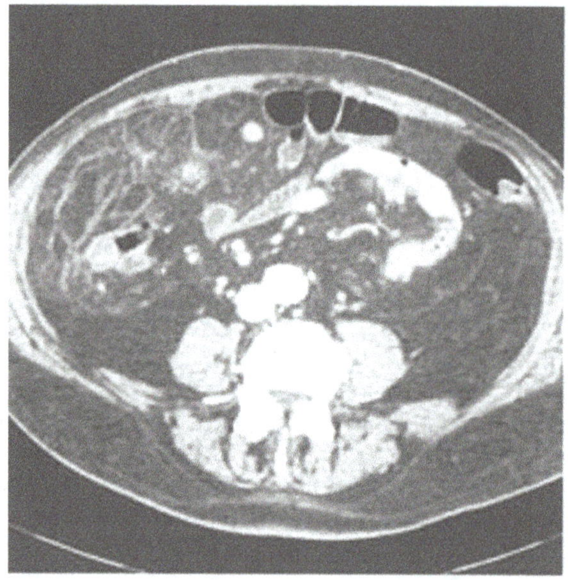

Figure 2 Computerized tomography (CT) scan shows the fat pattern. An omental vascular structure is seen at the center of concentrically layered streaks.

Discussion

POT is a rare pathological condition which presents with generic symptoms, and may mimic a variety of acute abdominal conditions such as cholecystitis, acute diverticulitis, appendicitis [6] and Meckel diverticulum

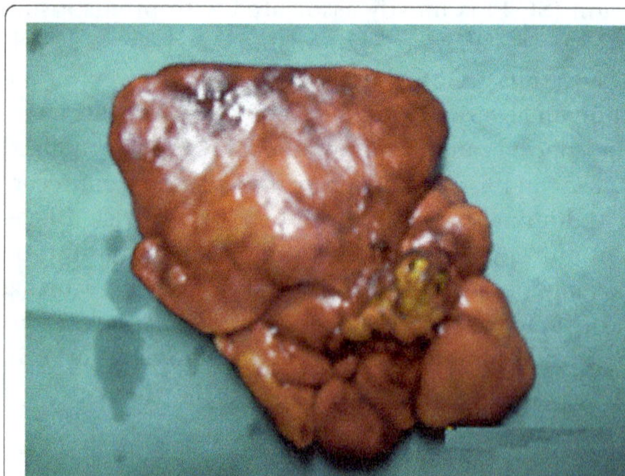

Figure 3 Example of POT. A normal appearing omentum was above the torsion point. You can see the vascular hanged and the torsion point with the distal thickened and congested omentum.

[7]. The pathogenesis of POT with infarction has not been established, however, some anatomical malformations and anomalies are recognized as predisposing factors to OT: presence in the great omentum of tongue-like projections and bifid and accessory omentum, anomalous vascular blood supply, other vascular anomalies that modify the weight of the omentum, vascular kinking, irregular omental pad, mostly in obese patients [8,9]. SOT is more common than POT and is associated with pre-existing abdominal pathologies, including cysts, tumours, foci of intra abdominal inflammations [10] and surgical wounds or scarring and hernial sacs [11]. Most cases of SOT occur in patients with inguinal hernia as reported by Morris et al. [2]. Mentioned in literature as precipitant factors are trauma of the abdominal wall, coughing, effect of lifting, bicycle racing, hard labour, ingestion of heavy meals, hyperperistalsys, violent purgation or the taxis of an hernia, causes of passive displacement of the omentum [12]. The OT determines the omentum twists around a pivotal point, usually in a clockwise direction. Engorgement of the tortuous veins that are more easily compressed may compromise venous return, and the distal omentum becomes congested and oedematous. Recovery may follow or the process may go on [2]. Resultant hemorrhagic extravasations create a characteristic serosanguineous fluid inside the great omentum and in the peritoneal cavity. As the torsion progresses, arterial occlusion leads to acute hemorrhagic infarction and eventual necrosis of the omentum occur [6]. Furthermore omental infarction can occur without torsion due to hypercoagulable state or vascular abnormalities predisposing to thrombosis [7]. Vasculitis or congestion of mesenteric veins may be caused by right sided heart failure [13,14]. The differential diagnosis between POT and SOT is difficult and has seldom been made during the operation. Helpful is US or CT scan. Usually US findings are evaluated as normal [7]. Some times US may show a complex mass or a mixture of solid material and hypoechoic zones. US is a diagnostic procedure useful to exclude other acute abdominal conditions. CT scan is an effective procedure in diagnosis of acute abdominal torsion [15-17]. Preoperative US or CT scan are mandatory and the preoperative diagnosis can be accurately accomplished by these procedures. With increased use of US and CT scan, preoperative diagnosis of POT may increased in frequency [18] and in selected cases can avoid surgery and lead to conservative treatment [19-21]. In practice, US and CT scan are often avoided only for economical reasons. CT scan of our patient showed an inhomogeneous irregular edge profile mass of 38×30×25 cm of omental appearance localized at the right side. Concentric distribution of fibrous and fatty folds converging radially toward the torsion with oedema of the fat tissue, of the mesentery and little fluid collection between the right muscle wall and the lower liver surface were shown. The same pattern of concentric linear streaks in the omental fat with high-attenuated vascular structure of omentum running perpendicular to the axial plane at the centre of a concentrically layered streaks was observed by Sakamoto et al. [22]. In their report, CT scan showed also a closed vascular pedicle. Balthazar et al. [15] showed effective also the MRI specially when OT is complicated by bleeding or development of an abscess [15]. Conversely, the radiography studies are ineffective in differential diagnosis between infarction of great omentum and infarction caused by torsion [9]. OT is usually diagnosed during explorative laparotomy that represents diagnostic and therapeutic procedure. Thus, laparoscopy is the first choice procedure for diagnosis and treatment of acute omental torsion [23]. This procedure permits definitive diagnosis, when US and imaging (CT and MRI) findings are unclear [24]. In all cases laparoscopy permits a correct diagnosis of omental infarction and surgical excision [25]. The minimally invasive access to the abdominal cavity without surgical incision evocates less pain than traditional procedure and permits a praecox discharge of the patient in the first postoperative day [26]. Furthermore, in cases of POT with extensive mass of omentum, the laparoscopic technique alone might require to long surgery time; in such cases the therapeutic management of choice is diagnostic laparoscopy proceeding to laparotomy [18], which can permit the omental excision with small abdominal incision.

Conclusions

POT is a rare pathological condition with generic symptoms that may mimic many acute abdominal conditions. The pathogenesis of POT has not been established. Anatomical malformations and vascular anomalies are predisposing factors.

SOT is a more common condition than POT, due to pre-existing abdominal pathology: cysts, tumours, abdominal inflammatory foci, postsurgical wounds and hernial sacs.

The symptoms and the laboratory findings of POT are not specific and mimic other pathological abdominal conditions, for these reasons they make loose time to make diagnosis and provoke increasing degree and duration of OT.

The differential diagnosis between POT and SOT is difficult and has seldom been made during the surgical operation. Helpful are US and/or CT scan. MRI can be effective when OT is accompanied by infarction or abscess.

Explorative laparotomy represents a diagnostic and definitive therapeutic procedure.

Nowadays laparoscopy is the first choice procedure for diagnosis and treatment of acute abdominal torsion.

In cases of POT with extensive mass of omentum, diagnostic laparoscopy followed by laparotomy could permit the omental excision with small abdominal incison.

Consent

The patient knew about this case report and he signed a consent statement. A copy of the written consent was in the patient medical record.

Acknowledgements

We would like to thank Emergency Operating Room staff, Emergency Surgery Department, Policlinico Umberto I, Roma, for providing us with the intra-operative cooperation.

Authors' contributions

JA drafted the manuscript and participated in the management of patient care. CC carried out a revision of the literature about the topic. OM participated in the management of patient care. MC contributed to write down the manuscript and participated in the management of patient care. NP reviewed the manuscript. DT reviewed the manuscript, carried out the surgery and participated in its design and coordination. All authors read and approved the final draft.

Competing interests

The authors declare that they have no competing interests.
All authors read and approved the final manuscript.

References

1. Eitel GG: **Rare omental torsion.** *New York Med Rec* 1899, **55**:715.
2. Morris JH: **Torsion of the Omentum.** *Arch. Surg* 1932, **1(24)**:40.
3. Adam JT: **Primary torsion of omentum.** *Am J Surg* 1973, **126**:102-105.
4. Barcia PJ, Nelson TG: **Primary segmental infarction of omentum with and without torsion.** *Am J Surg* 1973, **126**:328-331.
5. Barsky E, Schwartz AM: **Primary Omental Torsion.** *Am. J. Surg* 1937, **38**:356.
6. Karayiannakis AJ, Polychronidis A, Chatzigianni E, Simopoulos C: **Primary torsion of the great Omentum.** *Report of a case. Surgery Today* 2002, **32**:913-915.
7. Cianci R, Filippone A, Basilico R, Storto M: **Idiopatic segmental infarction of the greater Omentum diagnosed by unenhanced multidetector-row CT and treated successfully by laparoscopy.** *Emerg. Radiol* 2008, **15**:51-56.
8. Naffa LN, Shebb NS, Haddad M: **CT finding of omental torsion and infarction: case report and review of the literature.** *J. Clinical Imaging* 2003, **27**:116-118.
9. Steinauer-Gebauer AM, Yee Y, Lutolf ME: **Torsion of the greater omentum with infarction: the vascular sign.** *Clinical Radiol* 2001, 999-1002.
10. Leitner MJ, Jordan CG, Spinner MH, Reese EC: **Torsion, infarction and hemorrhage of the omentum as a cause of acute abdominal distress.** *Ann Surg* 1952, **135**:103-110.
11. Young TH, Lee HS, Tang HS: **Primary torsion of the greater omentum.** *Int Surg* 2004, **89(2)**:72-5.
12. Barbier C, Pradoura JM, Tortuyaux JM: **Diagnostic imaging of idiopathic segmental infarct of the greater omentum. Diagnostic and physiopathologic considerations.** *J. Radiol* 1998, **79**:1485.
13. Wiesner W, Keplan V, Bongartz G: **Omental infarction associated with right sided heart failure.** *Eur. Radiol* 2000, **10(7)**:1130-1132.
14. Stella DL, Schelleman TG: **Segmental inferction of the omentum secondary to torsion: ultrasound and computed tomography diagnosys.** *Australas Radiol* 2000, **44**:212-215.
15. Balthazar EJ, Lefkowitz RA: **Left sided omental infarction with associated omental abscess: CT diagnosis.** *J Comput Assist Tomogr* 1993, **17**:375-381.
16. Puylaert JB: **Right sided segmental infarction of the omentum: clinical, US and CT findings.** *Radiology* 1992, **185**:169-172.
17. Saito N, Yamazaki T, Hanawa M, Koyama T: **A case of primary torsion of the greater omentum.** *J Jpn Surg Association* 2004, **65**:810-813.
18. Breunung N, Strauss P: **A diagnostic challenge: primary omental torsion and literature review - a case report.** *World J Emerg Surg* 2009, **4**:40.
19. Matheos E, Vasileos K, Fragkiskos F, Kostas F, Kostac C: **Primary omental torsion: report of two cases.** *Surg Today* 2009, **36**:64-67.
20. Ayodeji N, Whitney Mc.B, Gustavo S: **Primary omental infarct: conservative US operative management in the era of ultrasound, computerized tomography and laparoscopy.** *J Pediatr Surg* 2009, **44**:953-956.
21. Albuz O, Ersoz N, Kilbas Z, Ozerhan IHakki, Harlak A, Altinel O, Yigit T: **Primary torsion of omentum: rare case of acute abdomen.** *Am J Emerg Med* 2010, **28**:115-117.
22. Sakamoto N, Ohishi T, Kurisu S, Horiguchi H, Arai Y, Sugimura K: **Omental torsion.** *Radiat Med* 2006, **24**:373-377.
23. Costi R, Cecchini S, Pardone B, Violi V, Roncaroni L, Sarli L: **Laparoscopic Diagnosis and Treatment of Primary Torsion of the Greater Omentum.** *Surg Laparosc Endosc Percutan Tech* 2008, **18(1)**:102-105.
24. Poujade O, Ghiles E, Senasli A: **Primary torsion of the greater omentum: case report- Review of literature. Diagnosis cannot always be performed before surgery.** *Surg. Laparosc Endosc Percutan Tech* 2007, **17**:54-55.
25. Sasmal PK, Tania O, Patle N, Khanna S: **Omental torsion and infarction: a diagnostic dilemma and its laparoscopic management.** *J Laparoendosc Adv Surg Tech* 2010, **20**:225-229.
26. Goti F, Hollmann R, Stieger R: **Idiopathic segmental infarction of the greater omentum successfully treated by laparoscopy: report of a case.** *Surg. Today* 2000, **30**:451-453.

Emergency right hemicolectomy for inflammatory cecal masses mimicking acute appendicitis

Hakan Guven[1], Bora Koc[1,3*], Fazil Saglam[1], Irem Akin Bayram[2] and Gokhan Adas[1]

Abstract

Background: Unexpected inflammatory cecal masses of uncertain etiology, encountered in the emergency surgical departments can be indistinguishable, and appropriate operative management of these cases is a dilemma for the surgeons.

Methods: Over a 30-months period between January 2009 and June 2011, a series of 3032 patients who live in sub-urban underwent emergency surgery for clinical diagnosis of acute appendicitis and ileocecal resection or right hemicolectomy for inflammatory cecal mass were performed in 48 patients.

Results: 28 men and 20 women from suburban between ages 16–73 presented with right iliac fossa pain. The major presenting symptom was pain in the right iliac fossa (100%). On physical examination; tenderness at or near the McBurney point was detected in 44 (91,6%) patients. The range of the leucocyte level was between 8.000 to 24.000 and mean level is 16.000. After initial laparoscopic exploration, ileocecal resection or right hemicolectomy was performed conservatively because of the uncertainty of the diagnosis. Overall 32 patients underwent ileocecal resection and 16 patients underwent right hemicolectomy. Pathology revealed appendicular phlegmon in 18 patients, perforated cecal diverticulitis in 12 patients, tuberculosis in 6 patients, appendiceal and cecal rupture in 4 patients, malign mesenquimal neoplasm in 4 patients, non-spesific granulomatous in 2 patients and appendecular endometriosis in 2 patients.

Conclusion: Most inflammatory cecal masses are due to benign pathologies and can be managed safely and sufficiently with ileocecal resection or right hemicolectomy. The choice of the surgical procedure depends on the experience of the surgical team.

Keywords: Appendicular mass, Right hemicolectomy, Ileocecal resection

Introduction

Appendectomy for appendicitis is the most commonly performed emergency operation in the world. Compared with younger patients, elderly patients with appendicitis often pose a more difficult diagnostic problem because of the atypical presentation, expanded differential diagnosis, and communication difficulty. These factors contribute to the disproportionately high perforation rate seen in the elderly [1].

An appendiceal mass is the end result of a walled-off appendiceal perforation and represents a pathological spectrum ranging from phlegmon to abscess [2]. This condition is a common surgical entity, encountered in 2%-6% of patients presenting with acute appendicitis [2-4]. It has been suggested that delays in presentation are responsible for the majority of perforated appendices or the other complications.

Malignancy and appendiceal inflammation frequently form masses which are virtually indistinguishable and surgeons are often challenged to determine the pathologic origin of masses [5]. There are many reports in the literature that have addressed this promiscuousness, and right hemicolectomy has been recommended because of the concern of possible malignancy [5-8]. The studies were carried out to evaluate the pathologies and surgical management of the inflammatory cecal masses in patients with suspected appendicitis. In this study, we aim to present the diversity of the inflammatory cecal masses mimicking acute appendicitis.

* Correspondence: drborakoc@hotmail.com
[1]Department of Surgery, Okmeydanı Training and Research Hospital, İstanbul, Turkey
[3]Department of Surgery, Başkent University, Oymacı sokak No: 7 Altunizade, İstanbul, Turkey
Full list of author information is available at the end of the article

Methods and results

A series of 3032 patients from suburban who underwent emergency surgery for clinical diagnosis of acute appendicitis at Bagcılar Training and Research Hospital and Okmeydanı Training and Research Hospital between January 2009 and June 2011 were evaluated retrospectively. 48 patients who had right-hemicolectomy or ileocecal resection for inflammatory cecal masses of uncertain etiology were included in our study. Right-hemicolctomy was performed as formal resection of the right colon including lymphatic drainage along the ileocolic and right colic arteries. The relevant case notes were subsequently retrieved from the medical records and the following data were obtained for each patient: age, gender, time duration between the onset of symptoms and admission to hospital, the history and the symptoms of the patient, signs at presentation, results of the imaging methods, type of surgery, pathology results, length of hospital stay and the outcomes. The present study was approval by Okmeydani Training and Research Hospital Ethics Committee.

28 men and 20 women between ages 16–73 years (mean age 43.1) presented with right iliac fossa pain (Table 1). All patients had localized tenderness leading to a preoperative diagnosis of acute appendicitis. None of the patients applied to the surgery department at the onset of symptoms. They generally preferred self-medication and initial consultation with quacks. Based on our experience in this community, it wasn't surprising for us to find out at least 4 days between the onset of symptoms and admission to hospital (Table 2).

The major presenting symptoms were pain in the right iliac fossa in 48 (100%), anorexia in 42 (87,5%), nausea and vomiting in 30 (62,5%), fever in 26 patients (54,2%) (Table 3). When we questioned the patients retrospectively; nausea and vomiting were the major onset symptoms; but the patients could endure this symptoms generally. On physical examination; all patients prefer to lie supine, with the thighs, particularly the right thigh, drawn up; while asked to move, they do so slowly and with caution. Tenderness is at or near the Mc Burney point in 44 (91,6%) patients. Direct rebound tenderness was present at the admission time in 42 patients (87,5%).

Table 1 Age range of patients (mean 43,1 years)

Age	Number of cases	%
10-20	4	8,3
20-30	8	16,6
30-40	4	8,3
40-50	12	24,9
50-60	12	24,9
>60	8	16,6
Total	48	100

Table 2 The time between onset of symptoms and admission to hospital

Day	Number of cases	%
0-1	0	0
1-2	0	0
2-3	0	0
3-4	0	0
4-5	6	12,5
5-6	10	20,8
6-7	18	37,5
>7	14	29,2

In addition, referred or indirect rebound tenderness was present in 42 (87,5%) patients. There was a firm, palpable mass in the right iliac fossa in 28 patients (58,3%) (Table 4).

White blood cells were clearly different for each patient. Leucocyte levels ranged between 8.000 to 24.000 and mean level was 16.000 (Table 5). There was no correlation between the onset of symptoms or time of admission to hospital and leucocyte levels. The surgery team preferred abdominal USG and abdominal CT for all patients before the surgery. The scanning methods showed inflammatory cecal masses in all patients, but the radiological team couldn't decide whether these masses were inflammatory or malignant (Figures 1, 2 and 3). As a result; preoperatively 48 patients (100%) were diagnosed as having appendiceal masses, none of the patients had an appendiceal abscess.

After initial laparoscopic exploration ileocecal resection or right hemicolectomy was performed via laparatomy. During the operation, 12 of these patients were suspected to have perforated cecal diverticulitis and underwent ileocecal Resection. 16 patients had an appendicular mass and ileocecal resection was performed because of the uncertainty of the diagnosis and technique difficulties (Figure 4). 4 patients had an appendicular and also cecal rupture in the initial exploration and ileocecal resection performed. In 16 patients malignancy was suspected; in 4 of them right hemicolectomy was performed due to a suspected cecal tumor and in 12 of them the diagnosis remained uncertain, but right hemicolectomy was performed due to the suspicious malignancy. Overall 32 patients underwent ileocecal resection and 16 patients underwent right hemicolectomy. Ileocecal resection was performed through

Table 3 Major presentation symptoms

Symptoms	Number of cases	%
Pain at the right iliac fossa	48	100
Anorexia	42	87,5
Nausea and vomiting	30	62,5
Fever	26	54,2

Table 4 Signs at presentation

Sign	Number of cases	%
Tenderness	44	91,6
Direct rebound	42	87,5
Indirect rebound	42	87,5
Palpable mass	28	58,3

extension of the Mc-Burney incision in 28 patients, but 4 patients had required a separate midline incision because of difficulty of exposure. Right hemicolectomy was performed through conversion to a midline incision in all 16 patients. Primary end-to-side ileocolic anastomosis was performed in all cases.

During surgery, the surgeons examined the specimens macroscopically and in 16 patients malignancy was suspected. The histopathologic diagnoses of these patients were tuberculosis in 4, appendiceal phlegmon in 4, non-spesific granulomatous in 2, appendecular endometriosis in 2 and malign mesenquimal neoplasm in 4 patients. Totally the histopathologic diagnosises were as follows, appendiceal phlegmon in 18, perforated cecal diverticulitis in 12, tuberculosis in 6, appendiceal and cecal rupture in 4 patients, malign mesenquimal neoplasm in 4 patients, non-spesific granulomatous in 2 and appendecular endometriosis in 2 patients (Table 6) (Figure 5).

There was no mortality and all of the patients were discharged in good health. There was only one complication of wound infection. The postoperative hospital stay duration was between 1 to 7 days, especially depending on the co-morbidity of the patients.

Discussion

Appendicitis is the most common cause of acute abdomen requiring emergency surgery. Only half of the patients present classical clinical diagnosis of appendix infection [1]. Sometimes inflammatory cecal masses or cancers mimick acute appendicitis and during the operation the surgeons can not distinguish the pathology. Inflammation and cancer frequently form masses which are hardly distinguishable, and surgeons are often challenged to determine the pathologic origin of an inflammatory mass. Such masses involving the cecum are relatively uncommon when one excludes those resulting from appendicitis. Because such lesions are rare they are often reported, many are found unexpectedly at emergency operations as lesions simulating appendicitis [9].

Table 5 White blood cell levels

Leucocyte	Number of cases	%
5.000-10.000	4	8,3
10.000-15.000	12	24,9
15.001-20.000	20	41,5
>20.000	12	24,9

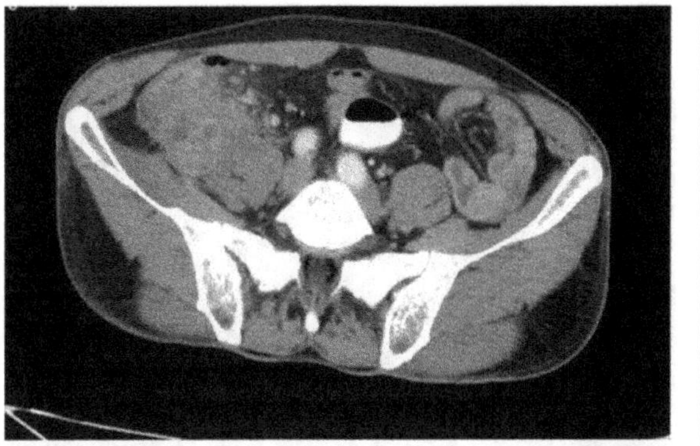

Figure 1 Cecal Diverticulitis: Axial pre-contrast CT image shows mesenteric inflammation adjacent to the distal ileum and cecum, minimal free peritoneal fluid and free air wall thickening and multiple small diverticula in the distal ileum.

Although most of the appendicular masses are benign and can be solved simplistically, a number of other conditions, some of them sinister, can be a dilemma for the surgeons. Such conditions including cecal diverticulitis, cecal carcinoma, ileocecal tuberculosis, non-specific granulomatous, appendicular endometriosis are more complex and should be managed and treated carefully. Sometimes in the emergency conditions the surgeon could not decide the exact diagnose and exclude malignancy. In our study, we could not exclude malignancy in 16 patients during the operative period.

Ultrasonography has been advocated as the diagnostic modality of choice, revealing the diagnosis in%72 of cases, but computerized tomography (CT) scan is superior [10]. In our experience we saw that ultrasonography could not guide us for the diagnosis in majority of the

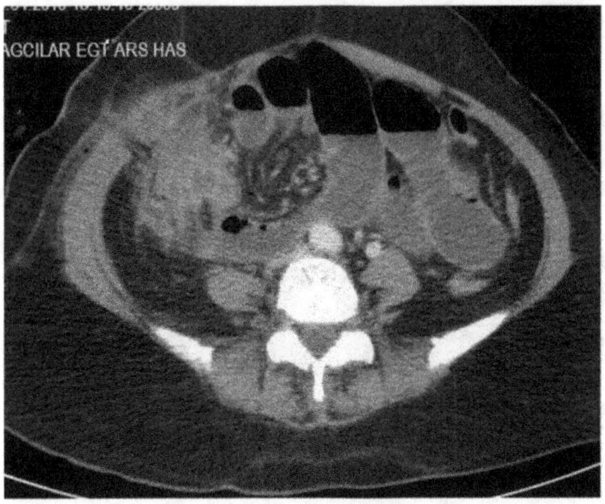

Figure 2 Small bowel and cecal tuberculosis: Contrast-enhanced CT scan shows wall thickening in several distal small bowel loops and cecum.

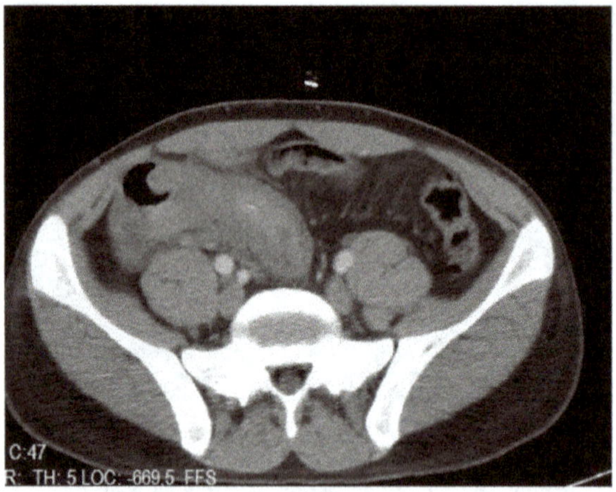

Figure 3 Non-spesific granulomatous: small segment in the terminal ileal wall thickening and inflammation in the adjacent fatty tissue and reactive lymph nodes.

Table 6 The final pathology

Findings	Number of cases	%
Appendiceal phlegmon	18	37,5
Perforated cecal diverticulitis	12	25,0
Tuberculosis	6	12,5
Appendiceal-cecal rupture	4	8,3
Malign mesenquimal neoplasm	4	8,3
Non-spesific granulomatous	2	4,2
Appendecular endometriosis	2	4,2

patients. We suggest that in overdue and suspicious cases CT should be the first choice for the diagnosis. Most of the authors described the relation between the leukogram and acute abdomen. We could not observe any correlation between onset of symptoms or the time of admission to hospital and laboratory tests especially leucocyte levels.

Some management issues has been surrounded with controversy with no general agreement among surgeons; a recent questionnaire study of 67 consultant and specialist register surgeons in the Mid-Trent region of England showed no agreed consensus on the management of appendiceal mass [11]. Most inflammatory cecal masses are due to benign pathologies and could be managed safely and sufficiently with ileocecal resection. Careful intraoperative assessment including examination of the resected specimen is essential to exclude malignancy, which would require right hemicolectomy [8-11]. In the present study, overall 32 patients underwent ileocecal resection and 16 patients underwent right hemicolectomy. 4 of the right hemicolectomies were performed for cecal tumor while 12 of them were performed for the suspicious malignancy. No malignancy was determined in these 12 patients.

Based on our experience in this community, it wasn't surprising that none of the patients admitted to hospital before 4 days after the onset of symptoms. Delayed admission to the hospital is common in our rural hospitals. It depends on numerous factors. Self-medication, especially anti-pyretics and analgesics is the most common one. Poverty, illiteracy, absence of health insurance and phobias are mainly responsible for the community indulging in self-medication. This postponement in admission to hospital by rural dwellers appears to be a common problem in most rural communities in the world. Harouna et al. [12] in a study of the current prognosis of appendicitis in the Niger Republic in 2000

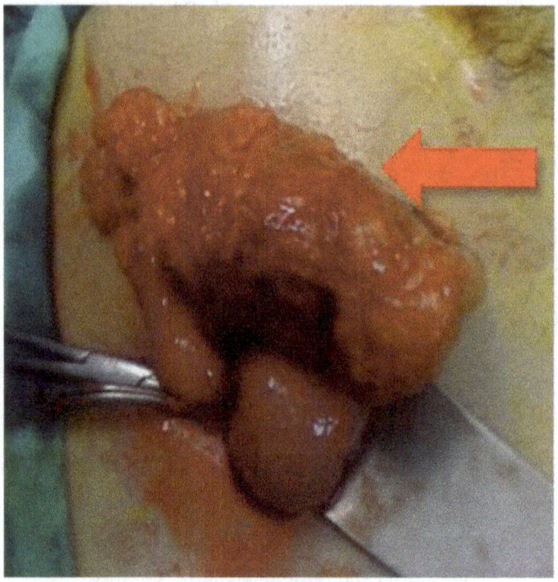

Figure 4 An unexpected ileocecal mass (red arrow). Final pathology of the specimen is malign mesenquimal tumor.

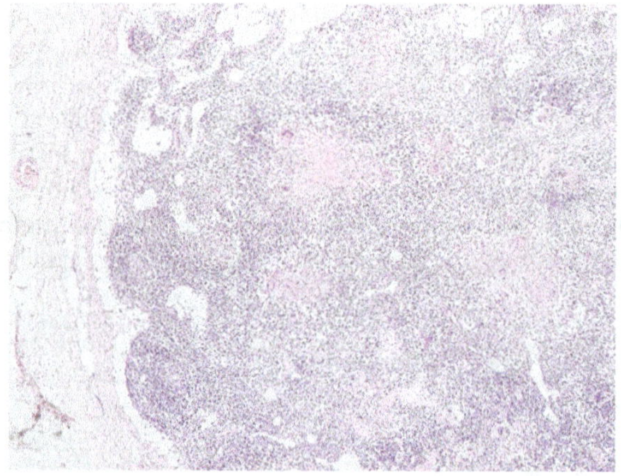

Figure 5 Ileocecal Tuberculosis. Tuberculous granulomatous lesions showing caseous necrosis in the centre, and a prominent cuff of lymphocytes and plasma cells at the periphery.

discussed this point and emphasized the deterioration of services offered by state health structures as one of the banes of health care services in Africa. The surgeons that work in rural hospitals should be aware of these delayed presentations. If a surgeon evaluates the case in emergency conditions as acute abdomen and cannot diagnosis the condition definitely, ileocecal and right hemicolectomy can be performed as a first choice for the suspicious malignancy.

Conclusions

Most inflammatory masses are caused by benign pathologies, and usually ileocecal resection is the procedure of choice. Rarely, when surgeons can not determine the pathology clearly and suspect malignancy they can prefer to perform right hemicolectomy or ileocecal resection. Because of the high incidence of appendiceal mass in our rural community, there is a need for all concerned to make sincere efforts to lower these figures.

Consent

Written informed consent was obtained from the patient for publication of this care report and any accompanying images. A copy of the written consent is available for review by the Editor-in-Chief of this journal.

Competing interests

The authors declare that they have no competing interests.

Authors' contributions

HG and BK took care of patient and wrote the initial draft. HG, BK, FS and GA operated the patent. BK, GA and IAB edited manuscript with literature review. All authors read and approved the final manuscript.

Acknowledgements

We thank to Irmak Bircan for discussion and suggestions about the diagnosis.

Author details

[1]Department of Surgery, Okmeydanı Training and Research Hospital, İstanbul, Turkey. [2]Faculty of Medicine, Department of Radiology, İstanbul University, İstanbul, Turkey. [3]Department of Surgery, Başkent University, Oymacı sokak No: 7 Altunizade, İstanbul, Turkey.

References

1. Bernard MJ, David HB: **The Appendix**. In *Schwartz's Principles of surgery*. 9th edition. Edited by Brunicardi F. McGraw-Hill; 2010:1267–1342. Chapter 30.
2. Okafor PI, Orakwe JC, Chianakwana GU: **Management of appendiceal masses in a peripheral hospital in Nigeria: review of thirty cases.** *World J Surg* 2003, **27:**800–803.
3. Nitecki S, Assalia A, Schein M: **Contemporary management of the appendiceal mass.** *Br J Surg* 1993, **80:**18–20.
4. Hogan MJ: **Appendiceal abscess drainage.** *Tech Vasc Interv Radiol* 2003, **6:**205–214.
5. William AM: **Inflammatory masses of the cecum.** *Ann Surg* 1967, **165:**697.
6. Kovalcik PJ, Simstein NL, Cross GH: **Ileocecal masses discovered unexpectedly at surgery for appendicitis.** *Am Surg* 1978, **44:**279.
7. Riseman JA, Wichterman K: **Evaluation of right hemicolectomy for unexpected cecal mass.** *Arch Surg* 1989, **124:**1043.
8. Tung-Ping Poon R, MBBS: **Inflammatory cecal masses in patients presenting with appendicitis.** *World J Surg* 1999, **23:**713–716.
9. Dale WA: **Colon lesions simulating acute appendicitis.** *J Tenn Med Assoc* 1963, **56:**351–356.
10. Willemsen PJ, Hoorntje LE, Eddes EH, Ploeg RJ: **The need for interval appendectomy after resolution of an appendiceal mass questioned.** *Dig Surg* 2002, **19:**216–220.
11. Ahmed I, Deakin D, Parsons SL: **Appendix mass: do we know how to treat it.** *Ann R Coll Surg Engl* 2005, **87**(3):191–195.
12. Harouna Y, Amadou S, Gazi M, *et al*: **Appendicitis in Niger: current prognosis.** *Bull Soc Pathol Exot* 2000, **93:**314–316.

3

Factors predicting mortality in emergency abdominal surgery in the elderly

Naoto Fukuda[1*], Joji Wada[1], Michio Niki[1], Yasuyuki Sugiyama[2] and Hiroyuki Mushiake[2]

Abstract

Objective: This study aimed to investigate clinical features of abdominal emergency surgery in elderly patients, and to determine factors predicting mortality in these patients.

Methods: The study population included 94 patients aged 80 years or older who underwent emergency surgery for acute abdominal diseases between 2000 and 2010. Thirty-six patients (38.3%) were male and fifty-eight patients (61.7%) were female (mean age, 85.6 years). Main outcome measures included background of the patient's physical condition (concomitant medical disease, and performance status), cause of disease, morbidity and mortality, and disease scoring system (APACHE II, and POSSUM). Prognostic factors affecting mortality of the patient were also evaluated by univariate analysis using Fisher's exact test and Mann–Whitney U–test, and by multivariate analysis using multiple logistic regression analysis.

Results: Of the 94 patients, 71 (75.5%) had a co-existing medical disease; most patients had hypertension (46.8%). The most frequent surgical indications were acute cholecystitis in 23 patients (24.5%), followed by intestinal obstruction in 18 patients (19.1%). Forty-one patients (43.6%) had complications during hospital stay; the most frequent were surgical site infection (SSI) in 21 patients (22.3%) and pneumonia in 12 patients (12.8%). Fifteen patients died (overall mortality, 16%) within 1 month after operation. The most common causes of death were sepsis related to pan-peritonitis in 5 patients (5.3%), and pneumonia in 4 patients (4.3%). Multiple logistic regression analysis showed that time from onset of symptoms to hospital admission and the POSSUM scoring system could be prognostic factors for mortality.

Conclusions: Mortality in elderly patients who underwent emergency surgery for acute abdominal disease can be predicted using the disease scoring system (POSSUM) and on the basis of delay in hospital admission.

Keywords: Abdominal surgical emergency, Elderly, Mortality, Morbidity

Introduction

One of the most notable events being seen in recent years in people living in developed countries is an increased life span. In Japan, average life expectancy has gradually increased to 79.59 years among men and 86.44 years among women in 2009. Japan may be one of the most eminent countries where many people live to an advanced age because more than 50% of Japanese people survive over 80 years. As average life expectancy lengthens, the number of geriatric patients who need emergency abdominal surgery will increase. Compared with elective surgery, emergency abdominal surgery is associated with increased morbidity and mortality, especially in elderly patients [1-6]. Thus, elderly patients with abdominal surgical emergency may be at risk for severe and life-threatening conditions because of medical comorbidities, insufficient screening, unrecognized symptoms, and inadequate overall access to the health care system [7]. In this study, geriatric patients were limited to those aged 80 years or older because of increasing life expectancy in Japanese people. The aim of the present study was to report our experience with emergency abdominal surgery in the elderly patients and to identify risk factors that have an impact on mortality in these patients.

* Correspondence: nf341206@hotmail.co.jp
[1]Department of Surgery, Kawasaki Kyodo Hospital, Kawasaki 210-0833, Japan
Full list of author information is available at the end of the article

Methods

Ninety-four patients ages 80 years or over who underwent emergency surgery for acute abdominal disease at our institutions between 2001 and 2010 were enrolled in this study. They included 36 men (38.3%) and 58 women (61.7%) ages 80–104 years (mean, 85.6 years). Of the 94 patients, 71 (75.5%) had co-existing medical diseases such as hypertension in 44 patients (46.8%), chronic heart disease in 17 (18.1%), chronic obstructive pulmonary disease (COPD) in 14 (14.9%), cerebrovascular disease and DM in 11 (11.7%) respectively, chronic renal failure in 6 (6.4%), and others in 12 (12.8%). Of the 71 patients with concomitant medical disease, 32 had 1 medical disease and 39 had 2 or more additional medical problems. The Eastern Cooperative Oncology Group (ECOG) performance status score [8], which reflects the daily living abilities of the patient was estimated for these patients and the results were as follows: 2 patients were with grade 0, 28 with grade 1, 48 with grade 2, 13 with grade 3, and 3 with grade 4 (Table 1). Of the 94 patients, 76 (80.9%) underwent emergency surgery within 48 hours after admission. The other18 patients (e.g., those with acute cholecystitis, intestinal obstruction due to adhesion) were first treated conservatively, and only when the conservative treatment failed did they undergo surgery.

Table 1 Of the 94 patients, 71 (75.5%) had co-existing medical diseases such as hypertension in 44 patients (46.8%), chronic heart disease in 17 (18.1%), chronic obstructive pulmonary disease (COPD) in 14 (14.9%), cerebrovascular disease and DM in 11 (11.7%) respectively, chronic renal failure in 6 (6.4%), and others in 12 (12.8%)

Variables	n (%)
Age 80-104 years (mean: 85.6)	
Gender	
Male	36 (38.3%)
Female	58 (61.7%)
Co-existing medical disease	
Hypertension	44 (46.8%)
Chronic heart disease	17 (18.1%)
COPD	14 (14.9%)
Cerebrovascular disease	11 (11.7%)
DM	11 (11.7%)
Chronic renal failure	6 (6.4%)
Others	12 (12.8%)
Performance status (ECOG)	
Grade 0	2 (2.1%)
Grade 1	28 (29.8%)
Grade 2	48 (51.1%)
Grade 3	13 (13.8%)
Grade 4	3 (3.2%)

The ECOG performance status score were as follows: 2 patients were with grade 0, 28 with grade 1, 48 with grade 2, 13 with grade 3, and 3 with grade 4.

Data regarding the patient's clinical features, surgical outcomes including morbidity and mortality, and follow-up information were obtained from a clinical database. We evaluated clinical factors that could be associated with mortality in abdominal emergency surgery in elderly patients. These parameters included age, gender, background of the patient's physical condition (concomitant medical disease, and ECOG performance status [8]), time from onset of symptom to hospital admission, and disease severity scoring system (APACHE II [9], and POSSUM [10]). Physiological Score (PS) and Operative Severity Score (OSS) in POSSUM scoring system [10] as well as APACHE II score [9] were analyzed as parameters of the disease scoring system. For statistical analysis, the patients were grouped into 2 categories with respect to age [≤85 years or >85 years (mean value)], comorbidity (negative or positive), ECOG performance status score (Grade0 or 1 vs. Grade2 or 3 or 4), and time from onset of symptom to hospital admission (<24 h or ≥24 h). Post-operative morbidity and mortality were defined as operation-related complications or death that occurred within 30 days after the operation. Univariate comparison between the groups were performed using the Fisher's exact test and Mann–Whitney U – test.

Covariates that remained significant through univariate analysis were selected for multivariate analysis. Multivariate analysis was performed using the multiple logistic regression analysis. The results were evaluated at a confidence interval of 95% and significance was set at $p < 0.05$.

This study was carried out in compliance with the Helsinki Declaration. Written informed consent was obtained from the patient for publication of this report and any accompanying images.

Results

Causes of acute abdomen

The most frequent surgical indications were acute cholecystitis in 23 patients (24.5%), followed by intestinal obstruction in 18 patients (19.1%). There were also 16 cases (17.0%) of incarcerated hernias, 14 cases (14.9%) of intestinal perforation, 10 cases (10.6%) of gastroduodenal perforation, 9 cases (9.6%) of acute appendicitis, 5 cases (5.3%) of volvulus, and 4 cases (4.3%) of other acute abdominal disease (Figure 1).

Intestinal obstruction was most often caused by adhesion (n = 14); two patients needed intestinal resection due to intestinal necrosis and perforation. Other etiologies of intestinal obstruction were colonic malignancy (n = 2), internal hernia (n = 1), and gallstone ileus (n = 1). Incarcerated hernias consisted of 9 cases of femoral hernias, 4 cases of inguinal hernias, 2 cases of obturator hernias, and 1 case of incisional hernia. Among the cases of intestinal perforation, 5 cases were small intestinal perforations and 9 cases were large intestinal perforations. The most common cause of intestinal perforation was incarcerated hernia (n = 4),

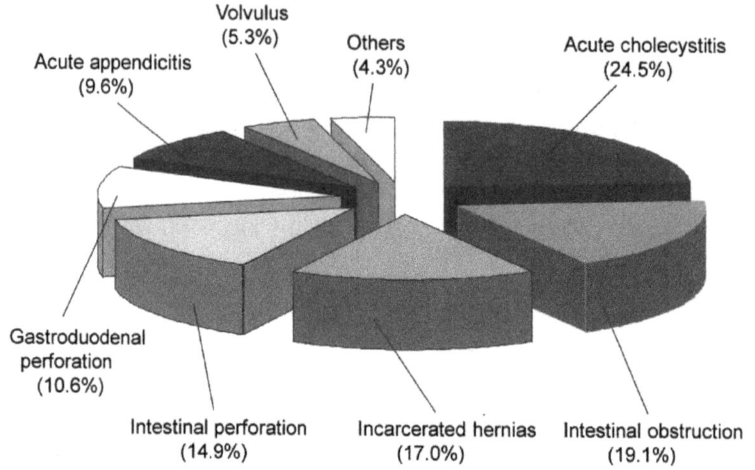

Figure 1 The most frequent surgical indications were acute cholecystitis in 23 patients (24.5%), followed by intestinal obstruction in 18 patients (19.1%). There were also 16 cases (17.0%) of incarcerated hernias, 14 cases (14.9%) of intestinal perforation, 10 cases (10.6%) of gastro-duodenal perforation, 9 cases (9.6%) of acute appendicitis, 5 cases (5.3%) of volvulus, and 4 cases (4.3%) of other acute abdominal disease.

followed by colon diverticulitis (n = 3). Gastro – duodenal perforations were found in 5 cases of perforated duodenal ulcer, 3 cases of perforated gastric ulcer, 1 case of duodenal perforation due to gallbladder cancer invasion, and 1 case of iatrogenic gastric perforation caused by guide-wire of a long tube using for intestinal obstruction.

Treatment

All patients were treated surgically. Seventy-six patients (80.9%) underwent emergency surgery within 48 hours after admission; the other 18 patients were first treated conservatively and then operated on more than 48 hours after admission. The most common operation was intestinal resection (n = 30), followed by cholecystectomy (n = 24), repair of intestinal adhesion (n = 15), and hernia repair (n = 14). Of the 30 patients treated with intestinal resection, large bowel resection was applied to 17 patients, and small bowel resection to 13 patients. Cholecystectomy was performed laparoscopically in 3 patients, and using laparotomy in 21 patients. There were only 3 cases of palliative surgery; 1 ileostomy for transverse colon perforation, 1 peritoneal lavage for acute pancreatitis, and 1 gastroduodenostomy for advanced gallbladder cancer. Twenty-three patients (24.5%) were followed in the intensive care unit after surgery. Of these, 20 patients needed mechanical ventilation for respiratory support.

Morbidity and mortality

Forty-one patients (43.6%) had post – operative morbidity. The most frequent complication was surgical site infection (SSI), which occurred in 21 patients (22.3%), followed by pneumonia in 12 patients (12.8%). Sepsis occurred in 5 patients (5.3%), DIC in 5 patients (5.3%), and ARDS, acute renal failure, anastomosis leakage, and urinary tract infection occurred in 2 patients (2.1%) respectively. Of the 12 cases of pneumonia, more than half (8 patients) were aspiration pneumonias. Fifteen patients (16.0%) died within 1 month after their operation. The most common causes of death were sepsis related to pan-peritonitis in 5 patients (5.3%), and pneumonia in 4 patients (4.3%). The other etiologies of mortality consisted of 2 cases of cancer, 1 multiple organ

Table 2 Forty-one patients (43.6%) had post-operative morbidity

	Patient (n = 94)	%
Morbidity	41	43.6
SSI	21	22.3
Pneumonia	12	12.8
DIC	5	5.3
Sepsis	5	5.3
ARDS	2	2.1
Acute renal failure	2	2.1
Anastomosis leakage	2	2.1
Urinary tract infection	2	2.1
Mortality	15	16.0
Sepsis	5	5.3
Pneumonia	4	4.3
Cancer	2	2.1
Multiple organ failure	1	1.1
Intraperitoneal bleeding	1	1.1
Renal failure	1	1.1
Suffocation	1	1.1

The most frequent complication was surgical site infection (SSI), which occurred in 21 patients (22.3%), followed by pneumonia in 12 patients (12.8%). Fifteen patients (16.0%) died within 1 month after their operation. The most common causes of death were sepsis related to pan-peritonitis in 5 patients (5.3%), and pneumonia in 4 patients (4.3%).

failure, 1 intraperitoneal bleeding due to DIC, 1 renal failure, and 1 suffocation. These complications are listed in Table 2.

Clinical factors affecting mortality

Clinical factors that might affect the mortality of elderly patients treated with emergency abdominal surgery were evaluated. Delay in hospital admission (more than 24 hours after onset of symptom), APACHE II score, and POSSUM score (PS, OSS) were identified as prognostic factors of these patients on univariate analysis (Table 3). Additionally, multivariate analysis using multiple logistic regression analysis demonstrated that delay in hospital admission ($p = 0.0076$) and POSSUM score (PS) ($p = 0.0301$) were effective prognostic factors of elderly patients who underwent emergency abdominal surgery (Table 4).

Discussion

As the increase of life expectancy has been observed in developed countries, especially in Japan, the number of geriatric patients with acute abdominal disease requiring emergency surgical treatment has increased in recent decades. Because physiological reserve is significantly diminished in the elderly, cardiovascular, pulmonary, endocrine, and renal comorbidities are more common in elderly patients. Previous studies [1,6,11-13] have shown that the incidence of comorbidity in the elderly with acute abdominal disease requiring emergency operation was more than 50%, ranging from 58 to 81.5%. Our study also revealed that the rate of having co-existing medical disease in the aged patient was 75.5%, and hypertension (46.8%) was the most common comorbidity, followed by chronic heart disease (18.1%), and COPD (14.9%). The presence of underlying chronic conditions may have an adverse effect on the prognosis in patients undergoing emergency surgery and may be responsible for the increased perioperative risk, and consequently, mortality. Ozkan [13] reported that all patients who died postoperatively had at least 1 comorbid condition, whereas comorbid conditions existed in 66.3% of the surviving patients in the study of emergency abdominal surgery in geriatric patients. On the other hand, Rubinfeld [14] showed that none of the comorbidities accurately predicted mortality in the patients aged 80 years and older who received an emergency major abdominal operation. Our study also revealed that comorbidity was not a significant prognostic factor for elderly patients with abdominal surgical emergency on univariate analysis ($p = 0.4715$).

According to the results, underlying medical disease may not affect the mortality of the elderly patient with acute abdominal disease requiring emergency operation, because appropriate management of medical comorbidities due to development of medical technology in recent decades may improve the prognosis of the elderly patient with underlying medical problems.

In the current study, the complication rate was as high as 43.6%, which is similar to those reported previously [1,4,6,15]. Surgical site infection (SSI) was the most frequent complication and occurred in 21 patients (22.3%), followed by pneumonia in 12 patients (12.8%). Arenal [6] reported that 48% of the patients had morbidity, the majority of which was wound infection (16.3%), followed by respiratory complications (11.4%) and cardiac complications (8.9%) in a study of 710 patients ages 70 years or older who underwent emergency surgery for intra-abdominal

Table 3 Delay in hospital admission (more than 24 hours after onset of symptom), APACHE II score, and POSSUM score (PS, OSS) were identified as prognostic factors of these patients on univariate analysis

	Alive (n = 79)	Dead (n = 15)	*P*
Age (mean: 85.6)			
≤85	41	10	
>85	38	5	0.2219
Gender			
Male	27	9	
Female	52	6	0.0567
Comorbidity			
negative	20	3	
positive	59	12	0.4715
PS(ECOG)			
Grade 0,1	28	2	
Grade 2, 3, and 4	51	13	0.0786
Time from onset of symptoms to hospital admission (hour)			
<24	51	4	
≥24	28	11	0.0074** (Fisher's exact test)
APACHE II (mean)	11.9	18.5	0.0002
POSSUM			
PS (mean)	30.1	38.6	0.0001**
OSS (mean)	13.9	17.2	0.0408* (Mann-Whitney U-test)

Table 4 Multivariate analysis using multiple logistic regression analysis demonstrated that delay in hospital admission (p=0.0076) and POSSUM score (PS) (p=0.0301) were effective prognostic factors of elderly patients who underwent emergency abdominal surgery

		Odds ratio	95% CI	*p*
Time from onset to hospital admission (>24 hr vs. 24 hr)		9.6039	1.8226-50.6079	0.0076**
APACHE II		1.1291	0.9223-1.3822	0.2395
POSSUM	PS	1.2013	1.0178-1.4178	0.0301*
	OSS	1.0202	0.8468-1.2292	0.8331

disorders. Thus, wound infection which is a local morbidity may be the most frequent complication after emergency operation for acute abdominal disease in elderly patient.

Among the systemic morbidities, cardio-pulmonary complications are more common in the elderly patients compared to younger patients because cardio – pulmonary function declines with aging. Our study also revealed that 12.8% of the patients had post – operative pneumonias, in which more than half of the cases were aspiration pneumonias. As swallowing ability is diminished in the elderly, especially those aged 80 years or more, we must pay more attention to aspiration pneumonia in the elderly patient after surgical treatment for acute abdominal disease.

Despite the relatively high incidence of morbidity (43.6%), the mortality of our patients was 16.0%. This result is similar or better than that of previously published reports, which ranged from 11 to 34% [4-6,13,14,16].

The most common causes of death in elderly patients in our study were sepsis related to pan-peritonitis (5.3%) and pneumonia (4.3%); these findings were similar to those of previous reports [13] in which post-operative pneumonia, cardiac complications and sepsis accounted for a large proportion of deaths in elderly patients. Cancer was reported to be the most common reason for death in elderly patients with abdominal emergency surgery in another study [4]. The different conclusions in that study might be explained by different patient populations, especially the number and percentage of patients with oncological emergency.

Many factors have been reported to be responsible for surgical mortality during acute abdomen in elderly patients. The most common factor was ASA score, which consists of 6 categories to evaluate the degree of a patient's sickness or physical status, and that was reported as an independent prognostic factor in 3 previous studies [6,13,14]. ASA score is ordinarily used to assess the patient's physical status before surgery by an anesthesiologist, whereas it is not commonly used by surgeons. The POSSUM scoring system developed by Copeland [10] in 1991 has since been applied to a number of surgical groups as surgical culture moves more towards outcome measures and providing the patient with as much information as possible to make fully informed decisions. The POSSUM scoring system has 2 main components: Physiological Score (PS) and Operative Severity Score (OSS). PS is based on 12 physiological parameters to evaluate a patient's physiological status before surgery, whereas OSS consists of 6 operative parameters accounting for the severity of the procedure. Since the ASA score is too simplistic and highly subjective compared to the APACHE II or POSSUM scoring system, we chose APACHE II and POSSUM (PS, OSS) as disease scoring systems instead of the ASA score in the study of prognostic factors for elderly patients who undergo emergency abdominal surgery. Consequently, the POSSUM score (PS) was identified as an effective prognostic factor in elderly patients who underwent emergency abdominal surgery on multivariate analysis. Since the PS in the POSSUM scoring system is objective and reflects the patient's overall condition, including his age, vital signs, blood chemistry, mental status and heart condition, it may be more effective than the ASA score for evaluating the prognosis of elderly patients with abdominal surgical emergencies. Another effective prognostic factor defined in the present study was delay in hospital admission (more than 24 hours after onset of symptoms).

The prognosis of the patient who was admitted more than 24 hours after onset of symptoms was significantly worsened than that of the patient who admitted within 24 hours on multivariate analysis ($p = 0.0076$). The difficulty in obtaining an accurate history and the mild character of symptoms due to decline in organ and tissue function in the aged patient have an effect on the findings, resulting in delayed diagnosis and a more complicated peri-operative period. Socioeconomic factors may also play a role because the elderly patient may not have adequate access to the health care system, which might be one of the reasons for delay in hospital admission. Because elderly patients with acute abdominal disease tend to have delayed diagnoses and surgical treatments, rapid access to the hospital, adequate diagnostic measures and decision-making should be required to prevent postoperative complications and to improve the prognosis.

Conclusions

POSSUM scoring system (PS) and delay in hospital admission may be prognostic factors for mortality in elderly patients who underwent emergency surgery for acute abdominal disease.

Competing interests

The authors declare that they have no competing interests.

Authors' contributions

Study Design/Data Collection/Analysis/Interpretation: FN. Manuscript Drafting: HM. Critical Review: YS. All authors read and approved the final manuscript.

Author details

[1]Department of Surgery, Kawasaki Kyodo Hospital, Kawasaki 210-0833, Japan. [2]Department of Surgery, Teikyo University School of Medicine, University Hospital, Mizonokuchi, Kawasaki 213-8507, Japan.

References

1. Kettunen J, Paajanen H, Kostiainen S: **Emergency abdominal surgery in the elderly.** *Hepatogastroenterol* 1995, **42**:106–108.
2. Karanikas ID, Liakakos TD, Koundourakis SS, Tzorakis SE, Dendrinos SS: **Emergency operations in the elderly: management and outcome.** *Int Surg* 1996, **81**:158–162.
3. Walsh TH: **Audit outcome of major surgery in the elderly.** *Br J Surg* 1996, **83**:92–97.
4. Miettinen P, Pasanen P, Salonen A, Lahtinen J, Alhava E: **The outcome of elderly patients after operation for acute abdomen.** *Ann Chir Gynaecol* 1996, **85**:11–15.

5. Van Geloven AAW, Biesheuvel TH, Luitse JSK, Hoitsma HFW, Obertop H: **Hospital admissions of patients aged over 80 with acute abdominal complaints.** *Eur J Surg* 2000, **166:**866–871.
6. Arenal JJ, Bengoechea-Beeby M: **Mortality associated with emergency abdominal surgery in the elderly.** *Can J Surg* 2003, **46:**111–116.
7. Edward AM, Kevin MS, Kimberly AD, Walter EL: **Factors predicting morbidity and mortality in emergency colorectal procedures in elderly patients.** *Arch Surg* 2009, **144:**1157–1162.
8. Oken MM, Creech RH, Tormey DC, Horton J, Davis TE, McFadden ET, Carbone PP: **Toxicity and response criteria of the Eastern Cooperative Oncology Group.** *Am J Clin Oncol* 1982, **5:**649–655.
9. Knaus WA, Draper EA, Wagner DP, Zimmerman JE: **APACHE II: a severity of disease classification system.** *Crit Care Med* 1985, **13:**818–829.
10. Copeland GP, Jones D, Walters M: **POSSUM: A scoring system for surgical audit.** *Br J Surg* 1991, **78:**356–360.
11. Feny G: **Acute abdominal disease in the elderly.** *Am J Surg* 1982, **143:**751–754.
12. Mcintyre R, Reinbach D, Cuschieri RJ: **Emergency abdominal surgery in the elderly.** *J R Coll Surg Edinb* 1997, **42:**173–178.
13. Ozkan E, Fersahoğlu MM, Dulundu E, Ozel Y, Yıldız MK, Topaloğlu U: **Factors affecting mortality and morbidity in emergency abdominal surgery in geriatric patients.** *Ulus Travma Acil Cerrahi Derg* 2010, **16:**439–444.
14. Rubinfeld I, Thomas C, Berry S, Murphy R, Obeid N, Azuh O, Jordan J, Patton JH: **Octogenarian abdominal surgical emergencies: Not so grim a problem with the acute care surgery model?** *J Tauma* 2009, **67:**983–989.
15. Monaco A, Verna C, Gastalgdi L, Moncelli G: **Emergency abdominal surgery in the aged.** *Minerva Chir* 1996, **51:**1043–1047.
16. Costamagna D, Pipitone Federico NS, Erra S, Tribocco M, Poncina F, *et al*: **Acute abdomen in the elderly. A peripheral general hospital experience.** *G Chir* 2009, **30:**315–322.

Early recognition of acute thoracic aortic dissection and aneurysm

I Michael Leitman[1*], Kei Suzuki[1], Aaron J Wengrofsky[1], Eyal Menashe[1], Michal Poplawski[1], Kar-Mun Woo[2], Charles M Geller[1], David Lucido[1], Thomas Bernik[1], Barbara A Zeifer[3] and Byron Patton[1]

Abstract

Background: Thoracic aortic dissection (TAD) and aneurysm (TAA) are rare but catastrophic. Prompt recognition of TAD/TAA and differentiation from acute coronary syndrome (ACS) is difficult yet crucial. Earlier identification of TAA/TAD based upon routine emergency department screening is necessary.

Methods: A retrospective analysis of patients that presented with acute thoracic complaints to the ED from January 2007 through June 2012 was performed. Cases of TAA/TAD were compared to an equal number of controls which consisted of patients with the diagnosis of ACS. Demographics, physical findings, EKG, and the results of laboratory and radiological imaging were compared. P-value of > 0.05 was considered statistically significant.

Results: In total, 136 patients were identified with TAA/TAD, 0.36% of patients that presented with chest complaints. Compared to ACS patients, TAA/TAD group was older (68.9 vs. 63.2 years), less likely to be diabetic (13% vs 32%), less likely to complain of chest pain (47% vs 85%) and head and neck pain (4% vs 17%). The pain for the TAA/TAD group was less likely characterized as tight/heavy in nature (5% vs 37%). TAA/TAD patients were also less likely to experience shortness of breath (42% vs. 51%), palpitations (2% vs 9%) and dizziness (2% vs 13%) and had a greater incidence of focal lower extremity neurological deficits (6% vs 1%), bradycardia (15% vs. 5%) and tachypnea (53% vs. 22%). On multivariate analysis, increasing heart rate, chest pain, diabetes, head & neck pain, dizziness, and history of myocardial infarction were independent predictors of ACS.

Conclusions: Increasing heart rate, chest pain, diabetes, head & neck pain, dizziness, and history of myocardial infarction can be used to differentiate acute coronary syndromes from thoracic aortic dissections/aneurysms.

Keywords: Acute coronary syndrome, Thoracic aorta, Aortic aneurysm, Aortic dissection

Introduction

Among the "big three" catastrophic illnesses that present with acute thoracic complaints (myocardial infarction/ ischemia, thoracic aortic dissection, and pulmonary embolism) [1] differentiating between thoracic aortic aneurysms (TAA)/thoracic aortic dissections (TAD) and myocardial ischemia presents a great clinical challenge to the emergency department. The incidence of TAA and TAD are 10.4 and 2.9-3.5 cases per every 100,000 persons per year, respectively [2]. Rupture is the cause of death in approximately one-third of affected patients admitted to the hospital, although the rate of nonfatal rupture might be considerably higher [3]. Forty to 50% of patients with dissection of the proximal aorta die within 48 hours if not diagnosed and properly treated, yet, it is misdiagnosed in as many as 30% of patients [4]. On the other hand, for type A aortic dissections, those who rapidly undergo surgical treatment in experienced tertiary centers have a one year survival rate of 96% to 97.6% and a three year survival of 88.3% to 90.5%. [5]. The overall survival among recipients of thoracic endovascular aortic repair (TEVAR) stent grafts is 96%, 86%, and 69% at 1-, 3-, and 5-year follow-up, respectively [6] and 74 - 97% after open surgery [7,8]. This highlights the importance of making a prompt diagnosis of TAA/TAD.

Helical thoracic CT scanning has a reported diagnostic sensitivity of 100% and a specificity of 98% for diagnosing

* Correspondence: mleitman@chpnet.org
[1]Departments of Surgery, Albert Einstein College of Medicine-Beth Israel Medical Center, 10 Union Square East, Suite 2M, New York, NY 10003, USA
Full list of author information is available at the end of the article

TAD [9]. With such accurate imaging modality, it becomes crucial to triage patients such that appropriate workup leads to prompt diagnosis in a timely manner. Making a distinction between TAD/TAA and acute coronary syndrome (ACS) is especially important as the work-up of ACS is significantly different.

The early identification of patients with these rare acute aortic conditions requires astute clinical intuition. This paper examines the presentation of such patients and compares them to a cohort of patients with acute chest complaints that did not have this condition. The aim of the study was to develop a profile of patients who would be identified early in their ED course with routine screening done on most ED patients. Such information will help expedite prompt confirmatory imaging, leading to prompt and effective medical and surgical treatment.

Patients and methods

This study was reviewed and approved by the Institutional Review Board - Human Research Committee (IRB# 106–12). A retrospective analysis of patients that presented with acute thoracic complaints to the ED from January 2007 through June 2012 was performed. Patients were identified by ED diagnosis of "aortic dissection" and "aortic aneurysm", which were further reviewed to select only those with thoracic aortic dissection and thoracic aortic aneurysm. In addition, emergency room and inpatient hospital medical records were reviewed using ICD-9 (International Statistical Classification of Diseases and Related Health Problems) codes (441.0 – 441.9) for thoracic aortic dissection and aneurysm. In total, the study group consisted of 136 patients. Equal number of control group consisting of patients with the diagnosis of acute coronary syndrome (ACS) (primary ICD-9 414.00 thru 414.05 or secondary codes of 411.81, 411.89, 413.0, 413.1 or 413.9) were randomly chosen from the same time period and included in the study as the control group.

Demographics, physical findings, EKG, and the results of laboratory and radiological imaging were compared. Statistical analysis was performed utilizing the method of Chi-squared for categorical data and Student's *t*-test for continuous data. A p-value of less than 0.05 was considered to be statistically significant. The data were subjected to univariate and multivariate analysis using logistic regression.

Results

During this 5 1/2-year time period, 136 patients with initial chest complaints were found to have acute TAA only (63 patients), TAD only (49 patients) or both (24 patients) on chest CT. These 136 patients with acute thoracic aortic disease represented 0.36% of the 37,778 patients that presented with acute chest pain during the study period. The classification of the aortic pathology is listed in Table 1. The demographics and past medical history for the study group (TAA/TAD) were compared to the control group (ACS) (Table 2). When compared to the control group, study group was older (average age 69 vs. 63 years, $P = 0.0034$), less likely to be diabetic (13% vs. 32%, $P < 0.0005$), more likely to have a history of TAA/TAD (34% vs. 8%, $P < 0.0001$), and less likely to have a history of myocardial infarction (2% vs. 15%, $P = 0.0002$).

Presenting symptoms for the two groups are demonstrated in Table 3. Study group was less likely to complain of chest pain (47% vs. 85%, $P < 0.0001$) and head and neck pain (4% vs. 17%, $P = 0.0007$). The pain for the study group was less likely characterized as tight/heavy in nature (5% vs. 37%, $P < 0.0001$). While the pain was more likely to be of sudden onset (11% vs. 2%, $P = 0.007$), it was less likely to be increasing in severity (23% vs. 2%, $P < 0.0001$). Study group was also less likely to experience shortness of breath (42% vs. 51%, $P = 0.01$), palpitations (2% vs. 9%, $P = 0.0335$) and dizziness (2% vs. 13%, $P = 0.0025$).

The physical exam and radiographic findings of the two study groups are listed in Table 4. Study group had a greater incidence of focal lower extremity neurological deficits (6% vs. 1%, $P = 0.04$), bradycardia (15% vs. 5%, $P = 0.0013$) and tachypnea (53% vs. 22%, $P < 0.0001$). For patients that had chest x-rays (107 patients (79%) for the study group and 126 patients (96%) for the control group), widened mediastinum was associated with TAA/TAD (52% vs. 45%, $P = 0.005$).

Laboratory results are listed in Table 5. Elevated serum blood urea nitrogen (BUN) level correlated with acute thoracic aortic disease in patients in whom this testing was obtained (70% vs. 47%, $P < 0.0001$). Patients with laboratory evidence of coagulopathy (elevated initial normalized ration (INR) (40% vs. 19%, $P = 0.0017$) or D-dimer (80% vs. 13%, $P = 0.06$)) were also more likely to have TAA/TAD. Serum troponin levels were higher in patients with ACS (34% vs. 18% $P = 0.04$).

Table 1 Classification of pathology

Thoracic aortic dissection (n = 25)	
DeBakey I	15 (60%)
DeBakey II	5 (20%)
DeBakey III	5 (20%)
Thoracic aortic aneurysm (n = 87)	
Class A	33 (38%)
Class B	9 (10%)
Class C	45 (52%)
Combined dissection and aneurysm (n = 24)	

Table 2 Demographics and past medical history

Variable	TAA/TAD[1]	Control	P-value
Total patients	**136 (%)**	**136 (%)**	
Mean Age (Range)	69 (33–95)	63 (31–94)	0.0034*
Gender	69 (33–95)	63 (31–94)	0.0034*
Male	80 (59)	78 (58)	0.81
Female	56 (41)	58 (42)	0.89
Past Med History			
Diabetes	18 (13)	43 (32)	0.0005*
Previous TAA/TAD	46 (34)	11 (8)	<.0001*
Myocardial Infarction	2 (2)	20 (15)	0.0002*
Hypertension	96 (71)	88 (65)	0.37
Aortic Valve Disease	7 (5)	2 (1)	0.18
Peripheral Vascular Disease	4 (3)	2 (1)	0.68
Congestive Heart Failure	15 (11)	13 (10)	0.84
Arrhythmias	2 (1)	0 (0)	0.48
COPD[2]	10 (7)	10 (13)	0.82
Marfan's Syndrome	3 (2)	0 (0)	0.25
Coronary Artery Disease	30 (22)	41 (30)	0.20
Atrial Fibrillation	7 (5)	7 (5)	0.78
Hyperlipidemia	4 (3)	3 (2)	1
Social History			
Smoking	46 (34)	52 (38)	0.53
Drug	18 (13)	17 (13)	1
Alcohol	33 (24)	31 (28)	0.89

[1]TAA=thoracic aortic aneurysm, TAD=thoracic aortic dissection.
[2]COPD=chronic obstructive pulmonary disease.
*Signifies statistical significance.

On multivariate analysis, decreasing heart rate, absence of chest pain, no history of diabetes, absence of head & neck pain, absence of dizziness, and no history of myocardial infarction were independent predictors of TAA/TAD (Table 6). There were no differences when the subgroups of patients with TAA or TAD were compared to each other (data now shown).

Discussion

An expeditious diagnosis of thoracic aortic pathology in the emergency department remains a great challenge, especially its differentiation from acute coronary syndrome (ACS) [2]. Previous studies have suggested that there are many presenting signs and symptoms for TAD/TAA but routine blood work and standard imaging have not been shown to be reliable nor reproducible [10-12]. Potential genetic markers [13] and biomarkers in rat models [14] have been proposed; however, there is a need for practical and cost effective tools that can be quickly obtained in the emergency department for the routine screening of patients with acute thoracic complaints. In the present study, we have identified factors that are typically present on admission and routine emergency medical screening.

Table 3 Pain characterization and presenting symptoms

Variable	TAA/TAD	Control	P-value
Total patients	**136 (%)**	**136 (%)**	
Location of Pain			
Chest	64 (47)	115 (85)	<0.0001*
Head and Neck	5 (4)	23 (17)	0.0007*
Abdominal	33 (24)	24 (18)	0.08
Extremity	15 (11)	18 (13)	0.71
Back	33 (24)	21 (15)	0.09
Type of Pain			
Pressure/Tight	4 (5)	34 (37)	<0.0001*
Squeezing	8 (10)	6 (7)	0.56
Heavy	1 (1)	7 (8)	0.11
Sharp	14 (18)	20 (22)	0.65
Migrating	27 (35)	34 (37)	0.38
No pain	22 (28)	0 (0)	<0.0001*
Duration			
Increasing	21 (23)	2 (2)	<0.0001*
Sudden	10 (11)	2 (2)	0.0165*
Persistent	7 (6)	13 (12)	0.43
Constant	36 (37)	31 (37)	0.14
Decreasing	2 (2)	4 (4)	0.84
Intermittent	21 (22)	32 (38)	0.38
Symptoms			
Shortness of Breath	48 (42)	70 (51)	0.01*
Palpitation	3 (2)	12 (9)	0.03*
Dizziness	3 (2)	17 (13)	0.0025*
Dysphagia	3 (3)	0 (0)	0.25
Chills	7 (5)	10 (7)	0.62
Fever	10 (7)	11 (8)	1
Nausea	33 (24)	42 (31)	0.28
Emesis	19 (14)	20 (15)	1
Diaphoresis	16 (12)	21 (15)	0.48
Constipation	5 (5)	1 (1)	0.22
Cough	16 (12)	21 (15)	0.48
Weakness	13 (10)	18 (13)	0.45
Altered Mental Status	9 (8)	4 (3)	0.26
Syncope	21 (15)	20 (15)	1
Wheezing	3 (3)	3 (3)	0.68

TAA = thoracic aortic aneurysm, TAD = thoracic aortic dissection.
*Signifies statistical significance.

The study group of 136 patients with thoracic aortic dissection (TAD) or aneurysms (TAA) represented a mere 0.36% of the population presenting with acute chest complaints, highlighting the difficulty in diagnosing this rare

Table 4 Physical examination and x-ray results

Variable	TAA/TAD	Control	P-value
Total patients	**136 (%)**	**136 (%)**	
Physical Exam			
Focal Neurological Deficit	8 (6)	1 (1)	0.04*
Heart Murmur	11 (8)	5 (4)	0.19
Aortic Regurgitation	2 (2)	0 (0)	0.48
Irregular Rhythm	5 (5)	2 (1)	0.44
Heart Rate			
Normal	92 (68)	115 (86)	0.03*
Tachycardia (>120/min)	20 (15)	12 (9)	0.19
Bradycardia (< 60/min)	24 (18)	7 (5)	0.002*
Respiratory Rate			
Normal	63 (47)	105 (78)	<0.0001*
Tachypnea (>24/min)	72 (53)	29 (22)	<0.0001*
Bradypnea (<8/min)	0 (0)	0 (0)	1
Temperature			
Normal	114 (91)	122 (95)	0.29
Hyperthermic (> 39 C)	8 (6)	4 (3)	0.35
Hypothermic (< 36 C)	3 (2)	2 (2)	1
Systolic Blood Pressure			
Normal	58 (44)	61 (46)	0.84
Hypertensive (> 180 mmHg)	64 (47)	65 (49)	0.92
Hypotensive (SBP < 80 mmHg)	11 (8)	8 (6)	0.62
Diastolic Blood Pressure			
Normal	78 (59)	90 (67)	0.22
Hypertensive (>120 mmHg)	41 (31)	34 (25)	0.37
Hypotensive (<60 mmHg)	14 (11)	10 (7)	0.50
Chest X-Ray			
Widened Mediastinum	41 (52)	26 (45)	0.005*
Tortuous Aorta	21 (27)	17 (29)	0.28
Cardiomegaly	17 (16)	15 (15)	0.49

TAA = thoracic aortic aneurysm, TAD = thoracic aortic dissection.
*Signifies statistical significance.

Table 5 Blood test results

Test	TAA/TAD (%)	Control (%)	P-value
White Blood Cell			
Normal	93 (70)	103 (77)	0.29
Low (<3 million cells/mcL)	8 (6)	9 (7)	1
High (>12 million cells/mcL)	31 (23)	22 (16)	0.20
Hemoglobin			
Normal	80 (60)	81 (60)	1
Low (<9 grams/dL)	47 (35)	47 (35)	1
High (>15 grams/dL)	7 (5)	6 (4)	1
Hematocrit			
Normal	75 (56)	78 (58)	0.81
Low (<27%)	51 (38)	49 (37)	0.89
High (>55%)	8 (6)	7 (5)	1
Blood Urea Nitrogen			
Normal	45 (34)	69 (51)	<.0001*
Low	2 (2)	1 (1)	1
High	85 (64)	64 (48)	<.0001*
Creatinine			
Normal	71 (56)	80 (62)	0.40
Elevated (>35 mg/dL)	55 (44)	49 (38)	0.47
Lactate			
Normal	6 (60)	7 (64)	0.65
Elevated (>2.5 mEq/L)	4 (40)	4 (36)	0.89
INR			
Normal	76 (60)	75 (81)	
Elevated (>1.5)	51 (40)	18 (19)	0.0017*
D-Dimer			
Normal	1 (20)	7 (88)	0.06
Elevated (> 250 ng/ml)	4 (80)	1 (13)	0.06
Troponin			
Normal	53 (82)	80 (66)	0.04
Elevated (>0.3 ng/mL)	12 (18)	41 (34)	0.04*

TAA = thoracic aortic aneurysm, TAD = thoracic aortic dissection.
*Signifies statistical significance.

entity. It would not have been possible to employ contrast-enhanced CT scans on all such patients, especially in an emergency department that sees more than 100,000 patients per year. Pain characteristics have been shown to be unreliable in a systematic review [2,15]. The present study shows that the sudden onset in nature was more likely associated with TAA/TAD. This is in concordance with previous report by Klompas et al. [4]. On the other hand, our finding of association with increasing intensity has not been reported in other studies and may explain the evolving nature of thoracic aortic disease. On multivariate analysis, chest pain, head and neck pain, and dizziness were identified to be independently associated with

Table 6 Multivariate analysis

Factor	Odd ratio	P-value	95% Confidence interval
Heart rate	0.97	0.01	0.96 – 0.99
Chest pain	0.24	< 0.001	0.11 – 0.51
Diabetes	0.29	0.004	0.13 – 0.67
Head & neck pain	0.17	0.008	0.05 – 0.63
Dizziness	0.08	0.002	0.02 – 0.39
Myocardial infarction	0.07	0.007	0.01 – 0.48

ACS. These all represent easily obtainable factors in routine history taking.

As expected, past medical history for the most part was not a useful tool in differentiating TAA/TAD from ACS, as both share similar comorbidities. For example, having a history of hypertension was not a useful tool in differentiating the two disease processes. However, history of diabetes and myocardial infarction was significantly associated with ACS, both in univariate and multivariate analysis, providing another easily obtainable factor in differentiating TAA/TAD from ACS. In fact, diabetes may have a protective association against the development of aortic disease [16]. Diabetes has been shown to decrease the progression of aortic disease by direct metabolic effects by the decreased secretion of metalloproteinases from these individuals [16]. The decreased production of inflammatory cells caused by hyperglycemia in mice has also been shown to inhibit vascular smooth muscle cell death, thereby thwarting the progression of aortic disease [17]. Diabeteic patients are also more likely to develop ACS because of the proatherosclerotic and pro-inflammatory states associated with diabetes [18]. Our data is consistent with these findings. Diabetic patients are more likely to experience ACS than TAA/TAD.

On physical exam, we found tachypnea, bradycardia, and lower extremity neurological deficits to be associated with TAD/TAA. Of particular importance, when heart rate was analyzed as a continuous variable, increasing heart rate was independently associated with ACS.

There has been much interest in the identification of useful blood tests to make the diagnosis of TAA/TAD. Elevated plasma D-dimer levels [19-21] and plasma smooth muscle myosin heavy chain protein [22] have shown some diagnostic promise but are not routinely obtained on initial presentation. A protocol for or obtaining routine plasma D-dimer studies was not used in the present study but has been advocated by others [23]. Plasma D-dimer levels were obtained in only 13 patients in the current study (5 in study group, 8 in control), yet elevated levels showed a trend for significance. D-dimer levels may also be elevated in a large variety of other conditions, including venous thromboembolism (VTE), atrial fibrillation, congestive heart failure, disseminated intravascular coagulation and routine post-operative recovery [24]. Routine analysis on screening may therefore remains controversial. An element of coagulopathy may be a component of thoracic aortic diseases, however, as patients that presented with acute thoracic aortic disease had an elevated initialed normalization ratio (INR) compared to the ACS group. This association between elevated INR and thoracic aortic disease has been reported elsewhere [25]. Elevated BUN was associated with TAD/TAD in univariate analysis, an association that has not been reported. This may represent the physiological changes in blood flow resulting from the acute aortic injury.

It is worthwhile to note that while elevated troponin was associated with ACS in the present study, 9% of TAD/TAA cohort also demonstrated elevated serum troponin levels. Patients have been reported to have acute thoracic aortic dissection with concomitant myocardial infarction and this confusion could result in a catastrophe [26]. Thrombolytic therapy for acute myocardial infarction would be contraindicated in patients with acute thoracic aortic disease. Further confusion may be caused by EKG analysis because it has been reported that 0.1-0.2% of patients with proximal TAD will have ST-elevation myocardial infarctions occur in the setting [27]. Luo reported on six patients with clear electrocardiographic and serological evidence of acute myocardial infarction and concomitant thoracic aortic dissection, underscoring the need to be continuously vigilant for acute thoracic aortic disease, even after the diagnosis of myocardial infarction is confirmed [28].

When present, the finding of a widened mediastinum was associated with TAD/TAA, as previously reported [29]. Because a widened mediastinum is difficult to interpret on a portable x-ray, a formal standing posterior-anterior chest x-ray for patients presenting with chest pain may be necessary. CT scanning is an effective screening modality [30] but cannot be utilized for all patients with acute thoracic complaints who present to busy ED's. Transthoracic echocardiography may also a useful imaging modality for the diagnosis of acute aortic syndromes. Some have reported it to be beneficial for screening [31] but it should not be used as the sole screening imaging technique [32].

Limitations of the study include the retrospective nature of the study design. A larger cohort of patients that presented with acute thoracic symptoms but were not found to have acute thoracic aortic dissection or aneurysm would have provided a statistically enhanced database to allow for the development of a risk prediction model. Such modeling would facilitate the use of the findings reported herein. In addition examining the missed diagnosis rate and delay in diagnosis in a prospective fashion using this model would validate the findings from this study.

Screening patients with acute chest pain in the emergency department for thoracic aortic dissection or thoracic aortic aneurysm presents a clinical challenge. In the current study, we identified increasing heart rate, presence of chest pain, head and neck pain, dizziness, diabetes, and history of myocardial infarction to be independently associated with ACS as opposed to TAA/TAD. These represent easily obtainable factors that can be used to screen patients to undergo prompt confirmatory imaging with CT of the chest.

Competing interests
The authors declare that they have no competing interests.

Authors' contributions
IML conceived of the study, and participated in its design and coordination and helped to draft the manuscript. KS participated in the design of the study, performed the statistical analysis and coordination and helped to draft the manuscript. AJW participated in the design of the study, performed the statistical analysis and coordination and helped to draft the manuscript. EM participated in the design of the study and coordination and helped to draft the manuscript. MP participated in the design of the study and coordination and helped to draft the manuscript. KMW conceived of the study, and participated in its design and coordination and helped to draft the manuscript. CMG conceived of the study, and participated in its design and coordination and helped to draft the manuscript. DL participated in the design of the study and performed the statistical analysis. TB conceived of the study, and participated in its design and coordination and helped to draft the manuscript. BAZ conceived of the study, and participated in its design and coordination and helped to draft the manuscript. BP participated in the design of the study and coordination and helped to draft the manuscript. All authors read and approved the final manuscript.

Acknowledgments
This has been presented at the Eighth Annual Academic Surgical Congress in Feb, 2013.

Author details
[1]Departments of Surgery, Albert Einstein College of Medicine-Beth Israel Medical Center, 10 Union Square East, Suite 2M, New York, NY 10003, USA. [2]Emergency Medicine, Albert Einstein College of Medicine-Beth Israel Medical Center, New York, NY, USA. [3]Radiology, Albert Einstein College of Medicine-Beth Israel Medical Center, New York, NY, USA.

References

1. Woo KM, Schneider JI: **High-risk chief complaints I: chest pain-the big three.** *Emerg Med Clin North Am* 2009, **27**(4):685–712.
2. Assar AN, Zarins CK: **Ruptured abdominal aortic aneurysm: a surgical emergency with many clinical presentations.** *Postgrad Med J* 2009, **85**:268–273.
3. Mehta RH, Suzuki T, Hagan PG, *et al*: **Predicting death in patients with acute type a aortic dissection.** *Circulation* 2002, **105**(2):200–206.
4. Klompas M: **Does this patient have an acute thoracic aortic dissection?** *JAMA* 2002, **287**(17):2262–2272.
5. Booher AM, Isselbacher EM, Nienaber CA, *et al*: **The IRAD classification system for characterizing survival after aortic dissection.** *Am J Med* 2013, **126**(8):730.
6. Ramanath VS, Oh JK, Sundt TM, *et al*: **Acute aortic syndromes and thoracic aortic aneurysm.** *Mayo Clin Proc* 2009, **84**(5):465–481.
7. Legras A, Bruzzi M, Nakashima K, *et al*: **Risk factors for hospital death after surgery for type A aortic dissection.** *Asian Cardiovasc Thorac Ann* 2012, **20**(3):269–274.
8. Tanaka M, Kimura N, Yamaguchi A, *et al*: **In-hospital and long-term results of surgery for acute type A aortic dissection: 243 Consecutive Patients.** *Ann Thorac Cardiovasc Surg* 2012, **18**:18–23.
9. Shiga T, Wajima Z, Apfel CC, *et al*: **Diagnostic accuracy of transesophageal echocardiography, helical computed tomography, and magnetic resonance imaging for suspected thoracic aortic dissection: systematic review and meta-analysis.** *Arch Intern Med* 2006, **166**(13):1350–1356.
10. Hiratzka LF, Bakris GL, Beckman JA, *et al*: **2010 ACCF/AHA/AATS/ACR/ASA/SCA/SCAI/SIR/STS/SVM guidelines for the diagnosis and management of patients with Thoracic Aortic Disease: a report of the American College of Cardiology Foundation/American Heart Association Task Force on Practice Guidelines, American Association for Thoracic Surgery, American College of Radiology, American Stroke Association, Society of Cardiovascular Anesthesiologists, Society for Cardiovascular Angiography and Interventions, Society of Interventional Radiology, Society of Thoracic Surgeons, and Society for Vascular Medicine.** *Circulation* 2010, **121**(13):266–369.
11. Isselbacher EM: **Thoracic and abdominal aortic aneurysms.** *Circulation* 2005, **111**:816–828.
12. O'Gara PT: **Aortic aneurysm.** *Circulation* 2003, **107**:43–45.
13. Kuang S-Q, Guo D-C, Prakash SK: **Recurrent chromosome 16p13.1 duplications are a risk factor for aortic dissections.** *PLoS Genet* 2011, **7**:e1002118.
14. Das D, Gawdzik J, Dellefave-Castillo L, *et al*: **S100a12 expression in thoracic aortic aneurysm is associated with increased risk of dissection and perioperative complications.** *J Am Coll Cardiol* 2012, **60**:775–785.
15. Chua M, Ibrahim I, Neo X, *et al*: **Acute aortic dissection in the ed: risk factors and predictors for missed diagnosis.** *Am J Emerg Med* 2012, **30**:1622–1626.
16. Prakash S, Pedroza C, Khalil Y, *et al*: **Diabetes and reduced risk for thoracic aortic aneurysms and dissections: a nationwide case–control study.** *J Am Heart Assoc* 2012, **1**:jah3–e000323.
17. Miyama N, Dua MM, Yeung JJ, *et al*: **Hyperglycemia limits experimental aortic aneurysm progression.** *J Vasc Surg* 2010, **52**:975–983.
18. Keller PF, Carballo D, Roffi M: **Diabetes and acute coronary syndrome.** *Minerva Med* 2010, **101**(2):81–104.
19. Weber T, Högler S, Auer J, *et al*: **D-dimer in acute aortic dissection.** *CHEST Journal* 2003, **123**:1375–1378.
20. Eggebrecht H, Naber CK, Bruch C, *et al*: **Value of plasma fibrin d-dimers for detection of acute aortic dissection.** *J Am Coll Cardiol* 2004, **44**:804–809.
21. Sutherland A, Escano J, Coon TP: **D-dimer as the sole screening test for acute aortic dissection: a review of the literature.** *Ann Emerg Med* 2008, **52**(4):339–343.
22. Suzuki T, Katoh H, Watanabe M, *et al*: **Novel biochemical diagnostic method for aortic dissection: results of a prospective study using an immunoassay of smooth muscle myosin heavy chain.** *Circulation* 1996, **93**:1244–1249.
23. Marill KA: **Serum d-dimer is a sensitive test for the detection of acute aortic dissection: a pooled meta-analysis.** *J Emerg Med* 2008, **34**(4):367–376.
24. Koracevic GP: **Pragmatic classification of the causes of high D-dimer.** *Am J Emerg Med* 2009, **27**(8):1016.e5–7.
25. Aboulafia DM, Aboulafia ED: **Aortic aneurysm-induced disseminated intravascular coagulation.** *Ann Vasc Surg* 1996, **10**(4):396–405.
26. Lentini S, Perrotta S: **Aortic dissection with concomitant acute myocardial infarction: from diagnosis to management.** *J Emerg Trauma Shock* 2011, **4**(2):273–278.
27. Ankel F: **Aortic dissection.** In *Rosen's emergency medicine: Concepts and clinical practice.* Edited by Marx JH, Walls RM. Philadelphia: PA, Mosby Elsevier Publishing; 2010:1088–1092.
28. Luo JL, Wu CK, Lin YH, *et al*: **Type A aortic dissection manifesting as acute myocardial infarction: still a lesson to learn.** *Acta Cardiol* 2009, **64**(4):499–504.
29. Lai V, Tsang WK, Chan WC, *et al*: **Diagnostic accuracy of mediastinal width measurement on posteroanterior and anteroposterior chest radiographs in the depiction of acute nontraumatic thoracic aortic dissection.** *Emerg Radiol* 2012, **19**(4):309–15.
30. Nathan DP, Boonn W, Lai E, *et al*: **Presentation, complications, and natural history of penetrating atherosclerotic ulcer disease.** *J Vasc Surg* 2012, **55**(1):10–5.
31. Shah BN, Ahmadvazir S, Pabla JS, *et al*: **The role of urgent transthoracic echocardiography in the evaluation of patients presenting with acute chest pain.** *Eur Jour Emerg Med* 2012, **19**(5):277–83.
32. Cecconi M, Chirillo F, Costantini C, *et al*: **The role of transthoracic echocardiography in the diagnosis and management of acute type A aortic syndrome.** *Am Heart J* 2012, **163**:112–8.

5

Abdominal damage control surgery and reconstruction: world society of emergency surgery position paper

Laura Godat, Leslie Kobayashi, Todd Costantini and Raul Coimbra*

Abstract

Damage control laparotomy was first described by Dr. Harlan Stone in 1983 when he suggested that patients with severe trauma should have their primary procedures abbreviated when coagulopathy was encountered. He recommended temporizing patients with abdominal packing and temporary closure to allow restoration of normal physiology prior to returning to the operating room for definitive repair. The term damage control in the trauma setting was coined by Rotondo et al., in 1993. Studies in subsequent years have validated this technique by demonstrating decreased mortality and immediate post-operative complications. The indications for damage control laparotomy have evolved to encompass abdominal compartment syndrome, abdominal sepsis, vascular and acute care surgery cases. The perioperative critical care provided to these patients, including sedation, paralysis, nutrition, and fluid management strategies may improve closure rates and recovery. In the rare cases of inability to primarily close the abdomen, there are a number of reconstructive strategies that may be used in the acute and chronic phases of abdominal closure.

Keywords: Trauma, Damage control, Abdominal compartment syndrome, Temporary abdominal closure

Introduction

The bloody lethal triad of hypothermia, acidosis, and coagulopathy has been the nemesis of trauma surgeons for decades. Many advances in the field of trauma have evolved around prevention and treatment of this clinical scenario. One useful technique is damage control laparotomy (DCL). DCL has 3 stages, an abbreviated initial operative procedure with temporary abdominal closure (TAC); continued resuscitation and management of physiologic and acid–base derangements, and definitive treatment and closure.

The first stage in DCL is control of hemorrhage and contamination followed by use of a TAC strategy [1]. The optimal TAC strategy should prevent evisceration, evacuate fluid, allow access to the abdominal cavity, and allow for expansion in order to prevent abdominal compartment syndrome (ACS) [2-4]. The second stage of DCL involves continuation of resuscitation, which should include judicious fluid administration with aggressive correction of coagulopathy, acidosis, and hypothermia. Additional management may include paralysis, early enteral nutrition, and diuresis. Lastly, once normal physiology has been restored, the patient should return to the operating room for definitive repair of injuries, followed by abdominal wall closure with reconstruction if possible in the same or in subsequent operative interventions.

DCL has been associated with improved outcomes and decreased mortality in severely injured trauma patients [5,6]. Because of this, DCL indications have been expanded to include abdominal sepsis, ACS, and prolonged or extensive elective surgery. This is a review of the current literature on DCL including recommendations regarding the indications for DCL, techniques of TAC, intensive care unit (ICU) management, and abdominal closure with reconstruction.

To our knowledge no randomized controlled trials (RCT) exist for the use of DCL, although there are many retrospective reviews and prospective observational trials demonstrating improved outcomes in both trauma and acute care surgery populations [2,7].

* Correspondence: rcoimbra@ucsd.edu
Division of Trauma, Surgical Critical Care, and Burns, University of California, San Diego, 200 West Arbor Dr., #8896, San Diego CA 92103-8896, United States of America

Review

Indications

The decision to switch from definitive treatment to damage control should be made early, ideally prior to entering the operative suite, as this has been associated with improved mortality [7]. In trauma patients, relative pre-operative indications for DCL include systolic blood pressure (SBP) <90 mmHg with penetrating torso, blunt abdominal, or severe pelvic trauma, and the need for resuscitative thoracotomy [1]. Other Emergency Department (ED) variables associated with increased use of DCL include SBP <60 mmHg, hypothermia, inappropriate bradycardia, and pH of <7.2 [8,9]. Intraoperative indications for DCL in trauma patients include "non-surgical" bleeding, pH ≤ 7.18, temperature ≤33°C, transfusion of ≥10 units of blood, total fluid replacement >12 L, and estimated blood losses of ≥5 L [5,6]. Platelet count, PT, aPTT, fibrinogen levels and thromboelastography findings can also be used to guide decision making if available [8].

In addition to the above indications, patients at high risk for ACS should be left open prophylactically at the time of laparotomy [10,11]. This includes patients requiring large volume resuscitation (>15 L or 10 Units of PRBCs), those with evidence of visceral edema, peak inspiratory pressures >40, or intra-abdominal pressure (IAP) >21 during attempted closure [12-16]. Patients with IAP >12 mmHg are considered to have intra-abdominal hypertension (IAH) which is graded from I to IV (Table 1). ACS is a syndrome of organ dysfunction; cardiac, renal or pulmonary associated with elevated IAP and reduced intra-abdominal blood flow [17]. If organ failure has developed patients require emergent decompressive laparotomy or revision of their TAC [12,13,17].

DCL has also been beneficial in general surgery patients with severe abdominal sepsis, including those with diverticulitis or necrotizing pancreatitis who require serial debridement as well as those with significant blood loss [12,18-22]. Patients with mesenteric ischemia or venous occlusive disease who require staged laparotomies due to questionable bowel viability may also benefit from DCL [23]. Advanced age is not a contraindication to DCL as good outcomes have been seen in the elderly [24,25].

Despite improvements in mortality seen in severely injured patients treated with DCL, there is evidence to suggest that it may worsen outcomes in patients who do not meet the indications described above [26]. A retrospective review of over 600 cases, found that low risk patients, identified as those with absence of shock, severe head or combined abdominal injury (Abbreviated Injury Scale <3) had significantly higher rates of infections, organ failure, pulmonary and bowel related complications compared to similar patients closed at the time of their first procedure [27].

Temporary abdominal closure methods

Because the abdomen is left open at DCL, the resultant wound requires a dressing or TAC. The ideal TAC should be easily and quickly applied, allow room for expansion, limit contamination, decrease bowel edema, protect the viscera, fascia and skin from damage, evacuate fluids, prevent adhesions, minimize loss of domain and be cost effective. The TAC should be easily changed, result in a high rate of closure and be associated with a low rate of complications, particularly enterocutaneous fistula (EC fistula) and mortality (Table 2).

The first series of DCLs used towel clips or running sutures for closure of the skin or fascia to provide a tamponade effect with peritoneal packing [5]. However, this type of closure frequently resulted in ACS [2,14,28,29], and it is no longer recommended. The next generation TACs were performed using a silo or Bogota bag where a non-permeable barrier; IV bag, bowel bag, steri-Drape or silastic cloth was sutured to the skin or fascia. Advantages are prevention of desiccation, swift application, ability to visualize the bowel and low cost. However, disadvantages include damage to the skin, loss of domain, and lack of effective fluid removal [2,30]. Primary closure rates vary from 12.2-82% [31,32]. EC fistula rates are generally low, reported at 0–14.4% [14,31-36] however ACS rates range as high as 33% [11,33,36]. This method has also largely been abandoned.

Vacuum assisted closure (VAC) devices are most commonly used today. Barker et al., coined the term "vacuum pack" (VP) in 1995; describing a 3 layer TAC;

Table 1 Grades of intra-abdominal hypertension

Grade	*IAP	Organ failure
I	12-15	Absent
II	16-20	Absent
III	21-25	Absent
IV	>25	Absent
**ACS	>20	Present

*IAP = Intra-abdominal pressure.
**ACS = Abdominal Compartment Syndrome.

Table 2 Methods of temporary abdominal closure (TAC)

Method of TAC	Primary closure rate	Mortality rate	Enterocutaneous fistula rate
Bogota Bag/Silo [14,31-36]	12.2-82%	19-58.4%	0-14.4%
Mesh/Wittman Patch [19,42,51,54,55,58]	18-93%	7.7-43%	0-26%
Vacuum Assisted Closure Device [38,39,41,44,45]	31-100%	14-44%	1.2-15%

consisting of a fenestrated polyethylene sheet between the abdominal viscera and parietal peritoneum, followed by a moist towel with closed suction drains covered with an occlusive adhesive drape [37]. This method is inexpensive, easily applied and changed, protects the viscera, prevents adhesions, removes exudate and prevents some loss of domain [2,37]. Commercially prepared negative pressure dressings are available and function similar to the VP. These are the V.A.C.©Abdominal Dressing system and the Abthera™ system. Both devices use three layers. The inner layer is a plastic covered sponge that is inserted into the gutters to protect the viscera and facilitate fluid removal, this is followed by a Micro or Macroporous sponge covered by an occlusive dressing that is attached to suction [38-40]. These techniques have been associated with a 31-100% primary closure rate [38-42]. EC fistula rates vary in the literature from 1.2%-15% [41-45], but are generally low. A prospective comparison of these two systems showed higher 30-day primary fascial closure rates and lower 30-day all-cause mortality with the Abthera™ system compared to the Barker VP [46].

Lastly, there are multiple TACs that interpose a graft material between the fascial edges. This can be absorbable such as vicryl or biologic mesh, non-absorbable such as polypropylene (PPE) or expanded polytetrafluoroethylene (ePTFE), or a Wittman patch. The material is initially applied loosely to allow for bowel expansion and prevent ACS. Serial examinations of the wound at the bedside or in the operating room must be done and the mesh is pleated or refastened to gradually pull the fascial edges together [47-49]. The primary benefit of these systems is their ability to maintain and recover fascial domain. Drawbacks include damage to the fascia, inability to prevent adhesions and difficulty with fluid management. EC fistula rates vary with type of graft material; as high as 7-26% with non-absorbable mesh [42,50-52], followed by 4.6-18% with absorbable mesh [49,53,54], and the Wittman patch which has the lowest reported rates of 0–4.2% [55-58]. Risk of ECF is reduced if omentum is interposed between the mesh and bowel [52]. Primary closure has been reported as late as >50 days after the initial damage control operation [49]. ACS rates associated with interposition grafts are seldom sited in the literature; most that did reported no incidences [48,53,54].

Resuscitation

The second stage of DCL is resuscitation focused on correction of physiologic derangements, acidosis, oxygen debt, coagulopathy and hypothermia [1]. Hemodynamic derangements due to hypovolemic shock should be reversed as quickly as possible with volume resuscitation. However, over use of crystalloids can result in third spacing worsening bowel edema, anastomotic leaks, ACS and multi-organ failure [59,60]. Accordingly, the use of massive transfusion protocols (MTP) has been recommended for DCL patients [60-62]. MTP's advocate using blood transfusion earlier in resuscitation, using blood and blood products instead of crystalloid or colloid, and the infusion of red cells, plasma, and platelets in a 1:1:1 ratio. There is evidence to suggest that MTP's and use of 1:1:1 transfusion ratios results in lower overall fluid requirements, blood utilization, and possibly improved mortality in patients with massive blood loss, severe injury and severe physiological derangements, such as are encountered in DCL patients [63,64]. In addition, fluid resuscitation should be guided by hemodynamic parameters such as stroke volume variance or pulse pressure differentials and central venous or left atrial pressures. Improved fluid management may decrease the incidence of ACS and promote early fascial closure [28,65,66]. There is also some evidence that the use of hypertonic fluids in the postoperative period may decrease time to primary closure and improve the primary closure rate [67]. Patients should be monitored for development of ACS and if exhibiting symptoms, the TAC should be removed and replaced with a looser device immediately [2].

Prophylactic antibiotics should be administered preoperatively when possible as infection rates increase if given intra or post operatively [68], and duration should be no longer than 24 hours [69].

It has been proposed that neuromuscular blockade (NMB) can help prevent retraction of the fascial edge and improve closure rates. However, the current evidence comparing NMB to simple sedation is equivocal [44,70]. Similarly diuresis is often suggested as a means to decrease bowel edema and facilitate fascial closure once patients have been resuscitated; however, there is no convincing data to suggest use of diuretics improves the rate or time to closure [71].

Nutrition is known to be a key component to the recovery of patients following severe injury. There are no RCT's of enteral nutrition in patients with an open abdomen; however multiple retrospective reviews and one prospective cohort study demonstrate safety of enteral nutrition within 36 hours to 4 days of DCL [72-75]. Two studies have demonstrated increased rates of fascial closure [72,73], and 3 demonstrated decreased infectious complications [72,73,75] with early enteral nutrition.

Closure and abdominal wall reconstruction

Initial return to the operating room should occur as soon as normal physiology has been restored and can vary from 6–72 hours from the time of the primary procedure [2]. Patients should also be taken back to the operating room if there is evidence of surgical bleeding concerning for missed or inadequately addressed injury. A survey from the Western Trauma Association found the majority of its members wait approximately 24 hours for first return to the operating room [2]. Once all injuries have been definitively addressed the abdomen should be closed. The American Association for the Surgery of Trauma studied factors contributing to primary closure and found that those who achieved primary closure were more likely to be women, had lower peak airway pressures, an injury severity score <15, lower lactate levels, higher pH, and lower blood loss. Those who were closed primarily also had fewer EC fistula, abscesses, ICU and ventilator days. Interestingly the volume of crystalloid given was <5 L and did not vary between groups. Overall closure rate was 59.1% [76].

A review of the literature suggest a bimodal distribution of patients with TAC, the first are able to be closed within 4–7 days and achieve a high rate of primary closure, the second group have a delayed (20–40 days) and much lower overall rate of closure [77]. Thus, if unable to close the abdomen within 7 days a progressive closure device may be necessary. This can be achieved using multiple devices, one of the most common; the Wittman patch is sewn to the fascial edges and prevents further loss of domain while slowly bringing the fascial edges together. Multiple studies of the Wittman patch have demonstrated a 78-93% fascial closure rate [55-58]. Modifications of the VAC closure with the addition of retention type sutures in the skin and fascia can significantly increase rates of primary closure to 88-100% [38,39], compared to serial VAC changes which have a primary closure rate of 31% [42]. Absorbable mesh can be used similarly to the Wittman patch, stitching it to the fascia and slowly bringing the fascial edges together during serial returns to the operating room as the visceral edema resolves with primary closure rates of 22-38% [42,50,51].

If unable to close the fascial defect with progressive closure techniques, the operative plan must shift gears to one of an expectant hernia (Figure 1). Patients with residual fascial defects should be covered with split thickness skin grafting once the viscera are fixed and granulation tissue is sufficient [42,50,51]. Because of the high risk of infection, synthetic graft material should be removed prior to skin grafting [49].

Formal reconstruction of the ventral hernia should be deferred until after the patient has fully recovered and is ready for another large operation. Timing of the definitive repair is not well studied, Jernigan et al., recommend 6–12 months but no longer as they found less need for prosthetic bridging and lower recurrence rate due to more tension free repair in patients operated on earlier than 12 months. Component separation may be required to span the defect; there are multiple methods for this procedure with good outcomes reported [51]. In clean fields, synthetic mesh may be utilized as a bridge if the patient cannot be closed primarily with or without component separation. Another option to close the fascial defect is to use a biologic material, such as human acellular dermal matrix (HADM). This has the benefit of being an option in a contaminated or infected field. As described by Scott et al., the HADM is fixed transfascially with 2-3 cm of underlay, with multiple pieces stitched together if necessary. The repair should be taut to reduce laxity. If the skin edges can be mobilized and closed, closed suction drains are left to manage the dead space; otherwise a non-adherent dressing is placed over the HADM and a negative pressure dressing is applied [78]. Two series looked at this method [78,79] and reported good outcomes, but with concern for recurrent hernia and eventration.

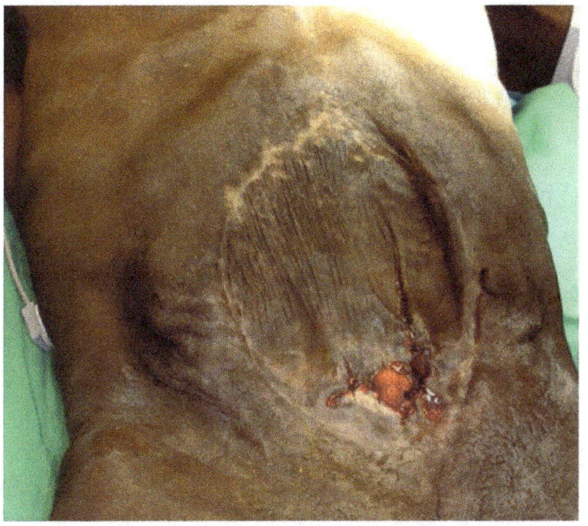

Figure 1 Example of a patient's abdominal wall with planned ventral hernia after vicryl mesh placement and split thickness skin grafting.

Recommendations

We recommend

1. Damage control laparotomy for trauma or acute general surgical patients under physiologic stress including; acidosis, hypothermia, hypocoagulable state, prolonged hypotension. Also, those requiring a "second-look" after ischemic or embolic events or intra-abdominal infections which may need additional debridement such as necrotizing pancreatitis.
2. Initial abdominal closure should employ a negative pressure dressing such as the "vacuum pack" method or its commercially available alternative.
3. After 5-7 days if the abdomen cannot be closed convert to the use of a bridging device which progressively brings the fascia together such as the Wittman patch or modified V.A.C.©.

We suggest

1. Unless otherwise contraindicated enteral nutrition should be started early.
2. In the absence of definite indication, prophylactic antibiotics should be limited to 24 hours.
3. Formal reconstruction if necessary should be delayed 6-12 months and tempered with a planned ventral hernia.

Abbreviations

DCL: Damage control laparotomy; TAC: Temporary abdominal closure; ACS: Abdominal compartment syndrome; ICU: Intensive care unit; RCT: Randomized controlled trials; SBP: Systolic blood pressure; ED: Emergency department; PRBCs: Packed red blood cells; IAP: Intra-abdominal pressure; IAH: Intra-abdominal hypertension; EC fistula: Enterocutaneous fistula; VAC: Vacuum assisted closure; VP: Vacuum pack; PPE: Polypropylene; ePTFE: expanded polytetrafluoroethylene; MTP: of massive transfusion protocols; NMB: neuromuscular blockade; HADM: Human acellular dermal matrix.

Competing interests

The Authors all declare that they have no competing interests.

Authors' contributions

All authors helped to draft the manuscript. All authors read and approved the final manuscript.

References

1. Wyrzykowski AD, Feliciano DV: **Trauma damage control.** In *Trauma.* 6th edition. Edited by Feliciano DV, Mattox KL, Moore EE. United States of America: The McGraw-Hill Companies, Inc; 2008:851–870.
2. Campbell A, Chang M, Fabian T, Franz M, Kaplan M, Moore F, Reed RL, Scott B, Silverman R: **Management of the open abdomen: from initial operation to definitive closure.** *Am Surg* 2009, **75:**S1–S22.
3. Barker DE, Green JM, Maxwell RA, Smith PW, Mejia VA, Dart BW, Cofer JB, Roe SM, Burns RP: **Experience with vacuum-pack temporary abdominal wound closure in 258 trauma and general and vascular surgical patients.** *J Am Coll Surg* 2007, **204:**784–792. discussion 792–783.
4. Aydin C, Aytekin FO, Yenisey C, Kabay B, Erdem E, Kocbil G, Tekin K: **The effect of different temporary abdominal closure techniques on fascial wound healing and postoperative adhesions in experimental secondary peritonitis.** *Langenbecks Arch Surg* 2008, **393:**67–73.
5. Stone HH, Strom PR, Mullins RJ: **Management of the major coagulopathy with onset during laparotomy.** *Ann Surg* 1983, **197:**532–535.
6. Sharp KW, Locicero RJ: **Abdominal packing for surgically uncontrollable hemorrhage.** *Ann Surg* 1992, **215:**467–474. discussion 474–465.
7. Hirshberg A, Wall MJ Jr, Mattox KL: **Planned reoperation for trauma: a two year experience with 124 consecutive patients.** *J Trauma* 1994, **37:**365–369.
8. Asensio JA, McDuffie L, Petrone P, Roldan G, Forno W, Gambaro E, Salim A, Demetriades D, Murray J, Velmahos G, *et al*: **Reliable variables in the exsanguinated patient which indicate damage control and predict outcome.** *Am J Surg* 2001, **182:**743–751.
9. Garrison JR, Richardson JD, Hilakos AS, Spain DA, Wilson MA, Miller FB, Fulton RL: **Predicting the need to pack early for severe intra-abdominal hemorrhage.** *J Trauma* 1996, **40:**923–927. discussion 927–929.
10. Offner PJ, de Souza AL, Moore EE, Biffl WL, Franciose RJ, Johnson JL, Burch JM: **Avoidance of abdominal compartment syndrome in damage-control laparotomy after trauma.** *Arch Surg* 2001, **136:**676–681.
11. Johnson JW, Gracias VH, Schwab CW, Reilly PM, Kauder DR, Shapiro MB, Dabrowski GP, Rotondo MF: **Evolution in damage control for exsanguinating penetrating abdominal injury.** *J Trauma* 2001, **51:**261–269. discussion 269–271.
12. Diaz JJ Jr, Cullinane DC, Dutton WD, Jerome R, Bagdonas R, Bilaniuk JW, Collier BR, Como JJ, Cumming J, Griffen M, *et al*: **The management of the open abdomen in trauma and emergency general surgery: part 1-damage control.** *J Trauma* 2010, **68:**1425–1438.
13. Cheatham ML, Malbrain ML, Kirkpatrick A, Sugrue M, Parr M, De Waele J, Balogh Z, Leppaniemi A, Olvera C, Ivatury R, *et al*: **Results from the international conference of experts on intra-abdominal hypertension and abdominal compartment syndrome. II. Recommendations.** *Intensive Care Med* 2007, **33:**951–962.
14. Raeburn CD, Moore EE, Biffl WL, Johnson JL, Meldrum DR, Offner PJ, Franciose RJ, Burch JM: **The abdominal compartment syndrome is a morbid complication of postinjury damage control surgery.** *Am J Surg* 2001, **182:**542–546.
15. Oelschlager BK, Boyle EM Jr, Johansen K, Meissner MH: **Delayed abdominal closure in the management of ruptured abdominal aortic aneurysms.** *Am J Surg* 1997, **173:**411–415.
16. Rasmussen TE, Hallett JW Jr, Noel AA, Jenkins G, Bower TC, Cherry KJ Jr, Panneton JM, Gloviczki P: **Early abdominal closure with mesh reduces multiple organ failure after ruptured abdominal aortic aneurysm repair: guidelines from a 10-year case-control study.** *J Vasc Surg* 2002, **35:**246–253.
17. Malbrain ML, Cheatham ML, Kirkpatrick A, Sugrue M, Parr M, De Waele J, Balogh Z, Leppaniemi A, Olvera C, Ivatury R, *et al*: **Results from the international conference of experts on intra-abdominal hypertension and abdominal compartment syndrome. I. Definitions.** *Intensive Care Med* 2006, **32:**1722–1732.
18. Garcia-Sabrido JL, Tallado JM, Christou NV, Polo JR, Valdecantos E: **Treatment of severe intra-abdominal sepsis and/or necrotic foci by an 'open-abdomen' approach. Zipper and zipper-mesh techniques.** *Arch Surg* 1988, **123:**152–156.
19. Wittmann DH, Aprahamian C, Bergstein JM: **Etappenlavage: advanced diffuse peritonitis managed by planned multiple laparotomies utilizing zippers, slide fastener, and velcro analogue for temporary abdominal closure.** *World J Surg* 1990, **14:**218–226.
20. Ozguc H, Yilmazlar T, Gurluler E, Ozen Y, Korun N, Zorluoglu A: **Staged abdominal repair in the treatment of intra-abdominal infection: analysis of 102 patients.** *J Gastrointest Surg* 2003, **7:**646–651.
21. Besselink MG, de Bruijn MT, Rutten JP, Boermeester MA, Hofker HS, Gooszen HG: **Surgical intervention in patients with necrotizing pancreatitis.** *Br J Surg* 2006, **93:**593–599.
22. Kafka-Ritsch R, Birkfellner F, Perathoner A, Raab H, Nehoda H, Pratschke J, Zitt M: **Damage control surgery with abdominal vacuum and delayed bowel reconstruction in patients with perforated diverticulitis Hinchey III/IV.** *J Gastrointest Surg* 2012, **16:**1915–1922.
23. Kaminsky O, Yampolski I, Aranovich D, Gnessin E, Greif F: **Does a second-look operation improve survival in patients with peritonitis due to acute mesenteric ischemia? A five-year retrospective experience.** *World J Surg* 2005, **29:**645–648.
24. Arhinful E, Jenkins D, Schiller HJ, Cullinane DC, Smoot DL, Zielinski MD: **Outcomes of damage control laparotomy with open abdomen management in the octogenarian population.** *J Trauma* 2011, **70:**616–621.
25. Subramanian A, Balentine C, Palacio CH, Sansgiry S, Berger DH, Awad SS: **Outcomes of damage-control celiotomy in elderly nontrauma patients with intra-abdominal catastrophes.** *Am J Surg* 2010, **200:**783–788. discussion 788–789.
26. Hatch QM, Osterhout LM, Podbielski J, Kozar RA, Wade CE, Holcomb JB, Cotton BA: **Impact of closure at the first take back: complication burden and potential overutilization of damage control laparotomy.** *J Trauma* 2011, **71:**1503–1511.
27. Martin MJ, Hatch Q, Cotton B, Holcomb J: **The use of temporary abdominal closure in low-risk trauma patients: Helpful or harmful?** *J Trauma Acute Care Surg* 2012, **72:**601–606. discussion 606–608.
28. Balogh Z, McKinley BA, Cocanour CS, Kozar RA, Holcomb JB, Ware DN, Moore FA: **Secondary abdominal compartment syndrome is an elusive early complication of traumatic shock resuscitation.** *Am J Surg* 2002, **184:**538–543. discussion 543–534.
29. Balogh Z, McKinley BA, Holcomb JB, Miller CC, Cocanour CS, Kozar RA, Valdivia A, Ware DN, Moore FA: **Both primary and secondary abdominal compartment syndrome can be predicted early and are harbingers of multiple organ failure.** *J Trauma* 2003, **54:**848–859. discussion 859–861.
30. Rutherford EJ, Skeete DA, Brasel KJ: **Management of the patient with an open abdomen: techniques in temporary and definitive closure.** *Curr Probl Surg* 2004, **41:**815–876.

31. Kirshtein B, Roy-Shapira A, Lantsberg L, Mizrahi S: **Use of the "Bogota bag" for temporary abdominal closure in patients with secondary peritonitis.** *Am Surg* 2007, **73:**249–252.
32. Doyon A, Devroede G, Viens D, Saito S, Rioux A, Echave V, Sauve M, Martin M, Poisson J: **A simple, inexpensive, life-saving way to perform iterative laparotomy in patients with severe intra-abdominal sepsis.** *Colorectal Dis* 2001, **3:**115–121.
33. Tremblay LN, Feliciano DV, Schmidt J, Cava RA, Tchorz KM, Ingram WL, Salomone JP, Nicholas JM, Rozycki GS: **Skin only or silo closure in the critically ill patient with an open abdomen.** *Am J Surg* 2001, **182:**670–675.
34. Brox-Jimenez A, Ruiz-Luque V, Torres-Arcos C, Parra-Membrives P, Diaz-Gomez D, Gomez-Bujedo L, Marquez-Munoz M: **Experience with the Bogota bag technique for temporary abdominal closure.** *Cirugia Espanola* 2007, **82:**150–154.
35. Foy HM, Nathens AB, Maser B, Mathur S, Jurkovich GJ: **Reinforced silicone elastomer sheeting, an improved method of temporary abdominal closure in damage control laparotomy.** *Am J Surg* 2003, **185:**498–501.
36. Howdieshell TR, Proctor CD, Sternberg E, Cue JI, Mondy JS, Hawkins ML: **Temporary abdominal closure followed by definitive abdominal wall reconstruction of the open abdomen.** *Am J Surg* 2004, **188:**301–306.
37. Brock WB, Barker DE, Burns RP: **Temporary closure of open abdominal wounds: The vacuum pack.** *Am Surg* 1995, **61:**30–35.
38. Cothren CC, Moore EE, Johnson JL, Moore JB, Burch JM: **One hundred percent fascial approximation with sequential abdominal closure of the open abdomen.** *Am J Surg* 2006, **192:**238–242.
39. Miller PR, Meredith JW, Johnson JC, Chang MC: **Prospective evaluation of vacuum-assisted fascial closure after open abdomen: Planned ventral hernia rate is substantially reduced.** *Ann Surg* 2004, **239:**608–614. discussion 614–606.
40. Suliburk JW, Ware DN, Balogh Z, McKinley BA, Cocanour CS, Kozar RA, Moore FA, Ivatury RR: **Vacuum-assisted wound closure achieves early fascial closure of open abdomens after severe trauma.** *J Trauma* 2003, **55:**1155–1160. discussion 1160–1151.
41. Barker DE, Kaufman HJ, Smith LA, Ciraulo DL, Richart CL, Burns RP: **Vacuum pack technique of temporary abdominal closure: A 7-year experience with 112 patients.** *J Trauma* 2000, **48:**201–206. discussion 206–207.
42. Bee TK, Croce MA, Magnotti LJ, Zarzaur BL, Maish GO 3rd, Minard G, Schroeppel TJ, Fabian TC: **Temporary abdominal closure techniques: a prospective randomized trial comparing polyglactin 910 mesh and vacuum-assisted closure.** *J Trauma* 2008, **65:**337–342. discussion 342–334.
43. Smith LA, Barker DE, Chase CW, Somberg LB, Brock WB, Burns RP: **Vacuum pack technique of temporary abdominal closure: A four-year experience.** *Am Surg* 1997, **63:**1102–1107. discussion 1107–1108.
44. Teixeira PG, Salim A, Inaba K, Brown C, Browder T, Margulies D, Demetriades D: **A prospective look at the current state of open abdomens.** *Am Surg* 2008, **74:**891–897.
45. Miller PR, Thompson JT, Faler BJ, Meredith JW, Chang MC: **Late fascial closure in lieu of ventral hernia: The next step in open abdomen management.** *J Trauma* 2002, **53:**843–849.
46. Cheatham ML, Demetriades D, Fabian TC, Kaplan MJ, Miles WS, Schreiber MA, Holcomb JB, Bochicchio G, Sarani B, Rotondo MF: **Prospective study examining clinical outcomes associated with a negative pressure wound therapy system and Barker's vacuum packing technique.** *World J Surg* 2013, **37:**2018–2030.
47. Acosta S, Bjarnason T, Petersson U, Palsson B, Wanhainen A, Svensson M, Djavani K, Bjorck M: **Multicentre prospective study of fascial closure rate after open abdomen with vacuum and mesh-mediated fascial traction.** *Br J Surg* 2011, **98:**735–743.
48. Vertrees A, Kellicut D, Ottman S, Peoples G, Shriver C: **Early definitive abdominal closure using serial closure technique on injured soldiers returning from Afghanistan and Iraq.** *J Am Coll Surg* 2006, **202:**762–772.
49. Vertrees A, Greer L, Pickett C, Nelson J, Wakefield M, Stojadinovic A, Shriver C: **Modern management of complex open abdominal wounds of war: a 5-year experience.** *J Am Coll Surg* 2008, **207:**801–809.
50. Mayberry JC, Burgess EA, Goldman RK, Pearson TE, Brand D, Mullins RJ: **Enterocutaneous fistula and ventral hernia after absorbable mesh prosthesis closure for trauma: the plain truth.** *J Trauma* 2004, **57:**157–162. discussion 163–153.
51. Jernigan TW, Fabian TC, Croce MA, Moore N, Pritchard FE, Minard G, Bee TK: **Staged management of giant abdominal wall defects: acute and long-term results.** *Ann Surg* 2003, **238:**349–355. discussion 355–347.
52. Brandt CP, McHenry CR, Jacobs DG, Piotrowski JJ, Priebe PP: **Polypropylene mesh closure after emergency laparotomy: morbidity and outcome.** *Surgery* 1995, **118:**736–740. discussion 740–731.
53. Tons C, Schachtrupp A, Rau M, Mumme T, Schumpelick V: **Abdominal compartment syndrome: prevention and treatment.** *Der Chirurg; Zeitschrift fur alle Gebiete der operativen Medizen* 2000, **71:**918–926.
54. Sugrue M, Jones F, Janjua KJ, Deane SA, Bristow P, Hillman K: **Temporary abdominal closure: a prospective evaluation of its effects on renal and respiratory physiology.** *J Trauma* 1998, **45:**914–921.
55. Weinberg JA, George RL, Griffin RL, Stewart AH, Reiff DA, Kerby JD, Melton SM, Rue LW 3rd: **Closing the open abdomen: improved success with Wittmann Patch staged abdominal closure.** *J Trauma* 2008, **65:**345–348.
56. Tieu BH, Cho SD, Luem N, Riha G, Mayberry J, Schreiber MA: **The use of the Wittmann Patch facilitates a high rate of fascial closure in severely injured trauma patients and critically ill emergency surgery patients.** *J Trauma* 2008, **65:**865–870.
57. Wittmann DH: **Staged abdominal repair: Development and current practice of an advanced operative technique for diffuse suppurative peritonitis.** *Acta Chirurgica Austriaca* 2000, **32:**171–178.
58. Hadeed JG, Staman GW, Sariol HS, Kumar S, Ross SE: **Delayed primary closure in damage control laparotomy: The value of the Wittmann patch.** *Am Surg* 2007, **73:**10–12.
59. Schnuriger B, Inaba K, Wu T, Eberle BM, Belzberg H, Demetriades D: **Crystalloids after primary colon resection and anastomosis at initial trauma laparotomy: Excessive volumes are associated with anastomotic leakage.** *J Trauma* 2011, **70:**603–610.
60. Cotton BA, Guy JS, Morris JA Jr, Abumrad NN: **The cellular, metabolic, and systemic consequences of aggressive fluid resuscitation strategies.** *Shock* 2006, **26:**115–121.
61. Cotton BA, Gunter OL, Isbell J, Au BK, Robertson AM, Morris JA Jr, St Jacques P: **Damage control hematology: the impact of a trauma exsanguination protocol on survival and blood product utilization.** *J Trauma* 2008, **64:**1177–1182. discussion 1182–1173.
62. Holcomb JB, Jenkins D, Rhee P, Johannigman J, Mahoney P, Mehta S, Cox ED, Gehrke MJ, Beilman GJ, Schreiber M, *et al*: **Damage control resuscitation: directly addressing the early coagulopathy of trauma.** *J Trauma* 2007, **62:**307–310.
63. Holcomb JB, Wade CE, Michalek JE, Chisholm GB, Zarzabal LA, Schreiber MA, Gonzalez EA, Pomper GJ, Perkins JG, Spinella PC, *et al*: **Increased plasma and platelet to red blood cell ratios improves outcome in 466 massively transfused civilian trauma patients.** *Ann Surg* 2008, **248:**447–458.
64. Lustenberger T, Frischknecht A, Bruesch M, Keel MJ: **Blood component ratios in massively transfused, blunt trauma patients–a time-dependent covariate analysis.** *J Trauma* 2011, **71:**1144–1150. discussion 1150–1141.
65. Wafaisade A, Maegele M, Lefering R, Braun M, Peiniger S, Neugebauer E, Bouillon B: **High plasma to red blood cell ratios are associated with lower mortality rates in patients receiving multiple transfusion (4</=red blood cell units < 10) during acute trauma resuscitation.** *J Trauma* 2011, **70:**81–88. discussion 88–89.
66. Cotton BA, Au BK, Nunez TC, Gunter OL, Robertson AM, Young PP: **Predefined massive transfusion protocols are associated with a reduction in organ failure and postinjury complications.** *J Trauma* 2009, **66:**41–48. discussion 48–49.
67. Harvin JA, Mims MM, Duchesne JC, Cox CS Jr, Wade CE, Holcomb JB, Cotton BA: **Chasing 100%: the use of hypertonic saline to improve early, primary fascial closure after damage control laparotomy.** *Trauma Acute Care Surg* 2013, **74:**426–430. discussion 431–422.
68. Fullen WD, Hunt J, Altemeier WA: **Prophylactic antibiotics in penetrating wounds of the abdomen.** *J Trauma* 1972, **12:**282–289.
69. Goldberg SR, Anand RJ, Como JJ, Dechert T, Dente C, Luchette FA, Ivatury RR, Duane TM: **Prophylactic antibiotic use in penetrating abdominal trauma: An Eastern association for the surgery of trauma practice management guideline.** *Trauma Acute Care Surg* 2012, **73:**S321–S325.
70. Abouassaly CT, Dutton WD, Zaydfudim V, Dossett LA, Nunez TC, Fleming SB, Cotton BA: **Postoperative neuromuscular blocker use is associated with higher primary fascial closure rates after damage control laparotomy.** *J Trauma* 2010, **69:**557–561.
71. Webb LH, Patel MB, Dortch MJ, Miller RS, Gunter OL, Collier BR: **Use of a furosemide drip does not improve earlier primary fascial closure in the open abdomen.** *J Emerg Trauma Shock* 2012, **5:**126–130.

72. Collier B, Guillamondegui O, Cotton B, Donahue R, Conrad A, Groh K, Richman J, Vogel T, Miller R, Diaz J Jr: **Feeding the open abdomen.** *JPEN J Parenter Enteral Nutr* 2007, **31:**410–415.
73. Burlew CC, Moore EE, Cuschieri J, Jurkovich GJ, Codner P, Nirula R, Millar D, Cohen MJ, Kutcher ME, Haan J, *et al*: **Who should we feed? Western trauma association multi-institutional study of enteral nutrition in the open abdomen after injury.** *Trauma Acute Care Surg* 2012, **73:**1380–1387. discussion 1387–1388.
74. Byrnes MC, Reicks P, Irwin E: **Early enteral nutrition can be successfully implemented in trauma patients with an "open abdomen".** *Am J Surg* 2010, **199:**359–362. discussion 363.
75. Dissanaike S, Pham T, Shalhub S, Warner K, Hennessy L, Moore EE, Maier RV, O'Keefe GE, Cuschieri J: **Effect of immediate enteral feeding on trauma patients with an open abdomen: protection from nosocomial infections.** *J Am Coll Surg* 2008, **207:**690–697.
76. Dubose JJ, Scalea TM, Holcomb JB, Shrestha B, Okoye O, Inaba K, Bee TK, Fabian TC, Whelan J, Ivatury RR: **Open abdominal management after damage-control laparotomy for trauma: a prospective observational American association for the surgery of trauma multicenter study.** *Trauma Acute Care Surg* 2013, **74:**113–120. discussion 1120–1122.
77. Regner JL, Kobayashi L, Coimbra R: **Surgical strategies for management of the open abdomen.** *Am J Surg* 2012, **36:**497–510.
78. Scott BG, Welsh FJ, Pham HQ, Carrick MM, Liscum KR, Granchi TS, Wall MJ Jr, Mattox KL, Hirshberg A: **Early aggressive closure of the open abdomen.** *J Trauma* 2006, **60:**17–22.
79. de Moya MA, Dunham M, Inaba K, Bahouth H, Alam HB, Sultan B, Namias N: **Long-term outcome of acellular dermal matrix when used for large traumatic open abdomen.** *J Trauma* 2008, **65:**349–353.

6

Post-traumatic diaphragmatic herniation of the liver, examined by positron emission tomography

Katsutoshi Sato[1*], Kazumasa Orihashi[3], Yoshiharu Hamanaka[1], Norimasa Mitsui[1], Shinji Hirai[1], Naru Chatani[1] and Takashi Nishisaka[2]

Abstract

We present a case of post-traumatic diaphragmatic herniation of the liver, which mimicked an intrathoracic tumor. After an automobile accident, the patient underwent thoracotomies for hemothorax and lung cancer in the right chest. Seven months later, computed tomography (CT) demonstrated a round tumor in the thorax adjacent to the right diaphragm with a higher density than the liver parenchyma. An intrathoracic tumor including a primary or metastatic lung cancer was suspected. However, positron emission tomography (PET) showed that the uptake of fluorine-18-fluorodeoxyglucose (FDG) was identical to that in the liver, and the tumor appeared to be contiguous with the liver. Thus, we suspected liver herniation. Core needle biopsy revealed liver cells without neoplastic tissue. Upon surgical exploration, herniation of the liver was found and repaired. PET was helpful in providing morphological and functional information leading to accurate diagnosis of liver herniation in this unusual case.

Keywords: Diaphragmatic herniation, Positron emission tomography: PET, Blunt trauma

Introduction

Diaphragmatic herniation of the liver following blunt trauma may develop long after the initial trauma and remain clinically silent. Unless a large portion of liver and/or other abdominal organs are herniated, it is often difficult to distinguish diaphragmatic herniation of the liver from an intrathoracic tumor [1]. Positron emission tomography (PET) imaging using fluorodeoxyglucose (FDG) labeled with the positron-emitter fluorine-18 provides useful information allowing differentiation of benign lesions from malignant ones. However, FDG is a nonspecific marker of malignancy, and uptake may be seen at sites of active inflammation [2], and also from normal metabolically active tissues, such as the liver [3,4]. We report a case of small diaphragmatic herniation of the liver with diagnostic PET and histological findings. We believe this is the first reported case in the literature of PET findings of herniated liver.

* Correspondence: satoktts@hiroshima-u.ac.jp
[1]Department of Thoracic Surgery, Hiroshima Prefectural Hospital, Hiroshima, Japan, Ujinakanda 1-5-54, Minami-ku, Hiroshima, 734-8530, Japan
Full list of author information is available at the end of the article

Case

A 68-year-old woman was involved in an automobile accident and was transferred to the emergency department at the Hiroshima Prefectural Hospital. Computed tomography (CT) on admission demonstrated traumatic aortic injury, multiple rib fractures, and bilateral hemopneumothoraces as well as a spiculated mass, 2 cm diameter with pleural indentation in segment 6 of the right lung. She underwent emergent repair of the descending aorta and right pleural drainage. On the fourth postoperative day, bloody drainage from the right chest suddenly increased in volume. The patient was taken back to the operating room and at right thoracotomy, a bleeding point was found on the surface of the diaphragm. Hemostasis was established by using polypropylene suture.

Four months later, the size of lung mass was unchanged, and PET showed little FDG uptake. Because malignancy was suspected and her general condition improved, she underwent surgical resection of the tumor. After meticulous dissection, the right lower lobe was partially resected, but systematic lobectomy and radical lymph node dissection was not feasible due to significant adhesion. Histological examination revealed a well-differentiated adenocarcinoma with clear tissue margins.

The follow-up CT at 3 months revealed another tumor in the right lower lobe adjacent to the diaphragm, which had not been recognized before. Twelve months after lung resection, a discrete ovoid mass 3.7 × 2.7 cm in diameter with slightly higher density than that of liver parenchyma was apparent (Figure 1). Subsequent PET showed FDG uptake in the lesion [the maximum standard uptake value (SUV max) was 3.1] (Figure 2). Metastasis of lung cancer or another heterogenic tumor was entertained as a diagnosis; however, the mass appeared to be contiguous with the liver, which had an identical FDG uptake level. Since liver herniation was suspected, percutaneous needle core biopsy of the mass was performed (Figure 3). The tissue contained only liver cells with inflammatory cell infiltration, and was diagnosed as liver herniation (Figure 4). Because the size of the mass had steadily increased, we elected to perform surgical repair. At operation, diaphragmatic herniation of the liver (3 cm in diameter) was found. The herniated portion of the liver appeared to be congested. As a polypropylene suture was found at the edge of the hernia hilus, we concluded that the hernia had originated from the motor vehicle trauma (Figure 5). The defect was repaired with interrupted sutures. The patient was discharged home after an uneventful recovery and has no evidence of recurrence after two years of follow-up.

Discussion

Traumatic rupture of the right diaphragm following blunt trauma is uncommon. The extent of herniation varies, from a small portion of liver, to the entire liver plus other abdominal organs. Small herniations are typically asymptomatic, and diagnosis can be delayed for many years [5-7]. The diagnosis can be made when a defect of the diaphragm and/or liver parenchyma is observed on imaging studies such as ultrasonography (US) [8], CT [9], isotopic liver tomogram [10] or magnetic resonance imaging (MRI) [11]. Herniation may be difficult to differentiate from an intrathoracic tumor, especially when only a small portion of the liver is herniated.

In our case, several factors contributed to the difficulty in making an accurate diagnosis of diaphragmatic hernia. These include small herniation of the liver, concomitant lung cancer with suboptimal resection, and elevated CT density in the herniated portion of the liver. At first, as an intrathoracic tumor or metastasis from a lung cancer was suspected, a PET study was performed. Identical FDG uptake in the intrathoracic lesion to that in the liver was seen, leading to a diagnosis of liver herniation. However, since the patient's previous lung cancer showed little FDG uptake, and other neoplasms could not be differentiated solely by PET findings, additional supportive evidence was needed to make a definite diagnosis. US and MRI could not be performed, because of difficulties with the patient's control of breathing during the examination. As the tumor was adherent to the chest wall, we decided to perform a needle biopsy. This provided a conclusive finding of liver cells without neoplastic tissue thus confirming the diagnosis of liver herniation. The CT findings could be explained by strangulation of the herniated liver likely inducing congestion, which was confirmed at operation. This might have led to the higher density in the herniated portion on CT.

Increased FDG uptake in PET is an important finding for differentiating benign lesions from malignant ones and is interpreted by calculation of the SUV [12]. However, FDG is a nonspecific marker of malignancy, and FDG uptake can be seen in normal metabolically-active tissue such as the liver [3,4], or may be caused by active inflammation, probably due to uptake by activated macrophages and inflammatory cells [13].

In this case, histological examination of the specimen by needle biopsy revealed inflammatory cell infiltration around normal liver cells and fibrosis of Glisson's sheath. Yoshimura et al. [14] reported a case in which a herniated liver was resected with histological findings similar to those in our case, without a history of viral and/or other hepatitis. This inflammatory response was likely caused by repeated and sustained mechanical stress upon the herniated portion of the liver. However,

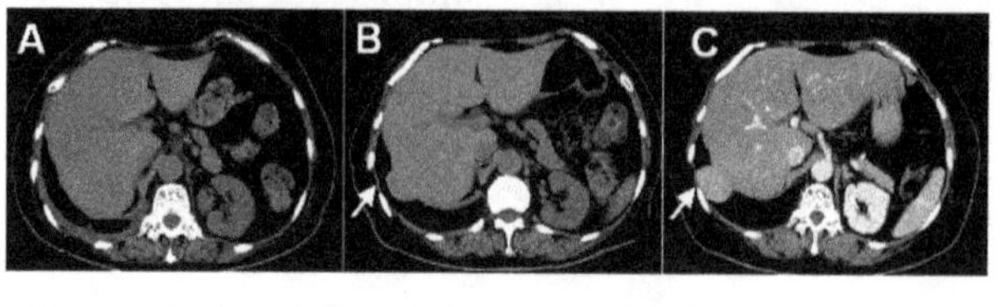

Figure 1 CT findings of the tumor. The mass in the right lung field with its inferior border abutting the diaphragm (arrow) increased in size over time. **A** At the first admission. **B** At 3 months, and **C** 12 months after the operation for lung cancer.

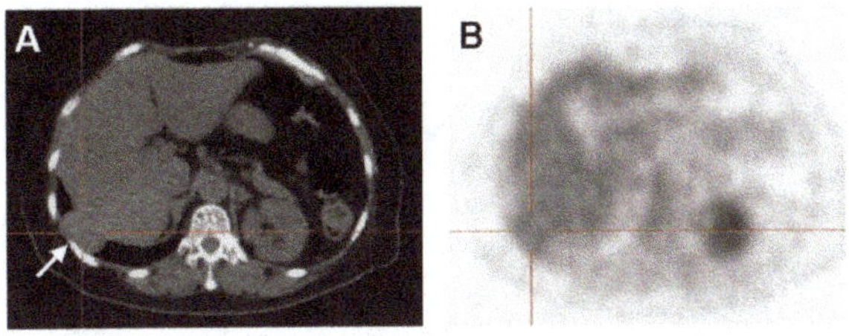

Figure 2 CT and corresponding PET findings of the tumor. **A** CT before the operation for liver herniation showed a 3.7 × 2.7 cm solid tumor (arrow). **B** The corresponding PET scan revealed the FDG uptake (SUV max was 3.1), which was equal to the level in liver parenchyma, and contiguous with the liver.

it did not show increased FDG uptake above the normal liver level on PET. It is likely that the inflammation might not have been severe enough to induce increased FDG uptake.

Since this report involves only one patient, and there are no other reports in the literature, we cannot assume that herniated liver always exhibits FDG uptake at the same level as liver parenchyma. Hepatic hernias should be included in the differential diagnosis of a right basal mass in the thorax, in the patient with a history of thoraco-abdominal trauma. Recently, PET study has been used frequently in the differential diagnosis of intrathoracic neoplasms. The authors believe that knowledge of this case will be important for diagnosis and decision-making in other cases of ambiguous intrathoracic masses.

Conclusion

We present a case of post-traumatic diaphragmatic herniation of the liver masquerading as an intrathoracic mass. Although the herniated liver had inflammatory cell infiltration, PET did not show increased FDG uptake above that of the normal liver level. In this case, PET information was helpful for diagnosing even a small liver herniation, due to its normal FDG uptake pattern, informing the subsequent management and repair of the diaphragmatic defect.

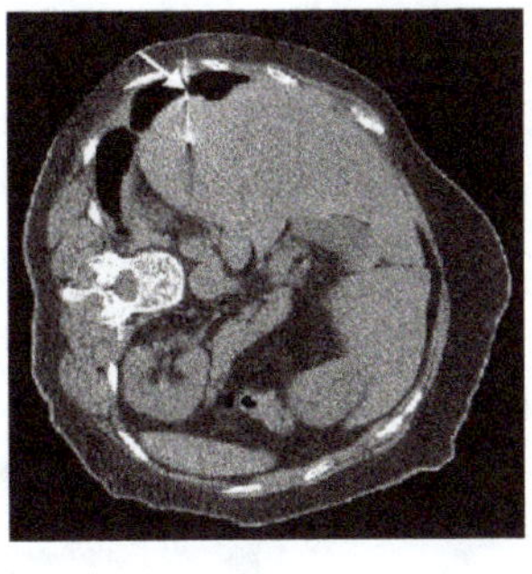

Figure 3 Percutaneous needle biopsy of the mass. The biopsy needle penetrated the mass (arrow).

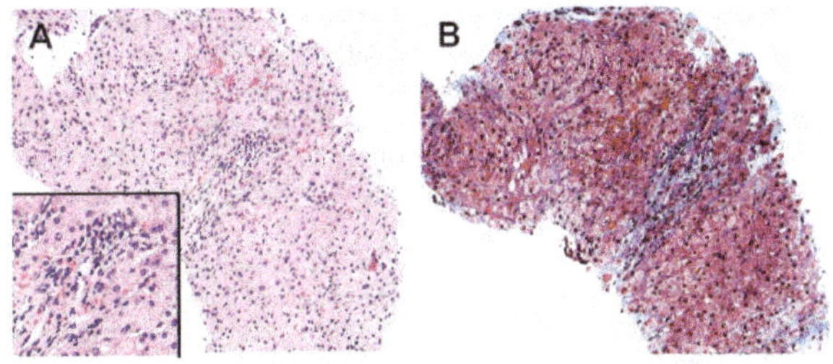

Figure 4 Histological findings of the tumor. Histological examination revealed inflammatory cell infiltration around normal liver cells and fibrosis of Glisson's sheath (H & E: **A** ×50; inset, ×100. Masson-Trichrome stain: **B** ×50).

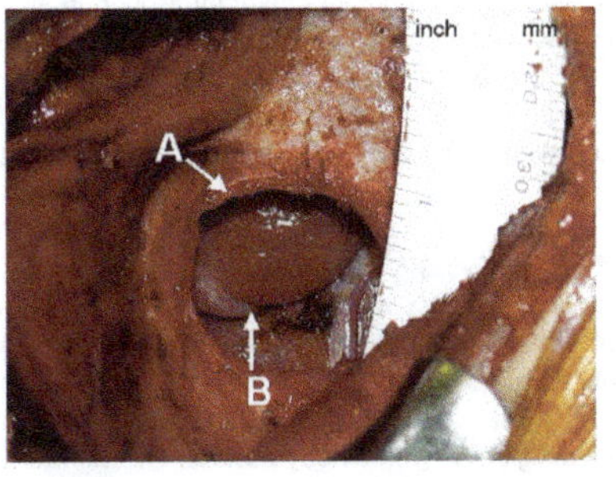

Figure 5 Intraoperative findings of the herniated liver. **A** A defect in the right diaphragm. **B** The herniated portion of the liver. The herniated liver surface was congested, compared with surrounding normal liver surface.

Consent

Written informed consent was obtained from the patient for publication of this Case report and any accompanying images. A copy of the written consent is available for review by the Editor-in-Chief of this journal.

Author details

[1]Department of Thoracic Surgery, Hiroshima Prefectural Hospital, Hiroshima, Japan, Ujinakanda 1-5-54, Minami-ku, Hiroshima, 734-8530, Japan. [2]Department of Pathology, Hiroshima Prefectural Hospital, Hiroshima, Japan, Ujinakanda 1-5-54, Minami-ku, Hiroshima, 734-8530, Japan. [3]Department of Cardiovascular Surgery, Hiroshima University Hospital, Hiroshima, Japan, Kasumi 1-2-3, Minami-ku, Hiroshima, 734-8551, Japan.

Authors' contributions

KS, NM, SH, NC and YH participated in the care of the patient, including the operative part.
TN participated in the pathology.
KS wrote the first draft of the manuscript.
KO and YH critically reviewed the manuscript.
All authors read and approved the final manuscript.

Competing interests

The authors declare that they have no competing interests.

References

1. Fanta CH, Kacoyanis GP, Koster JK, McFadden ER: **Pseudopseudotumor of the lung. Hepatic herniation into the right major fissure imitating a pseudotumor on chest roentgenogram.** *Chest* 1980, **78(2)**:346-48.
2. Valk PE, Pounds TR, Hopkins DM, Haseman MK, Hofer GA, Greiss HB, Myers RW, Lutrin CL: **Staging non-small cell lung cancer by whole-body positron emission tomographic imaging.** *Ann Thorac Surg* 1995, **60(6)**:1573-82.
3. Minamimoto R, Takahashi N, Inoue T: **FDG-PET of patients with suspected renal failure: standardized uptake value in normal tissues.** *Ann Nuc Med* 2007, **21(4)**:217-22.
4. Lin CY, Ding HJ, Lin CC, Chen CC, Sun SS, Kao CH: **Impact of age on FDG uptake in the liver on PET scan.** *Clin Imaging* 2010, **34(5)**:348-50.
5. Rashid F, Chakrabarty MM, Singh R, Iftikhar SY: **A review on delayed presentation of diaphragmatic rupture.** *World J Emerg Surg* 2009, **4**:32.
6. Vilallonga R, Pastor V, Alvarez L, Charco R, Armengol M, Navarro S: **Right-sided diaphragmatic rupture after blunt trauma. An unusual entity.** *World J Emerg Surg* 2011, **6**:3.
7. Peck WA: **Right-sided diaphragmatic liver hernia following trauma.** *Am J Roentgenol* 1957, **78(1)**:99-108.
8. Khan AN, Gould DA: **The primary role of ultrasound in evaluating right-sided diaphragmatic humps and juxtadiaphragmatic masses: a review of 22 cases.** *Clin Radiol* 1984, **35(5)**:413-18.
9. Israel RS, Mayberry JC, Primack SL: **Diaphragmatic rupture. Use of helical CT scanning with multiplanar reformations.** *Am J Roentgenol* 1996, **167(5)**:1201-3.
10. Mamay M, Michils A, De Vuyst P, Gevenois PA, Yernault JC: **Peripheral lung mass.** *Eur Respir J* 1990, **3(6)**:734-35.
11. Shanmuganathan K, Mirvis SE, White CS, Pomerantz SM: **MR imaging evaluation of hemidiaphragms in acute blunt trauma: experience with 16 patients.** *Am J Roentgenol* 1996, **167(2)**:397-402.
12. Saunders CA, Dussek JE, O'Doherty MJ, Maisey MN: **Evaluation of fluorine-18-fluorodeoxyglucose whole body positron emission tomography imaging in the staging of lung cancer.** *Ann Thorac Surg* 1999, **67(3)**:790-97.
13. Kubota R, Kubota K, Yamada S, Tada M, Ido T, Tamahashi N: **Microautoradiographic study for the differentiation of intratumoral macrophages, granulation tissues and cancer cells by the dynamics of fluorine-18-fluorodeoxyglucose uptake.** *J Nucl Med* 1994, **35(1)**:104-12.
14. Yoshimura Y, Nakano M, Okuno K, Koteda T, Nakatsuka S: **A case of diaphragmatic liver herniation simulating a pulmonary benign tumor.** *Nihon Kyoubu Shikkan Gakkai Zasshi (J Jpn Resp Society)* 1974, **12(11)**:691-95.

Endoscopic duodenal perforation: surgical strategies in a regional centre

Richard C Turner[1*], Christina M Steffen[2] and Peter Boyd[2]

Abstract

Background: Duodenal perforation is an uncommon complication of endoscopic retrograde cholangio-pancreatography (ERCP) and a rare complication of upper gastrointestinal endoscopy. Most are minor perforations that settle with conservative management. A few perforations however result in life-threatening retroperitoneal necrosis and require surgical intervention. There is a relative paucity of references specifically describing the surgical interventions required for this eventuality.

Methods: Five cases of iatrogenic duodenal perforation were ascertained between 2002 and 2007 at Cairns Base Hospital. Clinical features were analyzed and compared, with reference to a review of ERCP at that institution for the years 2005/2006.

Results: One patient recovered with conservative management. Of the other four, one died after initial laparotomy. The other three survived, undergoing multiple procedures and long inpatient stays.

Conclusions: Iatrogenic duodenal perforation with retroperitoneal necrosis is an uncommon complication of endoscopy, but when it does occur it is potentially life-threatening. Early recognition may lead to a better outcome through earlier intervention, although a protracted course with multiple procedures should be anticipated. A number of surgical techniques may need to be employed according to the individual circumstances of the case.

Keywords: Duodenum, Perforation, Endoscopy, Surgery, Necrosis

Background

Duodenal perforation is an uncommon complication of endoscopic retrograde cholangiopancreatography (ERCP) and a very rare complication of upper gastrointestinal endoscopy. Most series report a majority of non-life-threatening perforations which settle with conservative management [1,2]. There are few references specifically describing the surgical interventions required for the minority of iatrogenic duodenal perforations where surgery is indicated.

Five cases of iatrogenic duodenal perforation occurring between 2002 and 2007 at Cairns Base Hospital are presented for comparison, with reference to a review of ERCP at Cairns Base Hospital for the years 2005/2006. Further, a focused review of the literature was undertaken to inform discussion of the surgical management of such cases.

* Correspondence: richard.turner@utas.edu.au
[1]Department of Surgery, Hobart Clinical School, University of Tasmania, Hobart, Australia
Full list of author information is available at the end of the article

Methods

Cairns Base Hospital is a secondary referral hospital in Far North Queensland, Australia. It serves a catchment population of approximately 250 000, 15% of which identify as Indigenous Australian. Hospital surgical audit and endoscopy records for the period 2002–2008 were searched for cases of duodenal perforation following endoscopy or ERCP. Age, sex, indication for endoscopy/ERCP, timing or delay to diagnosis and definitive management, type of perforation, surgical management, complications, length of stay, and late morbidity were recorded for each case.

An audit of ERCP at Cairns Base Hospital for the two year period 2005/2006 was utilized to determine incidence of complications of ERCP and is presented in Tables 1 and 2.

For the focused literature review, a PubMed search was undertaken using the terms "duodenal perforation", "endoscopic" and "retroperitoneal necrosis". Case-based articles cited by reviews were secondarily sourced. Articles

Table 1 Complications of ERCP procedures for 2005–6 at Cairns Base Hospital (N = 211)

Complication	N (%)
Pancreatitis	9 (4.3%)
Cholangitis	7 (3.3%)
Bleeding	4 (1.9%)
Perforation	2 (0.95%)
Death	3 (1.4%)
Other: Stroke	1 (0.5%)
Total (with complications)	22 (12.3%)

Adapted from Cotton et al. 1991 [3].

with English language abstracts were considered, and excluded if endoscopy was not the cause of the perforation (rather a treatment) or if specific operative details were not reported. Similarly, only cases that underwent some form of surgical management were included.

Approval to access and analyze de-identified patient records for this study was given by the Human Research Ethics Committee of the Cairns and Hinterland Health Service District.

Results

Five patients sustaining iatrogenic duodenal perforation were identified. The clinical data pertaining to these are presented in Table 3. All four of the ERCP cases had an associated pre-cut sphincterotomy. No significant bleeding was noted, and no additional procedures such as lithotripsy or stenting were performed. In two cases, there was no specific evidence of choledocholithiasis, with the ERCP being intended solely for diagnostic purposes. Figure 1 shows a representative CT image from Case 2 prior to surgical intervention. Figure 2 illustrates the necrotic retroperitoneal material debrided via a right flank incision in Case 1.

In cases 1, 2 and 4, the actual duodenal perforation could not be identified at operation. This may have been due to a smaller size of the perforation and/or delay to surgery resulting in difficulty identifying the perforation.

Table 2 Indications for ERCP 2005–06, Cairns Base Hospital (N = 202)

Indication	N (%)
CBD stone (s)	115 (57%)
Cholangitis	6 (3%)
Malignant jaundice	29 (14%)
Stent change or unblocking	33 (16%)
Abdominal pain, abnormal LFTs, dilated duct	5 (2.5%)
Chronic pancreatitis	10 (10%)
Abnormal CT	1 (0.5%)
Bile leak	3 (1.5%)

Ongoing leakage in Case 2 necessitated subsequent pyloric exclusion and gastrojejunostomy. Case 5, where endoscopy alone was performed, is likely to have perforated through a duodenal diverticulum, which is a known risk factor for perforation both in endoscopy and ERCP [4-6]. This large perforation was obvious at the time and early operation enabled definitive repair. As integrity of the repair was demonstrated radiologically, the subsequent delayed extensive retroperitoneal necrosis presumably arose from the leakage that occurred in the few hours between injury and laparotomy for repair.

Timing of intervention was assisted by serial computerized tomography examination. In the four cases treated surgically, definitive intervention consisted of open surgical drainage with or without subsequent CT-guided percutaneous drainage of amenable collections. While open surgical drainage was immediately effective in all cases, percutaneous drainage as an initial intervention was not effective in Case 1, attributable to the large volumes of semi-solid necrotic material in the retroperitoneum of this patient. This is consistent with experience in pancreatic necrosectomy [7,8]. In contrast, percutaneous drainage was an effective modality for the smaller, less accessible but more fluid presacral collection in Case 5.

Retroperitoneal necrosis was progressive and in most cases multiple operations were required due to ongoing symptoms. An oblique right flank to right iliac fossa incision was performed in Cases 1 and 5 giving good access to the upper and lower right retroperitoneal space and to the presacral space. A feature of the three cases in males was involvement of the right inguinoscrotal tract, with Cases 2 and 5 requiring separate drainage of symptomatic inguinoscrotal collections. None had pre-existing hernias.

One patient (Case 4) died indirectly as a result of the perforation, from sepsis associated with vascular access. This patient had significant co-morbidities, being steroid-dependent for pulmonary interstitial fibrosis and rheumatoid arthritis. Of the four survivors, one recovered quickly with conservative management alone, but the other three endured long hospital stays, underwent multiple surgical and other procedures, and developed short-term and long-term complications as a result of the original perforation and its treatment.

Discussion

All cases in this series were managed by General Surgeons at a regional hospital, serving a population of 250 000 and geographically remote from larger facilities. The endoscopic procedures were performed by a Gastroenterologist and a General Surgeon, both of whom were formally trained and accredited in these skills. As upper endoscopy and now ERCP are readily available in larger regional centres, an awareness of this serious but fortunately rare

Table 3 Characteristics of endoscopically induced duodenal injuries, Cairns Base Hospital, 2002–2008

Case (year) Age/Sex	1 (2002) 51 male	2 (2004) 69 male	3 (2005) 42 female	4 (2006) 61 female	5 (2007) 72 male
Indication for ERCP/ endoscopy	Post-cholecystectomy pain	Choledocholithiasis	Post- cholecystectomy pancreatitis	Choledocholithiasis	Post-cholecystectomy pain
Post-procedure symptoms, signs	Severe abdominal pain, tachycardia	Severe abdominal pain	Mild abdominal pain	Abdominal pain	Abdominal pain
Type of perforation	Not identified	Not identified (Duodenal diverticulum)	Type 2 (see Results)	Not identified	Type 1 (see Results) (Duodenal diverticulum)
Delay to Diagnosis/ Intervention	48 hours then 5 weeks	5 days	Immediate diagnosis	Immediate diagnosis, surgery within 24 hours	Immediate diagnosis, surgery at 6 hours
Indications for surgery	a) Duodenal perforation	a) Duodenal perforation	Nil	a) Duodenal perforation	a) Large defect duodenum,
a) at diagnosis	b) Infected retroperitoneal necrosis/collections	b) Extensive retroperitoneal necrosis/collections Persistent duodenal leak			b) Extensive retroperitoneal necrosis/collections
b) subsequent	Duodenal stenosis, Necrosis of posterior caecal wall			b) Extensive retroperitoneal necrosis	a) Laparotomy, repair duodenum
Management	a) Laparotomy	a) Laparotomy	Conservative	a) Laparotomy, retroperitoneal washout, pyloric, exclusion, gastrojejunostomy, jejunal feeding tube	b) Open drainage/evacuation right retroperitoneal space x 2
a) on diagnosis	b) Attempted percutaneous drainage	b) 7 x debridement of necrosis	(no surgery)		Drainage right scrotum
b) subsequent	2 x Open drainage procedure right retroperitoneal space	Open drainage right inguinoscrotal tract			
	Right hemicolectomy, end ileostomy and mucous fistula	Pyloric exclusion, gastrojejunostomy			
Complications of treatment	Deep vein thrombosis	Gastroparesis, UTI, CVL infection, wound infection, left brachial plexopathy	Nil	Necrotising fasciitis right thigh/abdomen	Right inguinal haematoma Incisional hernia Seroma
Length of stay (days)	99	132	4	6	63
Case fatality	No	No	No	Yes	No
Residual disability	Residual presacral collection and sinus to right iliac fossa	Retained CBD stones removed 2007	Nil	Died	Nil

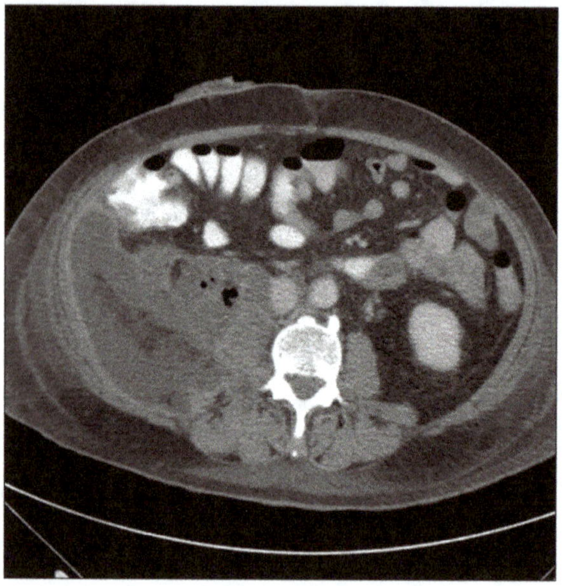

Figure 1 CT image showing extensive retroperitoneal necrosis prior to surgical intervention (Case 2).

complication and its clinical course is useful for General Surgeons faced with its management. Certainly Case 5, undertaken with the benefit of specific experience gained in the management of Case 1, does seem to have had a better quality outcome, with shorter length of stay, fewer procedures, and fewer complications.

While duodenal perforation at endoscopy alone is extremely rare, the rate during ERCP is significantly higher, estimated to be between 0.4 and 1% [9]. The rate of 0.95% in the audited series from Cairns Base Hospital is within these limits (Table 1). The indications for ERCP at our institution are shown in Table 2. It should be noted that two patients in the series had the uncommon indication of post-cholecystectomy pain. During the time period of this series, no other imaging modalities for the common bile duct were readily available. Despite the excellent standards set for training and quality assurance, ERCP, particularly when associated with sphincterotomy, still incurs a definite risk of complication, and its indications should be primarily interventional [10]. The emerging availability in regional centres of less invasive diagnostic modalities such as MRCP and endoscopic ultrasound (EUS) should reduce exposure to the risk of duodenal perforation in this group, [11,12] as has indeed been the case at our institution since 2007. Where these are not available, consideration should be given to transferring patients to centres where they are, particularly when there is no therapeutic intent at the outset.

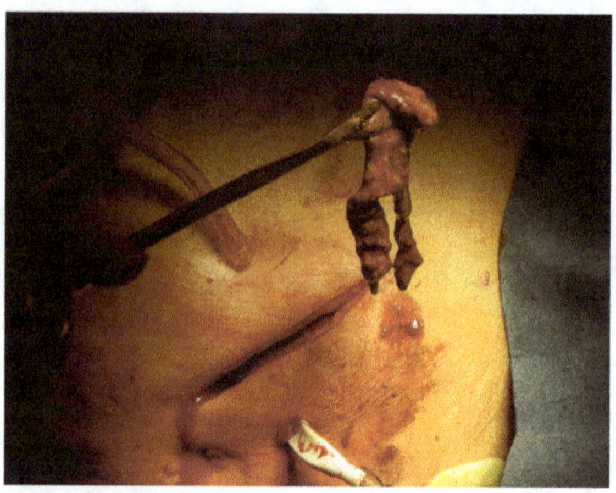

Figure 2 Necrotic retroperitoneal tissue debrided via right flank incision (Case 1).

Four types of duodenal perforation have been described – Type 1: lateral duodenal wall, Type 2: peri-Vaterian duodenum, Type 3: bile duct, and Type 4: tiny retroperitoneal perforations caused by the use of compressed air during endoscopy. Most perforations are Type 2, due to concomitant endoscopic sphincterotomy, and may be suitable for a trial of conservative management [13-15]. In our series, Case 3 was documented as a Type 2 perforation. Case 5 was documented as a Type 1 perforation, and Cases 1, 2, 4 were most likely this, based on the ensuing clinical course. Type 1 perforations have the most serious consequences and typically require complex and invasive treatment. They are mostly caused by the endoscope itself and may result in considerable intra- or extraperitoneal spillage of duodenal fluid (a mixture of gastric juice, bile and pancreatic juice), the latter causing rapid, extensive, and ongoing necrosis of the right retroperitoneum. The patient becomes intensely catabolic with fevers, raised inflammatory markers, leucocytosis, and nutritional depletion. Without surgical intervention death is likely from a combination of massive auto-digestion, nutritional depletion and sepsis. Delay in diagnosis increases the likelihood of a fatal outcome [16,17].

Various management algorithms for duodenal injuries have been proposed, largely focusing on early diagnosis and the decision for surgical management [18-21]. Indications for surgery have been well described. If a Type 1 injury is noted at endoscopy or on subsequent imaging (eg. extravasation of contrast), immediate operative intervention is generally mandated. Failure of conservative management due to signs of progressive systemic inflammatory response syndrome (SIRS) is a relative indication for operation. Guidelines for specific operative strategies in the face of ERCP-related duodenal injury and retroperitoneal necrosis have been proposed, but are often based on evidence derived from individual case reports or case series, or from experience in the trauma setting [22,23]. Due to its uncommon nature, prospective comparative studies to determine the optimal procedure for

Table 4 Reports in the literature of Type 1 and 2 duodenal injuries caused by endoscopic procedures

Case/series	N =	Range of management strategies for:			Average days in hospital	Case fatality (%)
		Duodenal injury	Retroperitoneal necrosis	Underlying pathology		
Stapfer et al. 2000 [13]	8	Pyloric exclusion and gastro-jejunostomy	Drain placement	Cholecystectomy	62.9	2 (25%)
		Tube duodenostomy		CBD exploration		
		Duodeno-antrectomy		Hepatico-jejunostomy		
Preetha et al. 2003 [25]	13	Primary repair	Not described	Cholecystectomy	23.8	3 (23.1%)
		Pyloric exclusion and gastro-jejunostomy		CBD exploration		
		T-tube		Hepatico-jejunostomy		
		Bowel decompression				
Kalyani et al. 2005 [26]	1	Jejunal serosal patch	Not required	Nil required	>15	0 (0%)
Melita et al. 2005 [27]	1	Nil required	CT-guided abscess drainage	Nil required	Not specified	0 (0%)
Wu et al. 2006 [18]	10	Primary repair	Drain placement	Cholecystectomy	31.4	4 (40%)
		Omental patch	Open abscess drainage	CBD exploration		
		Duodenostomy	Percutaneous abscess drainage	Cholecysto-jejunostomy		
Fatima et al. 2007 [28]	22	Primary repair	Drain placement	Choledocho-jejunostomy	16	3 (13.6%)
		Omental patch				
Knudson et al. 2008 [29]	12	Primary repair	Drain placement	Hepatico-jejunostomy	4.5	0 (0%)
		T-tube	Open abscess drainage			
		Omental patch				
		Duodenostomy tube				
		Gastrostomy				
		Jejunostomy tube				
		Pyloric exclusion				
Mao et al. 2008 [30]	3	Nil required	Drain placement	Cholecystectomy	50	0 (0%)
				CBD exploration		
				T-tube		
Angiò et al. 2009 [31]	1	Kocherization and primary repair	Not described	CBD exploration	23	0 (0%)
Avgerinos et al. 2009 [19]	15	Primary repair	Not described	Choledocho-duodenostomy	42	3 (20%)
		Omental patch				
		Pyloric exclusion				
		Gastro-enterostomy				
Morgan et al. 2009 [32]	10	Primary repair gastrojejunostomy	Drain placement		Not available	1 (10%)
Dubecz et al. 2012 [33]	4	Primary repair	Not described	Hepatico-jejunostomy	23	0 (0%)
		T-tube				
Ercan et al. 2012 [21]	13	Primary repair	Percutaneous abscess drainage	Cholecystectomy	10.2	6 (46.2%)
		Pyloric exclusion	Open abscess drainage	CBD exploration		
		Gastro-enterostomy		T-tube		
Caliskan et al. 2013 [34]	9	Primary repair	Not described	CBD exploration	22.6	4 (44.4%)
		Duodenostomy		T-tube		
		Pyloric exclusion, gastro-jejunostomy		Pancreatico-duodenectomy		

endoscopically induced duodenal perforation have yet to be published [24].

Published case series and reports regarding possible surgical management options for endoscopically induced Type 1 and 2 duodenal injuries are summarized in Table 4 [13,18,19,21,25-34]. In general, operative procedures are tailored to conditions encountered at the time of laparotomy, as well as to any underlying pathology that preceded or was the indication for the endoscopic procedure. Primary repair of a breach in the duodenal wall may be possible where the injury is diagnosed early and there is limited contamination of surrounding tissues. Kocherization is usually needed to facilitate this, along with debridement of any devitalized tissue. Additional operative variations worthy of consideration include repair in one or two layers, transverse or longitudinal closure, and augmentation with a jejunal serosal [35] or omental patch. For patients deemed to be at high risk for leak or fistula formation, a number of additional protective measures have been proposed [24,36]. Tube decompression involves placement of a trans-mural trans-parietal duodenostomy or jejunostomy tube [37]. There are concerns that this engenders additional trauma to the gastrointestinal tract and may not provide adequate decompression. Duodenal diverticulation is a complex procedure that involves duodenal repair, distal Billroth II gastrectomy, placement of a decompressive duodenostomy tube, and peri-duodenal drainage [38]. This is obviously time-consuming and is often inappropriate for haemodynamically unstable patients. A less onerous procedure is pyloric exclusion, which entails primary duodenal repair, pyloric suture or stapling via greater curvature gastrotomy, and gastrojejunostomy using the gastrotomy incision [39]. In certain circumstances, it may be suitable to perform a duodenojejunostomy, preferably with Roux-en-Y reconstruction [40]. Such a maneuver would obviously be predicated on a stable patient and a duodenum wall that is amenable to sutures. It is clear that the General Surgeon must have a variety of techniques in his/her repertoire in order to adapt to the situation at hand.

The other important issue to contend with in duodenal injuries is the management of retroperitoneal necrosis or sepsis. In most cases where laparotomy is performed, some degree of debridement and placement of drains is undertaken. This may be all that can be done if primary duodenal repair is not feasible, or the perforation cannot be localized amid the devitalized tissue. As illustrated by our own case series, repeated drainage procedures are often necessary if signs of recurrent sepsis develop. As has been noted by other authors, [41] males are also at risk of developing sepsis of the inguinoscrotal tract. Percutaneous drainage of any recurrent collections may be attempted using radiological guidance, unless the semi-solid nature of the debris necessitates an open approach. The technique of video-assisted retroperitoneal debridement, [42] as validated for infected necrotizing pancreatitis, may be of use, but there have been no reports of its application in this context.

Conclusion

Retroperitoneal necrosis due to duodenal perforation is a rare but serious complication of ERCP. Early recognition based on risk factors and clinical suspicion may lead to a better outcome, although a protracted course with multiple and various types of procedures should be anticipated. Urgent interventions typically involve debridement and drainage, duodenal repair where feasible, and if indicated, duodenal diversion or other protective procedures. Familiarity with a number of possible surgical strategies is desirable due to the need to adapt to individual circumstances. Surgical management plans should also take into account any underlying pathology that was the initial indication for the endoscopic procedure, although definitive procedures may not be feasible at first operation. The use of ERCP for purely diagnostic purposes should only be considered where less invasive imaging modalities are not possible.

Abbreviations

CBD: Common bile duct; CVL: Central venous line; CT: Computerized tomography; ERCP: Endoscopic retrograde cholangiopancreatography; EUS: Endoscopic ultrasound; LFTs: Liver function tests; MRCP: Magnetic resonance cholangiopancreatography; SIRS: Systemic inflammatory response syndrome; UTI: Urinary tract infection.

Competing interests

The authors declare that they have no competing interests.

Authors' contributions

RT contributed clinical cases to the series, co-wrote the manuscript and attended to reviewer comments. CS contributed clinical cases to the series and co-wrote the manuscript. PB provided the summary data of institutional endoscopy outcomes and edited the first draft of the manuscript. All authors read and approved the final manuscript.

Author details

[1]Department of Surgery, Hobart Clinical School, University of Tasmania, Hobart, Australia. [2]Department of Surgery, Cairns Base Hospital, Cairns & Hinterland Health Service District, Cairns, Australia.

References

1. Enns R, Eloubeidi MA, Mergener K, Jowell PS, Branch MS, Pappas TM, Baillie J: **ERCP-related perforations: risk factors and management.** *Endoscopy* 2002, **34**(4):293–298.
2. Kayhan B, Akdoğan M, Sahin B: **ERCP subsequent to retroperitoneal perforation caused by endoscopic sphincterotomy.** *Gastrointest Endosc* 2004, **60**(5):833–835.
3. Cotton PBLG, Vennes J, Geenen JE, Russell RC, Meyers WC, Liguory C, Nickl N: **Endoscopic sphincterotomy complications and their management: an attempt at consensus.** *Gastrointest Endosc* 1991, **37**(3):383–393.
4. Christensen M, Matzen P, Schulze S, Rosenberg J: **Complications of ERCP: a prospective study.** *Gastrointest Endosc* 2004, **60**(5):721–731.
5. Miller RE, Bossart PW, Tiszenkel HI: **Surgical management of complications of upper gastrointestinal endoscopy and esophageal dilation including laser therapy.** *Am Surg* 1987, **53**(11):667–671.

6. Ames JT, Federle MP, Pealer KM: **Perforated duodenal diverticulum: clinical and imaging findings in eight patients.** *Abdom Imaging* 2009, **34**(2):135–139.
7. Slavin JGP, Sutton R, Hartley M, Rowlands P, Garvey C, Hughes M, Neoptolemos J: **Management of necrotizing pancreatitis.** *World J Gastroenterol* 2001, **7**(4):476–481.
8. Freeny PC, Hauptmann E, Althaus SJ, Traverso LW, Sinanan M: **Percutaneous CT-guided catheter drainage of infected acute necrotizing pancreatitis: techniques and results.** *Am J Roentgenol* 1998, **170**(4):969–975.
9. Habr-Gama A, Waye JD: **Complications and hazards of gastrointestinal endoscopy.** *World J Surg* 1989, **13**(2):193–201.
10. Cotton PB: **Is your sphincterotomy really safe–and necessary?** *Gastrointest Endosc* 1996, **44**(6):752–755.
11. Vandervoort J, Soetikno RM, Tham TC, Wong RC, Ferrari APJ, Montes H, Roston AD, Slivka A, Lichtenstein DR, Ruymann FW, *et al*: **Risk factors for complications after performance of ERCP.** *Gastrointest Endosc* 2002, **56**(5):652–656.
12. Halme L, Doepel M, von Numers H, Edgren J, Ahonen J: **Complications of diagnostic and therapeutic ERCP.** *Ann Chir Gynaecol* 1999, **88**(2):127–131.
13. Stapfer M, Selby RR, Stain SC, Katkhouda N, Parekh D, Jabbour N, Garry D: **Management of duodenal perforation after endoscopic retrograde cholangiopancreatography and sphincterotomy.** *Ann Surg* 2000, **232**(2):191–198.
14. Suissa A, Yassin K, Lavy A, Lachter J, Chermech I, Karban A, Tamir A, Eliakim R: **Outcome and early complications of ERCP: a prospective single center study.** *Hepatogastroenterology* 2005, **52**(62):352–355.
15. Williams EJ, Taylor S, Fairclough P, Hamlyn A, Logan RF, Martin D, Riley SA, Veitch P, Wilkinson ML, Williamson PR, *et al*: **Risk factors for complication following ERCP; results of a large-scale, prospective multicenter study.** *Endoscopy* 2007, **39**(9):793–801.
16. Bharathi R, Rao P, Ghosh K: **Iatrogenic duodenal perforations caused by endoscopic biliary stenting and stent migration: an update.** *Endoscopy* 2006, **38**(12):1271–1274.
17. Doerr RJ, Kulaylat MN, Booth FV, Corasanti J: **Barotrauma complicating duodenal perforation during ERCP.** *Surg Endosc* 1996, **10**(3):349–351.
18. Wu HM, Dixon E, May GR, Sutherland FR: **Management of perforation after endoscopic retrograde cholangiopancreatography (ERCP): a population-based review.** *HPB (Oxford)* 2006, **8**(5):393–399.
19. Avgerinos DV, Llaguna OH, Lo AY, Voli J, Leitman IM: **Management of endoscopic retrograde cholangiopancreatography: related duodenal perforations.** *Surg Endosc* 2009, **23**(4):833–838.
20. Machado NO: **Management of duodenal perforation post-endoscopic retrograde cholangiopancreatography. When and whom to operate and what factors determine the outcome? A review article.** *JOP* 2012, **13**(1):18–25.
21. Ercan M, Bostanci EB, Dalgic T, Karaman K, Ozogul YB, Ozer I, Ulas M, Parlak E, Akoglu M: **Surgical outcome of patients with perforation after endoscopic retrograde cholangiopancreatography.** *J Laparoendosc Adv Surg Tech A* 2012, **22**(4):371–377.
22. Carrillo EH, Richardson JD, Miller FB: **Evolution in the management of duodenal injuries.** *J Trauma Inj Infect Crit Care* 1996, **40**(6):1037–1046.
23. Degiannis E, Boffard K: **Duodenal injuries.** *Br J Surg* 2000, **87**(11):1473–1479.
24. Lai CH, Lau WY: **Management of endoscopic retrograde cholangiopancreatography-related perforation.** *Surgeon* 2008, **6**(1):45–48.
25. Preetha M, Chung YF, Chan WH, Ong HS, Chow PK, Wong WK, Ooi LL, Soo KC: **Surgical management of endoscopic retrograde cholangiopancreatography-related perforations.** *ANZ J Surg* 2003, **73**(12):1011–1014.
26. Kalyani A, Teoh CM, Sukumar N: **Jeiunal patch repair of a duodenal perforation.** *Med J Malaysia* 2005, **60**(2):237–238.
27. Melita G, Currò G, Iapichino G, Princiotta S, Cucinotta E: **Duodenal perforation secondary to biliary stent dislocation: a case report and review of the literature.** *Chir Ital* 2005, **57**(3):385–388.
28. Fatima J, Baron TH, Topazian MD, Houghton SG, Iqbal CW, Ott BJ, Farley DR, Farnell MB, Sarr MG: **Pancreaticobiliary and duodenal perforations after periampullary endoscopic procedures: diagnosis and management.** *Arch Surg* 2007, **142**(5):448–454.
29. Knudson K, Raeburn CD, McIntyre RCJ, Shah RJ, Chen YK, Brown WR, Stiegmann G: **Management of duodenal and pancreaticobiliary perforations associated with periampullary endoscopic procedures.** *Am J Surg* 2008, **196**(6):975–982.
30. Mao Z, Zhu Q, Wu W, Wang M, Li J, Lu A, Sun Y, Zheng M: **Duodenal perforations after endoscopic retrograde cholangiopancreatography: experience and management.** *J Laparoendosc Adv Surg Tech A* 2008, **18**(5):691–695.
31. Angiò LG, Sfuncia G, Viggiani P, Faro G, Bonsignore A, Licursi M, Soliera M, Galati M, Putortì A: **Management of perforations as adverse events of ERCP plus ES. Personal experience.** *G Chir* 2009, **30**(11–12):520–530.
32. Morgan KA, Fontenot BB, Ruddy JM, Mickey S, Adams DB: **Endoscopic retrograde cholangiopancreatography gut perforations: when to wait! When to operate!** *Am Surg* 2009, **75**(6):477–483.
33. Dubecz A, Ottmann J, Schweigert M, Stadlhuber RJ, Feith M, Wiessner V, Muschweck H, Stein HJ: **Management of ERCP-related small bowel perforations: the pivotal role of physical investigation.** *Can J Surg* 2012, **55**(2):99–104.
34. Caliskan K, Parlakgumus A, Ezer A, Colakoglu T, Törer N, Yildirim S: **Surgical management of endoscopic retrograde cholangiopancreatography related injuries.** *Hepatogastroenterology* 2013, **60**(121):76–78.
35. McInnes WD, Aust JB, Cruz AB, Root HD: **Traumatic injuries of the duodenum: a comparison of primary closure and the jejunal patch.** *J Trauma* 1975, **15**:847–853.
36. Jansen M, Du Toit DF, Warren BL: **Duodenal injuries: surgical management adapted to circumstances.** *Injury* 2002, **33**(7):611–615.
37. Stone HH, Fabian TC: **Management of duodenal wounds.** *J Trauma* 1979, **19**:334–339.
38. Berne CJ, Donovan AJ, White EJ, Yellin AE: **Duodenal diverticulization for duodenal and pancreatic injury.** *Am J Surg* 1974, **127**:503–507.
39. Vaughan GD, Frazier OH, Graham DY, Mattox KL, Petmechy FF, Jordan GL: **The use of pyloric exclusion in the management of severe duodenal injuries.** *Am J Surg* 1977, **134**:785–790.
40. Cukingnan RA, Culliford AT, Worth MH: **Surgical correction of a lateral duodenal fistula with the Roux-Y technique.** *J Trauma* 1975, **15**:519–523.
41. Klipfel AA, Schein M: **Retroperitoneal perforation of the duodenum and necrotizing extension to the scrotum.** *Surgery* 2003, **133**(3):337–339.
42. Horvath K, Freeny P, Escallon J, Heagerty P, Comstock B, Glickerman DJ, Bulger E, Sinanan M, Langdale L, Kolokythas O, *et al*: **Safety and efficacy of video-assisted retroperitoneal debridement for infected pancreatic collections: a multicenter, prospective, single-arm phase 2 study.** *Arch Surg* 2010, **145**(9):817–825.

8

Mean platelet volume as a potential prognostic marker in patients with acute mesenteric ischemia

Fatih Altintoprak[1*], Yusuf Arslan[2], Omer Yalkin[2], Yener Uzunoglu[2] and Orhan Veli Ozkan[1]

Abstract

Introduction: We investigated prognostic parameters of patients who underwent surgical intervention for acute mesenteric ischemia by evaluating demographic characteristics and laboratory data on admission.

Methods: The hospital records of 30 patients who underwent surgical interventions due to acute mesenteric ischemia between January 2008 and December 2012, were reviewed retrospectively. The records were investigated with regard to demographic data, the presence of co-morbid diseases, presenting complaints, time elapsed between symptom onset and hospital admission, laboratory findings at admission, findings at surgical exploration, surgical methods used, and treatment outcomes. The patients were divided into two groups, according to death (Group 1) or survival (Group 2), and the two groups were compared in terms of the specified parameters.

Results: Of the patients, 15 were male (50%) and 15 female (50%); their mean age was 71.4 (29–94) years. Abdominal pain was the chief complaint in all patients (100%) and mean time from pain onset to hospital admission was 21 (1–72) h. In abdominal exploration, total small bowel (SB) ischemia and necrosis was found in 6 (20%) patients and other patients had subtotal SB, segmental SB, segmental SB with colon, or isolated colon ischemia. Treatment in 15 patients (50%) ended in mortality. Mean age ($p = 0.038$), urea ($p = 0.002$), AST ($p < 0.001$), ALT ($p < 0.001$), mean platelet volume (MPV; $p = 0.002$), and amylase ($p = 0.022$) levels in Group 1 were significantly higher versus Group 2, whereas Ca ($p = 0.024$) and albumin ($p = 0.002$) levels were significantly lower.

Conclusions: In this study, unlike other parameters that have been shown to be of prognostic significance in mesenteric ischemia, MPV values at presentation were higher among non-survivors than survivors.

Keywords: Acute mesenteric ischemia, Mean platelet volume, Prognosis

Introduction

Acute mesenteric ischemia (AMI) can result from vascular occlusive or non-occlusive conditions. Non-occlusive mesenteric ischemia is caused by conditions such as hypovolemia, sepsis, and cardiogenic shock, whereas the underlying cause of ischemia in 70–80% of cases with AMI is the occlusion of the superior mesenteric artery, caused by embolism or thrombosis [1]. Irreversible changes in the bowel mucosa occur within 6 h in the case of acute arterial occlusion, leading to the disruption of the mucosal barrier, which subsequently allows bacterial translocation, peritonitis, sepsis, and rapid progression to multiple organ failure. Bowel ischemia and necrosis develop rapidly due to a lack of sufficient time to develop collateral circulation, particularly in cases with embolism.

Despite advances in diagnosis, treatment, and post-operative care in recent years, AMI still has a high mortality rate, ranging between 40 and 70% [2]. The most important causes of the high mortality include delayed presentation, non-specific clinical findings, lack of simple biochemical parameters that could be routinely used to diagnose the condition early, and time loss while performing tests for differential diagnosis in patients who are not immediately suspected to have AMI at presentation [3]. From a different perspective, if it is impossible to diagnose AMI in the early period in most patients, it becomes more

* Correspondence: fatihaltintoprak@yahoo.com
[1]Department of General Surgery, Faculty of Medicine, Sakarya University, Sakarya, Turkey
Full list of author information is available at the end of the article

important that parameters be determined that would be useful to predict the disease course at the time of diagnosis.

The aim of the present study was to evaluate the outcomes of surgical treatment over a period of 5 years in patients who underwent surgery with a diagnosis of AMI and to investigate the parameters of prognostic significance.

Materials and methods

The hospital records of 30 patients who underwent surgical intervention due to acute mesenteric ischemia in the Department of General Surgery, Sakarya University Faculty of Medicine between January 2008 and December 2012 were reviewed retrospectively. The records were investigated regarding demographic data, presence of co-morbid diseases, presenting complaints, time elapsed between symptom onset and hospital admission, laboratory findings at admission, findings at surgical exploration, surgical methods used, and treatment outcomes. The patients were divided into two groups, according to death (Group 1) or survival (Group 2), and they were compared in terms of the specified parameters.

Among the parameters in complete blood counts, leukocytes (WBC), hematocrit (Htc), hemoglobin (Hb), mean platelet volume (MPV), and total platelet count (PC) were evaluated. Among the biochemical parameters, urea, creatinine, sodium (Na), potassium (K), calcium (Ca), chlorine (Cl), aspartate amino transferase (AST), alanine amino transferase (ALT), gamma glutamyl transferase (GGT), alkaline phosphatase (ALP), total bilirubin, albumin, and amylase were evaluated.

Survivors in whom more than 2 years had elapsed since their operation were contacted by phone to obtain their latest condition.

In total, 21 variables were compared between the groups. Student's *t*-test and Fischer's exact test were used for comparison between subgroups. Statistical analyses were performed using the SPSS software (ver. 16.0; SPSS, Inc., Chicago, IL, USA). P values < 0.05 were considered to indicate statistical significance.

Results

Of the patients, 15 were male (50%) and 15 female (50%); their mean age was 71.4 (29–94) years. Of the patients, 22 (73.3%) had a history of comorbid disease and cardiovascular disorders were the most common ($n = 16$; 72.7%). Abdominal pain was the chief complaint in all patients (100%) and mean time from pain onset to hospital admission was 21 (1–72) h. All patients underwent computed tomography (CT) of the abdomen and the use of intravenous contrast agent was avoided in 5 (16.6%) patients due to impaired renal function (creatinine > 2.5).

Hemogram and biochemical analysis results of all patients are presented in Table 1.

Table 1 Hemogram and biochemical analysis results of all patients

Parameters	All patients (n = 30)	Death (n = 15)	Survival (n = 15)	p
Hematocrit (%)	40.3	38.7	41.9	>0.05
Hemoglobin (g/dl)	13.4	12.8	14.0	>0.05
Leukocyte (/μL)	16.043	18.046	14.040	>0.05
Platelet (/μL)	256.563	240.193	272.933	>0.05
MPV	8.4	9.01	7.80	0.002
Urea	76.3	102.9	51.4	0.002
Creatinine (mg/dL)	1.52	1.67	1.06	>0.05
Na	136.6	136.3	137.3	>0.05
K	4.2	4.4	3.9	>0.05
Ca	8.1	7.6	8.6	0.024
Cl	102.5	101.0	103.8	>0.05
AST (U/L)	55.63	89.9	21.3	<0.001
ALT (U/L)	60.5	100.1	20.8	<0.001
GGT	35.5	36.7	34.7	>0.05
ALP	84.6	81.0	88.9	>0.05
T.Bilirubin	1.3	1.6	0.9	>0.05
Albumin	3.2	2.6	3.8	0.002
Amylase	137.6	214.0	73.0	0.022

In the abdominal exploration, 6 (20%) patients were found to have diffuse small bowel (SB) ischemia and necrosis, and 17 (56.6%) had subtotal (> 100 cm) SB ischemia; of the 17, 8 (47.0%) had right colonic ischemia. Five (16.6%) patients only had segmental SB ischemia and necrosis (<100 cm) and 1 (3.3%) patient had isolated right-sided colonic ischemia and necrosis. The operation was terminated without performing further intervention in patients suffering from diffuse SB ischemia and necrosis (total necrosis), whereas various resections were performed in the remaining 23 patients (76.6%): 9 (9/23; 39.1%) patients underwent subtotal SB resection, 8 (8/23; 34.7%) underwent subtotal SB resection plus right hemicolectomy, 5 (5/23; 21.7%) underwent segmental SB resection, and 1 (1/23; 4.3%) patients underwent a right hemicolectomy.

One patient (3.3%) was admitted to the hospital 1 h after the onset of abdominal pain and CT scans showed occlusion of the superior mesenteric artery (SMA). This patient subsequently underwent an embolectomy due to the presence of subtotal ischemic changes (dark color in the affected organs, decreased peristalsis, no pulses in the small mesenteric arteries) in the SB but without necrosis.

Demographic features and exploration findings of the patients are presented in Table 2.

The treatment resulted in mortality in 15 patients (50%) (6 of them had total necrosis and underwent only exploratory laparotomy) and there were 15 survivors (50%),

Table 2 Demographic features and exploration findings

Parameters	All patients (n = 30)	Death (n = 15)	Survival (n = 15)	p
Age		78.07	64.80	0.038
Co-morbid disease	22	12	10	>0.05
Diffuse SB ischemia	5	5	—	
Diffuse SB + colon ischemia	1	1	—	
Subtotal SB ischemia	10	4	6	
Subtotal SB + colon ischemia	8	4	4	
Segmental SB ischemia	5	1	4	
Segmental SB + colon ischemia	—	—	—	
Isolated colon ischemia	1	—	1	
Colon ischemia (+)	10	5	5	>0.05

discharged after a mean follow-up of 5 days [3-12]. In a mean follow-up period of 21 months (3–49), 2 (13.3%) patients died for reasons other than recurrence of mesenteric ischemia. Among the remaining 13 patients, only 1 (1/13; 7.6%) patient, who initially underwent an embolectomy, was re-admitted due to the recurrence of mesenteric ischemia at 13 months, and the patient subsequently underwent a subtotal SB resection.

In comparisons of the non-survivors (group 1, $n = 15$) and survivors (group 2, $n = 15$), mean age ($p = 0.038$), urea ($p = 0.002$), AST ($p = 0.001$), MPV ($p = 0.002$), and amylase ($p = 0.022$) levels in Group 1 were significantly higher than in Group 2, whereas Ca ($p = 0.024$) and albumin ($p = 0.002$) levels were significantly lower. No significant difference was found between the groups in terms of other parameters.

Discussion

Acute mesenteric ischemia is among those rare clinical conditions for which no significant improvement has been achieved in the prognosis, despite advances in diagnosis and treatment. Severe abdominal pain with a sudden onset and indistinct physical examination findings are common traits that could be considered to be classic for AMI. However, this is not straightforward and requires experience to consider the diagnosis of AMI based on this clinical picture. Time, which is the strongest and the most valuable factor affecting prognosis, has already been lost in late-presenting patients [4]. The need for radiological imaging of a mesenteric vascular tree for a definitive diagnosis (using multi-slice CT, multi-detector row CT angiography, or conventional angiography), and the fact that these methods are not always readily available consume valuable time in patients presenting at an early stage [1]. In the current study, only one patient (time to admission = 1 h) did not show transmural ischemia and treatment other than surgical resection was possible.

Various biochemical parameters have been investigated for diagnosing acute mesenteric ischemia earlier. Leukocytosis, metabolic acidosis, elevated serum amylase levels, high lactate (L and D stereoisomers), and high D-dimer levels can be found in the presence of AMI. Studies have shown that these findings are not useful in the early diagnosis of AMI and can even be elevated in acute abdominal conditions other than AMI due to their low sensitivity [5-9]. Based on the assumption that mucosa-derived enzymes could be used in the early diagnosis of AMI, considering that ischemia begins from the mucosa, several enzymes, such as intestinal fatty acid binding protein and alpha-glutathione S transferase, have been tested in some studies, which reported limited utility [10]. Leukocytosis, metabolic acidosis, and elevated amylase levels were common findings in the current study; however, these were considered to be expected results considering the long mean time to presentation. D-dimer and mucosa-derived enzymes are not routinely studied in patients presenting to our clinic with abdominal pain.

Predictive factors affecting mortality in patients with AMI upon admission to the hospital have been analyzed in various studies, which yielded different results for many parameters. Aliosmanoglu et al. [11] reported a positive correlation between mortality and leukocytosis, whereas Mamode et al. [12] reported a correlation with leukopenia. Sitges-Serra et al. [13] associated high urea-creatinine levels with poor prognosis, and Aktekin et al. [3] reported that the same parameters were higher in survivors. Acosta-Merida et al. [14] reported an association between hyperamylasemia and massive necrosis, whereas Unalp et al. [15] did not report any association between hyperamylasemia and poor prognosis. Huang et al. [16] reported an association between elevated aspartate aminotransferase (AST) levels and the mortality, and Aktekin et al. [3] reported an association with elevated alanine aminotransferase (ALT) levels. In the current study, urea, AST, ALT, and amylase levels in Group 1 were found to be significantly higher than Group 2, whereas Ca and albumin levels were significantly lower. These results are predictable, considering that late presentation was a common feature of the patients.

Many studies have described advanced age and colonic ischemia accompanying small bowel ischemia as factors indicating poor prognosis [14-17]. In the current study, the mean age in Group 1 was higher than Group 2, consistent with literature reports. However, accompanying colonic ischemia had no effect on prognosis. This could be explained by the small number of patients presenting with colon involvement in the current study compared with in previous reports.

Platelets play a critical role in the regulation of blood flow and thrombogenic cascades. MPV is a marker of the size and activation of platelets, and elevated levels of MPV reflect increased production and activation of platelets. Large platelets possess higher metabolic and enzymatic activity, and show higher thrombogenic potential [18]. Several molecules released from activated platelets, such as P-selectin and thromboxane A2, contribute to thrombus formation; activated platelets also attach to endothelium and up-regulate the expression of adhesions molecules [19]. It was thought that increased MPV could be associated with increased vascular inflammation and thrombogenicity, and a direct association has been shown between increased MPV and acute thrombotic events, such as acute myocardial infarction, unstable angina, and stroke [20-22]. Furthermore, increased MPV was found to be an independent predictor factor of mortality in ischemic vascular events, recurrent myocardial infarction, and coronary artery disease [23].

No published study has examined the relationship between MPV and AMI. AMI is a cardiovascular disease in origin, although its consequences affect predominantly the gastrointestinal system. As a matter of course, a relationship between AMI and increased MPV is considered to indicate increased thrombogenic activity. In the current study, MPV in Group 1 was significantly higher than in Group 2.

However, it would not be appropriate to consider that this result indicates that "increased MPV is a predictive factor for prognosis in AMI," because a high MPV is found in other atherosclerosis-related conditions (such as diabetes mellitus, hypertension, hypercholesterolemia, smoking, and obesity) [24]. High mean age and the presence of co-morbid conditions related to the cardiovascular system in most of our patients suggest that these patients might have had a high MPV before the development of AMI.

Considering the significantly higher MPV in Group 1 in the current study: 1) MPV could be used to predict the potential for vascular damage in other organs, such as the liver and kidneys (that is, to identify candidate multi-organ failure patients), and 2) because it reflects a tendency for thrombosis, MPV could be useful to justify re-operation when a second-look decision could not be made otherwise.

In conclusion, AMI continues to have a high mortality rate despite advances in diagnosis, treatment, and post-operative care. MPV can be beneficial in predicting patients with poor prognosis and in the planning of re-operations.

Competing interests

The authors declare that they have no competing interests.

Authors' contributions

FA, YA and OVO contributed to study design. YA, OY and YU contributed to data collection. FA and YA contributed to data analysis and writing. All authors read and approved the final manuscript.

Author details

[1]Department of General Surgery, Faculty of Medicine, Sakarya University, Sakarya, Turkey. [2]Department of General Surgery, Research and Educational Hospital, Sakarya University, Sakarya, Turkey.

References

1. van den Heijkant TC, Aerts BA, Teijink JA, Buurman WA, Luyer MD: **Challenges in diagnosing mesenteric ischemia.** *World J Gastroenterol* 2013, **19**(9):1338–1341.
2. Kassahun WT, Schulz T, Richter O, Hauss J: **Unchanged high mortality rates from acute occlusive intestinal ischemia: six year review.** *Langenbecks Arch Surg* 2008, **393**(2):163–171.
3. Aktekin A, Emir S, Saglam A: **Factors affecting mortality in acute mesenteric obstruction.** *Ulus Travma Acil Cerrahi Derg* 2009, **15**(3):217–221.
4. Klar E, Rahmanian PB, Bücker A, Hauenstein K, Jauch KW, Luther B: **Acute mesenteric ischemia: a vascular emergency.** *Dtsch Arztebl Int* 2012, **109**(14):249–256.
5. Block T, Nilsson TK, Björck M, Acosta S: **Diagnostic accuracy of plasma biomarkers for intestinal ischaemia.** *Scand J Clin Lab Invest* 2008, **68** (3):242–248.
6. Chiu YH, Huang MK, How CK, Hsu TF, Chen JD, Chern CH, Yen DH, Huang CI: **D-dimer in patients with suspected acute mesenteric ischemia.** *Am J Emerg Med* 2009, **27**(8):975–979.
7. Oldenburg WA, Lau LL, Rodenberg TJ, Edmonds HJ, Burger CD: **Acute mesenteric ischemia: a clinical review.** *Arch Intern Med* 2004, **164** (10):1054–1062.
8. Acosta S, Björck M: **Acute thrombo-embolic occlusion of the superior mesenteric artery: a prospective study in a well defined population.** *Eur J Vasc Endovasc Surg* 2003, **26**(2):179–183.
9. Demir IE, Ceyhan GO, Friess H: **Beyond lactate: is there a role for serum lactate measurement in diagnosing acute mesenteric ischemia?** *Dig Surg* 2012, **29**(3):226–235.
10. Evennett NJ, Petrov MS, Mittal A, Windsor JA: **Systematic review and pooled estimates for the diagnostic accuracy of serological markers for intestinal ischemia.** *World J Surg* 2009, **33**(7):1374–1383.
11. Aliosmanoglu I, Gul M, Kapan M, Arikanoglu Z, Taskesen F, Basol O, Aldemir M: **Risk factors effecting mortality in acute mesenteric ischemia and mortality rates: a single center experience.** *Int Surg* 2013, **98:**76–81.
12. Mamode N, Pickford I, Leiberman P: **Failure to improve outcome in acute mesenteric ischaemia: seven-year review.** *Eur J Surg* 1999, **165**(3):203–208.
13. Sitges-Serra A, Mas X, Roqueta F, Figueras J, Sanz F: **Mesenteric infarction: an analysis of 83 patients with prognostic studies in 44 cases undergoing a massive small-bowel resection.** *Br J Surg* 1988, **75**(6):544–548.
14. Acosta-Merida MA, Marchena-Gomez J, Cruz-Benavides F, Hernandez-Navarro J, Roque-Castellano C, Rodriguez-Mendez A, Alonso-Alvarado A, Hernandez-Romero J: **Predictive factors of massive intestinal necrosis in acute mesenteric ischemia.** *Cir Esp* 2007, **81**(3):144–149.
15. Unalp HR, Atahan K, Kamer E, Yasa H, Tarcan E, Onal MA: **Prognostic factors for hospital mortality in patients with acute mesenteric ischemia who undergo intestinal resection due to necrosis.** *Ulus Travma Acil Cerrahi Derg* 2010, **16**(1):63–70.
16. Huang HH, Chang YC, Yen DH, Kao WF, Chen JD, Wang LM, Huang CI, Lee CH: **Clinical factors and outcomes in patients with acute mesenteric ischemia in the emergency department.** *J Chin Med Assoc* 2005, **68**(7):299–306.
17. Aouni F, Bouhaffa A, Baazaoui J, Khelifi S, Ben Maamer A, Houas N, Cherif A: **Acute mesenteric ischemia: study of predictive factors of mortality.** *Tunis Med* 2012, **90**(7):533–536.
18. Kamath S, Blann AD, Lip GY: **Platelet activation: assessment and quantification.** *Eur Heart J* 2001, **22**(17):1561–1571.
19. Celik T, Yuksel UC, Bugan B, Iyisoy A, Celik M, Demirkol S, Yaman H, Kursaklıoglu H, Kilic S, Isik E: **Increased platelet activation in patients with slow coronary flow.** *J Tromb Trombolysis* 2010, **29**(3):310–315.
20. Isik T, Ayhan E, Uyarel H, Ergelen M, Tanboga IH, Kurt M, Korkmaz AF, Kaya A, Aksakal E, Sevimli S: **Increased mean platelet volume associated with extent of slow coronary flow.** *Cardiol J* 2012, **19**(4):355–362.

21. Unal EU, Ozen A, Kocabeyoglu S, Durukan AB, Tak S, Songur M, Kervan U, Birincioglu CL: **Mean platelet volume may predict early clinical outcome after coronary artery bypass grafting.** *J Cardiothorac Surg* 2013, **8**(1):91.
22. Slavka G, Perkmann T, Haslacher H, Greisenegger S, Marsik C, Wagner OF, Endler G: **Mean platelet volume may represent a predictive parameter for overall vascular mortality and ischemic heart disease.** *Arterioscler Thromb Vasc Biol* 2011, **31**(5):1215–1218.
23. Chu SG, Becker RC, Berger PB, Bhatt DL, Eikelboom JW, Konkle B, Mohler ER, Reilly MP, Berger JS: **Mean platelet volume as a predictor of cardiovascular risk: a systematic review and meta-analysis.** *J Thromb Haemost* 2010, **8**(1):148–156.
24. Guvenç TS, Hasdemir H, Erer HB, Ilhan E, Ozcan KS, Calik AN, Cetin R, Eren M: **Lower than normal mean platelet volume is associated with reduced extent of coronary artery disease.** *Arq Bras Cardiol* 2013, **100**(3):255–260.

9

The role of emergency surgery in hydatid liver disease

Ali I Yahya*, Hussen E Shwereif, Mustafa A Ekheil, Ahmed S Thoboot, Kalid A Algader, Fatma O Gyaed and Abdsalem S Aldarat

Abstract

Hepatic hydatid disease is very common in Libya. In Zliten hospital, we operated 400 patients with hepatic hydatid cysts over period of 20 years. All patients were symptomatic. Their ages varied from 3 to 85 years including 215 female and 185 male patients. Their symptoms varied from abdominal pain to abdominal mass 67 patients were admitted through Accident and Emergency Department with acute presentations including fever, skin rash, jaundice and shock with acute abdominal pain. Those 67 patients had necessary investigations, resuscitation and underwent emergency surgery. The hepatic cysts in all patients were excised, and the obstructive jaundice was cleared in those patients with obstructive jaundice. Unfortunately, one of the patients died two days after the surgery because of multiple organ failure (MOF) Morbidity was wound Infection, bile leak and recurrence rate were all reported in our series.

Keywords: Liver, Hydatid disease, Emergency surgery

Introduction

Hydatid is a disease caused by tape worm called ecchinococcous granulosis and ecchinococcous multilocularis. Hydatid disease is endemic in some regions in the world and Libya is one of the endemic countries of hydatid disease among the Middle East countries. This disease is common in sheepherder regions. Thus people who live thereare accidentally infected. Dogs are the definitive host and sheep is the intermediate host. Human gets the infection by eating contaminated vegetables by dogs' waste or by direct contact with dogs. Infection rate is higher in places where dogs are fed with infected carcasses and offal. Liver is the commonest organ involved in human as well as lung, kidneys,spleen, bones and soft tissues. Symptoms depend on the size of the cyst, the organ involved and the complications from the cyst.

The diagnosis of hydatid liver disease depends on history and clinical examination. Using imaging investigations is very valuable to confirm the diagnosis including ultrasound scan and CT scan. While serological investigations are not needed in endemic area, surgical intervention is the main way to treat hepatic hydatid cysts.

* Correspondence: aliyahyaz60@hotmail.com
General surgery department, Zliten Teaching Hospital and Edwaw District Hospital, Zliten, Libya

Methods and materials

The files of the patients were reviewed retrospectively. Four hundred patients were operated at the general surgery department at Zliten hospital while sixty seven patients were operated as emergency because of their acute presentations, the research was approved by the research and ethical committee in the hospital.

67 patients were admitted through Accident and Emergency Department. One of them was shocked and admitted to the surgical ICU. All the patients came from endemic areas of hydatid disease. Routine investigations were done including complete blood count, blood group, blood sugar, urea and electrolytes. Liver function tests and ultrasound scan were done for all patients. CT scan was also performed for most of the patients. All the patients had intravenous fluid, antibiotics, analgesia and hydrocortisone.

All patients had laparotomy at same day. The operations were done under general anesthesia through right subcostal incision. Precautions were taken to prevent spillage of the cyst content. Intraoperative ultrasound was done routinely for all patients to find out the exact number of cysts. The duration of surgeries varied from one and half an hour to three hours. All the cysts were excised.

Results

Group A - 45 patients were presented with abdominal pain and obstructive jaundice. Blood tests showed high bilirubin and alkaline phosphates while other blood tests were normal. The ultrasound showed hepatic hydatid cysts.

23 patients were with single big cyst with no daughter cysts. All cysts were near to the hilum with size ranges from 10 to 15 cm. In 9 patients, the cysts were in the left lobe and in the other 14 patients, they were in the right lobe. Bile ducts were normal in size.

In 22 patients, the ultrasound showed cysts with multiple daughter cysts. In twenty one of them, the cysts were in the right lobe and in one patient, the cyst was in the left lobe. The size of cysts ranges from 8 to 15 cm. MRCP was done for two patients and it showed clear communication between the cyst and the biliary tree. Preoperative ERCP was done for one patient who was in septicemia and renal impairment. 23 patients, with their cysts near the hilum, were excised and the fluid in the cyst was clear. There were no bile and no daughter cysts but only single endocyst. There was no bile duct communication and the cyst cavity was completely closed.

22 patients were with cysts at the right and the left lobe of the liver. Those cysts contain multiple daughter cysts. Some of them contain bile stained fluid. After removal of all daughter cysts, there were communications with bile ducts. With the use of the Fogarty catheter, daughter cysts and membranes came out. We flushed the bile ducts with huge amount of saline and the communication was closed with 2/0 PDS.

Group B - Two patients (one is male 18 years and the other is female 24 years old) were presented with swelling at anterior abdominal wall. Both the swellings were tender red, ultrasound findings in both patients showed that hydatid cyst liver communicating with the abdominal swellings which were cystic. Both patients had laparotomy and excision of the hydatid cysts and the abscess track. Both patients cured and discharged in good conditions.

Group C - Six patients were admitted with skin rashes all over the body. Two of them were males and the others were females ageing between 16 to 25 years. General conditions were stable and their blood pressure was within normal. On abdominal examination, there was guarding and tenderness all over the abdomen. The ultrasound examination showed huge hydatid cysts in the liver and all were in the right lobe with free fluid in the abdomen. 6 patients underwent urgent laparotomy and excision of the hydatid cysts. There was leak from the cysts into the abdominal cavity, but patients improved and discharged in good conditions.

Group D - One patient was admitted to Intensive Care Unit with shock. On examination, patient looked sick, pale and tachycardiac with low BP. Abdomen was guarding and rigid. The patient had resuscitation including IV fluid, IV hydrocortisone and IV analgesia. He had routine investigation and the ultrasound scan showed hydatid cyst liver in the left lobe with a lot of fluid in the abdomen. The patient had laparotomy and there was a big hydatid cyst at the left lobe which was ruptured. With excision of the cyst and cleaning of the abdominal cavity, the patient improved and discharged in good conditions.

Group E - Ten patients were admitted with abdominal pain and fever. They had ultrasound scan which showed hydatid cysts of the liver. In seven patients, the cysts were at the right lobe and in three patients at the left lobe. Laparotomy was performed for all of them. The cysts were full of pus, and the cyst cavity was completely cleared. Drain was inserted and the patients were covered with antibiotics. Patients improved and discharged in good conditions.

Group F - A female Patient was 35 years old was admitted with dyspnea and chest pain. On clinical examination, the patient looked pale and dyspnic with rapid pulse and decrease air entry on the right side of the chest.

X-ray of the chest showed that the right side was pleural effusion. The ultrasound of the abdomen showed huge hydatid cyst in the right lobe of the liver with a lot of daughter cysts in the right chest cavity. The CT scan of abdomen and chest confirmed the finding of hydatid cyst liver ruptured into chest. The patient had routine investigations and urgent surgery. The finding was a huge cyst in the right lobe of the liver full of daughter cysts and bile, ruptured into the chest cavity. Wound extended into the right thoracotomy and the hepatic cyst was excised and the fistula closed washing the pleural cavity. Drains were inserted and common bile duct was cleared from daughter cysts. The patient discharged in good conditions.

Group G - Two patients had laparotomy for hepatic hydatid cyst (one of them was male 18 years and the other was female 25 years old). The male Patient was diagnosed with huge right hepatic lobe hydatid cyst. MRCP showed big communication with cyst and the patient was not jaundiced. He had a laparotomy and excision of the cyst. The communication with bile duct was closed and the patient discharged in good conditions. After 10 days from the surgery, the patient came back to the hospital with abdominal pain. He looked dehydrated, sick and hypotensive. Routine investigations showed leucocytosis and raised bilirubin 3.3 mg with a slight increase of alkaline phosphates. The ultrasound showed that the abdomen was full of fluid. The patient had IV fluid, IV antibiotics and laparotomy was done. The abdomen was full of bile and it was cleaned completely. There was a leak from the cyst cavity and a big drain was inserted into the cyst cavity. Then the abdomen was closed and the patient improved and discharged in good conditions.

The female patient had laparotomy for the hydatid cyst liver. After three days, she developed severe abdominal pain. On examination, the abdomen was guarding and tender. The ultrasound showed plenty of fluid in the abdomen. The patient was sick and urgent laparotomy was done to her. The abdomen was full of bile, it was washed with plenty of saline and a big drain was inserted in the cyst cavity. And the patient improved and discharged in good conditions.

Sixty seven patients with hepatic hydatid cysts were admitted to our surgery ward with acute presentations included obstructive jaundice which was 11.25% of the total hydatid liver cysts operated in our institute. Six patients were presented with skin rash and acute abdominal pain was 1.25% of the total patients admitted and operated in Zlien hospital. Two patients were treated in the hospital with abdominal wall abscess which is fistula with hydatid liver cyst which was 0.5%. While ten patients were presented with liver abscess which was 2% of the total patients treated. One patient was presented with anaphylactic shock and another patient with bilipleaural fistula. Whereas another two patients were presented with peritonitis followed hepatic hydatid cyst excision. Those sixty seven patients underwent resuscitation and routine necessary investigations. All of them had urgent surgery and hepatic cysts were excised. One of the patients died after two days from the surgery due to multiple organ failure. The main hospital stay is 6 days. The morbidity noticed among 400 operated patients. 6% of them suffered from bile leak, 4% with wound infection and 2% with recurrence (Figure 1).

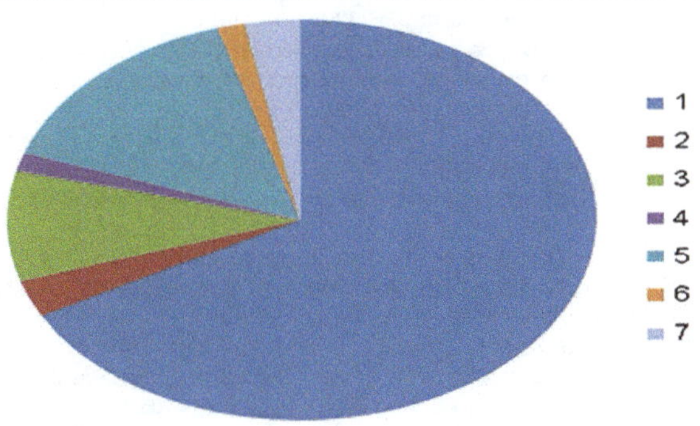

Figure 1 Distribution of patients presentations. A-45 patients with obstruction jaundice. B-2 patients with abdominal wall abscess. C-6 patients admitted with skin rash. D-One patient with anaphylactic shock. E-10 patients with liver abscess. F-1 patient with biliopleural fistula. G-2 patients with biliary peritonitis following hepatic hydatid cystectomy. Group A=1, Group B=2, Group C=3, Group D=4, Group E=5, Group F=6, Group G=7.

Discussion and conclusion

Sixty seven patients with hepatic hydatid cysts were admitted through Accident and Emergency Department of Zliten hospital with acute symptoms. They were operated urgently and their presentations were as follow:

A. 45 patients with obstruction jaundice.
B. 2 patients with abdominal wall abscess.
C. 6 patients with skin rash.
D. 1 patient with anaphylactic shock.
E. 10 patients with liver abscess.
F. 1 patient with biliopleural fistula.
G. 2 patients with biliary peritonitis following hepatic hydatid cystectomy.

Liver is the commonest organ gets infected by ecchinococous granulosis. The cyst can be asymptomatic discovered on routine ultrasound examination of the abdomen, or symptomatic like abdominal mass or abdominal pain [1-6]. Hepatic cyst can be seen or discovered as organized cyst during investigations or other abdominal operations. In endemic areas, any patient, comes with the right upper abdominal mass, is considered infected with hydatid cyst liver until it is proved otherwise. Surgery is the main treatment for hepatic hydatid cyst. Most of our patients were treated electively. Sixty seven patients (67) with acute symptoms were operated urgently to avoid complication such as rupture which was reported in the literatures of the patients [7-14]. Different nonsurgical treatment was performed like pair technique in different centers, but none of our patients was candidate for pair technique [15-22]. Medical treatment like albendazole (antihelmentic) is used in treatment of hepatic hydatid cysts. Some centers used the medical treatment and good results were observed. But in our center, we did not report significant benefits of medical treatment. We used albendazole preoperative and postoperative to prevent recurrence and antihelmintic. Medical treatment is not beneficial for patients with acute presentation where time makes difference in management. We also used medical treatment postoperatively for our patients to prevent recurrence. Sixty seven patients who came to the Accident and Emergency Department had routine investigations and ultrasound scan, and they were treated by urgent laparotomy through the right Kocher incision. Patients of group A, with obstructive jaundice, the obstruction was done by compression on bile duct from outside and obstruction from inside by daughter cysts and parasitic membrane [23-25]. None of the patients had preoperative ERCP [26]. Only four of them had ERCP postoperatively for continuous bile leak through the drain. ERCP will not cure them but it will only clear the bile ducts from intraductal obstruction by daughter cysts or parasitic membrane and will relief the jaundice before surgery. The patient will still need surgery to cure him or her from the disease. We explored the common bile duct through the communication with the cyst for those in whom the obstructive jaundice is intraductal. But those in whom the obstruction is extra ductal the obstruction is cleared with excision of the cyst. We reviewed the literatures of the patients. Most of the patients underwent ERCP before surgery. Patients of group B suffered from abdominal wall swelling due to fistulization of superficial laying hepatic hydatid cyst. Rare presentation was also reported in literatures of patients [27,28] with biliocutaneous fistula. Patients of group C were presented with skin rash and abdominal pain due to leakage of parasitic fluid into the abdominal cavity which induced anaphylactic reaction due to antigen antibody reaction. Those patients had minimal leak where they did not go into anaphylactic shock. All of them had intravenous fluid and hydrocortisone and underwent urgent laparotomy and excision of hydatid cyst. While patients of group D were presented with anaphylactic shock due to hydatid cyst. But this was very rare. Among four hundred patients operated in our institution, only three patients had anaphylactic shock, two of them had the shock during surgery and the other patient was case reported as emergency presentation. The three patients were saved with use of intravenous adrenaline and intravenous fluid. Patients of group E were presented with liver abscess and secondary infection by bacteria. Liver abscess was expected because of high temperature [29,30] patients were sick and dehydrated. The ultrasound showed that the cyst contents were thick. Liver abscess was confirmed by surgery. All the patients had antibiotics and only three of them had blood transfusion because of low hemoglobin. The patient of group F had very rare presentation. The hepatic hydatid cyst infiltrated the diaphragm and opened in the pleura. Patients of group G had urgent surgeries. The two patients had biliary peritonitis after hepatic hydatid cyst surgery. They were diagnosed clinically and underwent urgent surgery. The usual time of surgery varies from one hour to 3 hours and the patients had excision of the cyst and closure of the cyst cavity. But none of them had liver resection although they had big drain inserted around the cyst area which left for 3 to 5 days. Emergency surgery gives quick answer to patient with acute complain. Only one patient died. She had obstructive jaundice and died because of multiple organ failure. We reported morbidity includes bile leak, wound infection, recurrence. Hospital stay was longer for patients who had emergency surgery in comparison to elective surgery.

Conclusion

Hepatic hydatid disease can be asymptomatic or symptomatic with usual symptoms either abdominal pain or abdominal mass. We reviewed our patients admitted and treated in Zliten institution. Most of them were admitted and treated electively 67 patients were admitted through the Accident and Emergency Department. Those patients were sick and they had the investigations and treatment done urgently. They were presented with different acute presentations such as obstructive jaundice, skin rashes, anaphylactic shock, abdominal wall abscess, liver abscess, peritonitis and biliopleural fistula. All of them had urgent surgeries and could not be treated by medical or PAIR treatment. As usual, the complications from emergency surgery were expected to be more. But in this research, the rate of complications were not much different from the patients operated electively. This is due to emergency surgery done at the right time for the right patient.

Competing interests

The authors declare that they have no competing interests.

Authors' contribution

All authors read and approved the final manuscript.

References

1. Grosso G, Gruttadauria S, Biondi D, *et al*: **Worldwide Epidemiology of Liver Hydatidosis Including the Mediterranean Area.** *World J Gastroenterol* 2012, **18**(13):1425–1437.
2. Kjossev K, Losanoff J: **TNRC Classification for Liver Hydatid Cysts.** *Int Surg* 1998, **83:**311–313.
3. Kjossev K, Losanoff J: ***Response*** **to Comment on 'Classification of Hydatid Liver Cysts'.** *J Gastroenterol Hepatol* 2007, **22**(4):604.
4. Kjossev K, Losanoff J: **Classification of Hydatid Liver Cysts.** *J Gastroenterol Hepatol* 2005, **20**(3):35.
5. Kjossev K: *Classification, Staging and Surgical Treatment.* Sofia Bulgaria: PhD Dissertation 2012:165.
6. Dakkak A: **Echinococcosis/Hydatidosis: A Severe Threat in Mediterranean Countries.** *Vet Parasitol* 2010, **174**(1–2):2–11.
7. Akcan A, Akyildiz H, Artis T, *et al*: **Peritoneal Perforation of Liver Hydatid Cysts Clinical Presentation, Predisposing Factors, and Surgical Outcome.** *World J Surg* 2007, **31**(6):1284–1291.
8. Dumnici A, Papiu H, Olariu T: **Acute Surgical Abdomen Produced by an Abdominalized Infected Gigantic Hydatid Cyst. Case Reports. English Abstract.** *J Article Chirurgia (Bucur)* 2004, **99**(3):181–184.
9. Durif S, Marinkovic Z, Febvre C, *et al*: **Hydatid Liver Disease Revealed by Surgical Acute Abdominal Syndrome. Case Reports, English Abstract, Journal Article.** *Arch Pediatr* 2005, **12**(11):1617–1619.
10. Gogia N, Sharma R, Gamangatti S, *et al*: **Hepatic Hydatid cysts with biliary, and peritoneal rupture and transdiaphragmatic migration. Case reports, Journal article.** *Trop Gastroenterol* 2006, **27**(2):93–96.
11. Ghesquière F, Mourot N, Olivero de Rubiana JP, *et al*: **Surgery of Hepatic Hydatic Cyst. Per-operative Complications. Possibility of Anaphylactic Etiology. Case Reports, English Abstract, Journal Article.** *Anesth Analg (Paris)* 1979, **36**(11–12):561–563.
12. Daradkeh S, EL-Muhtaseb H, Farah G: **Predictors of Morbidity and Mortality in the Surgical Management of Hydatid Cyst of the Liver.** *Arch Surg* 2007, **392:**35–39.
13. Kang MJ, Lee SH, Kim SJ, *et al*: **A Case of Multiple Intraperitoneal Cysts From Ruptured Hepatic Hydatid Cysts. Case Reports, English Abstract, Journal Article.** *Korean J Gastroenterol* 2007, **50**(3):203–206.
14. Ozturk G, Aydinli B, Yildirgan MI, *et al*: **Posttraumatic Free Intraperitoneal Rupture of Liver Cystic Echinococcosis: a Case Series and Review of Literature.** *Journal Article* 2007, **194**(3):313–316.
15. Haddad M, Al Awar G, Jalbout R, Kanj V, Elkattah R, Faraj W, Khalifeh MJ: **New Trends in the Management of Hepatic Echinococcusgranulosus.** *Libya* 2011, **59**(3):154–159.
16. Filippou D, Tselepis D, Filippou G, Papadopoulos V: **Advances in LiverEchinococcosis: Diagnosis and Treatment.** *Clin Gastroenterol Hepatol* 2007, **5**(2):152–159.

17. Dziri C, Haouet, Fingerhut A: **Treatment of Hydatid Cyst of the Liver: WhereIs the Evidence?** *World J Surgery* 2004, **28**(8):731–736.
18. **Liver Echinococcosis, Consensus Statement of The National Conference, Sofia.** 2003.
19. Papadimitriou J, Mandrekas A: **The Surgical Treatment of Hydatid Disease of the Liver.** *Br J Surg* 2005 XII, **57**(6):431–433.
20. Nunnari G, Pinzone M, Gruttadauria S, *et al*: **Hepatic Echinococcosis: clinical and the Rapeutic Aspects.** *World J Gastroenterol* 2012, **18–13:**1448–1458.
21. Mandal S, Mandal M: **Human cystic echinococcosis: epidemiologic, zoonotic, clinical, Diagnostic and Therapeutic Aspects.** *Asian Pac J Trop Me* 2012, **5**(4):253–260.
22. Ivanov G: *Modern Approach in Diagnosis and Surgical Treatment of Liver. Echinococcosis in children and Adults.* Varna, Bulgaria: PhD Dissertation; 2012:182.
23. Lu SF, Li JZ: **Cases of Hydatid Disease of the Common Bile Duct. Journal Article.** *Zhongguo Ji Sheng Chong Xue Yu Ji Sheng Chong Bing ZaZhi* 2000, **18**(3):185.
24. Manterola C, Barroso M, Vial M, Bustos L, Muñoz S, Losada H, Bello N, Hernández F, Carrasco R: *Liver Abscess of Hydatid Origin: Clinical Features and Results of Aggressive Treatment.* 2003.
25. Prousalidis J, Kosmidis C, Kapoutzis K, *et al*: **Intrabiliary Rupture of Hydatid Cysts of the Liver. Journal Article.** *Am J Surg* 2009, **197**(2):193–198.
26. Târcoveanu E, Vasilescu A, Moldovanu R, Vlad N, Rusu V, Stanciu C: **Unusual Forms of Liver Abscesses.** *Rev Med Chir Soc Med Nat Las*, **112**(3):688–697.
27. Coyle WJ: **ERCP in Hepatic Hydatid Disease. [Comment, Journal Article].** *Gastroenterol Rep* 2004, **6**(4):272.
28. Florea M, Barbu ST, Crisan M, *et al*: **Spontaneous External Fistula of a Hydatid Liver Cyst in a Diabetic Patient. Case Reports, Journal Article.** *Chirurgia (Bucur)* 2008, **103**(6):695–698.
29. Losada H, Bello N, Hernández F, Carrasco R: *Liver Abscess of Hydatid Origin: Clinical Features and Results of Aggressive Treatment.* 2003.
30. Manterola C, Barroso M, Vial M, Bustos L, Muñoz S, Losada H, Bello N, Hernández F, Carrasco R: **Liver Abscess of Hydatid Origin: Clinical Features and Results of Aggressive Treatment.** *ANZ J Surg* 2003, **73**(4):220–224.

Italian Biological Prosthesis Work-Group (IBPWG): proposal for a decisional model in using biological prosthesis

Federico Coccolini[1], Ferdinando Agresta[2], Andrea Bassi[3], Fausto Catena[4], Feliciano Crovella[3], Roberto Ferrara[5], Francesco Gossetti[6], Domenico Marchi[7], Gabriele Munegato[8], Paolo Negro[6], Micaela Piccoli[7], Gianluigi Melotti[7], Massimo Sartelli[9], Michele Schiano di Visconte[8], Mario Testini[10], Paolo Bertoli[1], Michela Giulii Capponi[1], Marco Lotti[1], Roberto Manfredi[1], Michele Pisano[1], Elia Poiasina[1], Eugenio Poletti[1] and Luca Ansaloni[1*]

Abstract

Introduction: Indications for repair of abdominal hernia are well established and widely diffused. Controversies still exist about the indication in using the different prosthetic materials and principally about the biological ones.

Material and methods: In February 2012, the Italian Biological Prosthesis Work-Group (IBPWG), counting a background of 264 biologic implants, met in Bergamo (Italy) for 1-day meeting with the aim to elaborate a decisional model on biological prosthesis use in abdominal surgery.

Results: A diagram to simplify the decisional process in using biologics has been elaborated.

Conclusion: The present score represents a first attempt to combine scientific knowledge and clinical expertise in order to offer precise indications about the kind of biological mesh to use.

Keywords: Biological prosthesis, Work-group, Indication, Cross-linked, Non-cross-linked, Surgery, Reconstruction, Infection, Tissue loss, Mesh

Introduction

Prosthetic abdominal wall surgical repair is a common procedure [1,2]. Actually, about one million prostheses per year for abdominal wall repair are used worldwide [3]. Since the first description of a mesh use for abdominal wall repairing [4] plenty of new material have been introduced, first synthetic, but later biologic. Indications for repair are well established and widely diffused [5]. However controversies still exist about the indication in using the different materials and principally about the biological ones. More than a dozen of biological prosthesis (BP) are currently available (Table 1). All of them are derived from human or mammalian tissues [6]. It has already been noted the major variability among human dermis prosthesis than among the animal ones in terms of mechanical and physical properties [6]. In fact xenograft products are obtained from a more uniform animal population with similar age and life histories, this allows producers to obtain more consistent implants than from humans donors [6].

BP, independently from the origin, could be further and basically divided into two main groups: cross-linked and non-cross-linked. The difference between these two groups is the proceeding the cross-linked are submitted to. The introduction of chemical cross-linking between the collagen chains, strengthens the prosthesis reducing the efficacy of bacterial and host collagenase enzymes, thus the implant is less prone to degradation in vivo [7,8].

On the basis of either the presence or not of the cross-linking, biological prosthesis are divided into two subgroups: the partially remodeling (over time) and the completely remodeling ones. The partially remodeling (cross-linked) prosthesis are made of porcine or human dermal collagen and bovine pericardium collagen [6]. The completely remodeling (not cross-linked) ones are

* Correspondence: lansaloni@ospedaliriuniti.bergamo.it
[1]General and Emergency Surgery Department, Ospedali Riuniti, Bergamo, Italy
Full list of author information is available at the end of the article

Table 1 Biological prosthesis currently on the market

Name	Manufacturer	Tissue source	Material	X-linking
Alloderm	LifeCell	Human	Acellular dermis	No
AlloMax	Bard	Human	Acellular dermis	No
Flex HD	Ethicon/MTF[¥]	Human	Acellular dermis	-
DermaMatrix	MTF[¥]	Human	Acellular dermis	No
Permacol	Covidien	Porcine	Acellular dermis	Yes
CollaMend	Davol/Bard	Porcine	Acellular dermis	Yes
Strattice	KCI/LifeCell	Porcine	Acellular dermis	No
XenMatrix	Brennan Medical	Porcine	Acellular dermis	No
Surgisis	Cook	Porcine	Small intestine submucosa	No
Surgisis Gold	Cook	Porcine	Small intestine submucosa	No
Lyosis	Cook	Porcine	Lyophilized small intestine submucosa	No
FortaGen	Organogenesis	Porcine	Small intestine submucosa	Yes
SurgiMend	TEI bioscience	Bovine	Fetal dermis	No
Periguard	Synovis	Bovine	Pericardium	Yes
Veritas	Synovis	Bovine	Pericardium	No
Tutomesh	Tutogen	Bovine	Pericardium	No
Tutopatch	Tutogen	Bovine	Pericardium	No

[¥] MTF: Muscoloskeletal Transplant Foundation.

principally made of swine intestinal sub-mucosa, swine dermis, human dermis, fetal bovine dermis and bovine pericardium. The differences in remodeling times should be kept in mind when these materials are chosen for abdominal wall repair [6]. Each type of prosthesis allows and encourages host tissue ingrowth, although different prostheses can feature different clinical attributes. Thanks to the presence of additional linkages the partially remodeling ones resist better and for a longer period to mechanical stress. Moreover BP have the lowest adhesiogenic potential among all prosthetic materials available for intra-peritoneal use [9]. Post-operative pain and discomfort have been demonstrated to be inferior when biological prosthetic materials are used in groin hernia repair [10]. Implants would act as a scaffold inside which the host tissue cells and fibroblasts can replicate. They also provide resistance to tension and stress by supporting the abdominal wall until it is fully recovered. Times of remodeling range between a few months and few years [11]. It depends on prosthesis characteristics and host tissues properties.

Surgeons have not widely assumed the capability to manage with BP. The way to consider them should be completely different from the standard synthetic meshes. These last ones are as a "patch to apply on a hole"; essentially they trigger a foreign body host response leading to encapsulation of the prosthesis with intense fibrous reaction. On the contrary BP activate a remodeling process in which the host remodels the prosthesis and his own tissues by producing new healthy tissue. By using BP the surgeon starts a real tissue engineering process [12]. The scarcity of knowledge about BP is also due to the lack of high-evidence level literature about the topic. For this reason the Italian Chapter of the European Hernia Society has founded the Italian Register of Biological Prosthesis (IRBP) to archive and study the BP use in Italy. A similar registry associated with the European Hernia Society, the European Register of Biological Prosthesis (ERBP), is currently recruiting cases all over Europe [3].

To give an answer to the many different questions about the BP use in abdominal surgery we promoted a meeting of the Italian Biological Prosthesis Work-Group (IBPWG) constituted by surgeons with a wide experience in abdominal surgery either in elective or in emergency setting and in the use of BP. The purpose of the summit was mainly to give a few simple and reproducible indications about the correct use of BP in abdominal wall surgery keeping into consideration the two main challenges: the infected fields and the loss of tissue.

Material and methods

In February 2012, the IBPWG met in Bergamo (Italy) for 1-day summit with the aim to elaborate a decisional model on BP use in abdominal surgery. The group is constituted by general surgeons, all with extensive experience in abdominal wall surgery either in elective or in emergency setting, added to a wide experience in the use of BP (at the time of the meeting the participants had collectively implanted 284 BP).

Results

A diagram to simplify the decisional process in using BP has been elaborated (Figures 1, 2). It keeps into consideration the different kind of BP, the infection of the surgical field and the tissue loss.

The diagram suggests the type of BP that should be used by combining these three variables together on the basis of scientific literature and expert opinions.

Discussion

Complex abdominal hernia repair represents a significant challenge for surgeons. Complex hernia could be differently defined. The complexity of hernias could derive from contamination/infection, tissue loss, dimensions, anatomic position and clinical or pharmacological data.

For sure the introduction of tension-free techniques, thanks to the use of prosthetic materials, has greatly facilitated the duty. On one hand prosthetic techniques have been demonstrated to reduce the recurrence rate, on the other hand they introduced a series of new variables to take into consideration when repairing abdominal wall defects: actually prosthetic infection, dislocation, chronic pain, shrinkage, adhesions formation, fistula formation and skin erosion complicate the decision process in abdominal wall repair surgery. With the introduction of resorbable materials some of these factors have been eliminated with an increased recurrence rate as a counterpart. BP has completely changed the way to face the abdominal hernia surgery. They introduced the tissue engineering in field of the surgical practice [12]. The implant of biologic materials elicits a cascade of events leading to new healthy tissue deposition and prosthesis remodeling. It also allows to blood, growth and pro-/anti-inflammatory factors and drugs to reach the surgical field during the first phases of healing process. This for sure enhances the effect against potential or definite contamination/infection. Moreover the adhesiogenic power of BP is absolutely lower than the one of the other synthetic materials [13,14]. On the contrary there are a few doubts about the intra-peritoneal use of BP from the biomechanical point of view. It has been demonstrated that the best integration is reached if they are placed pre-peritoneally with a greater incorporation strength, less adhesion area and lower adhesion scores compared with intra-peritoneal placement [15]. Given that the long-term persistence of the prosthesis is crucial, some authors stated that the BP durability has a direct impact on the recurrence rate [16]. However durability depends on the implant intrinsic properties and also on the environment into which the BP are placed [16]. It has been demonstrated in animal models as the tensile strength is different between cross-linked and non-cross-linked meshes during the first months after the implant. However it reaches similar values after 12 months with the two kind of implants [8]. Moreover the strength of the repair sites doesn't change over time. This might indicate that new tissue is deposited in the repair site as the scaffold is degraded, preventing the site from weakening over time [8]. Another factor that should be kept into account in choosing which kind of BP to use is the demonstration that non-cross-linked material exhibits more favourable remodeling characteristics [8]. This has a great importance when BP are used as bridging or alternatively as

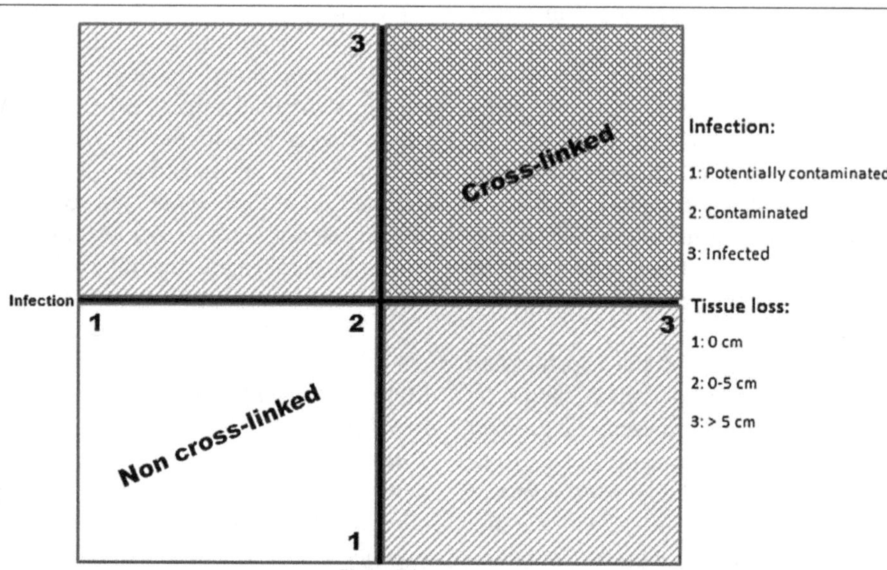

Figure 1 Decisional model diagram: the product of the infection and the loss of tissue scores gives as a result the value which indicate the kind of biological prosthesis to use.

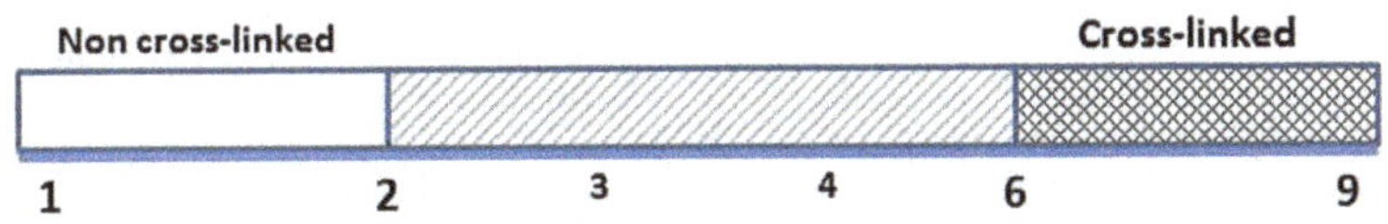

Figure 2 Decisional line: the different results indicate the kind of biological prosthesis to use.

reinforcement. In fact discordant data have been published about the use of BP to bridge wide defects [16]. Few different non-randomized studies have been published reporting recurrence rate ranging between 100% and 0% if the prosthesis are placed respectively either as a bridge or not [16-19]. Even if high-quality comparative data about BP exist in animal models, only clinical reports of a restricted number of cases are reported for humans. Moreover only the recurrence rate is registered as outcome in almost all studies. Other data regarding the use of BP as wound classification, contamination risk/grade, associated therapy or comorbidity are seldom reported. These data are needed to completely assess the usefulness, the efficacy and the versatility of BP. All reported data derived by retrospective uncontrolled series of limited number of patients. The methodology is seldom reported and/or poorly described. Moreover the time to recurrence is rarely evaluated [16]. One last observation is that the different studies reported data about non-homogeneous cohorts of patients. Different surgical techniques, different surgeons' skill and expertise in using BP and different hernia sites are often mixed together. These inconsistencies are probably due to the poorness of cases for each single centre. No definitive evidence based conclusions could be obtained from the literature. The majority of surgeons stated that they use BP in "difficult" situations, especially those with contaminated or infected field [16,20,21].

The present decisional model suggests, at the best of our knowledge, the way to apply scientific knowledge to the clinical practice in order to choose which type of BP use in abdominal wall defects repair. This should always be a dynamic process mediated by the surgeon decisional capability. We resumed the principal variables to keep in mind in deciding the kind of BP to use. Infection has been divided into three possible grades:

- 1: potentially contaminated
- 2: contaminated
- 3: infected

The same three steps division has been adopted for the tissue loss:

- 1: no tissue loss (only reinforcement)
- 2: 0–5 cm defect
- 3: >5 cm defect

By combining together these variables (multiplication) we obtained a score which determine the necessity to use either a cross-linked or a non-cross-linked BP (Figures 1, 2).

Operating field has been divided into three groups. In a previous grading system by the Ventral Hernia Working Group (VEWG) the four grade of risk for surgical site occurrences have been differentiated by considering also the comorbidity of the patients [5]. Clinical conditions are to be kept in mind in evaluating the use of prosthesis but in the present decisional model the principal aim is to help the surgeon to decide whether use cross-linked or non-cross-linked BP.

Undefined situations still exist. Cases with a score between 2 and 6 represent all that patients with a big tissue loss and a potential/low grade infection or vice-versa cases with an high grade infection and a low or null tissue loss. These cases need a cautious evaluation by the surgeon to establish if the priority has to be given to the tissue loss or to the grade of infection. The VEWG score could help in deciding. Infected fields with no residual loss of tissue don't represent an absolute indication for BP use. On the contrary a small tissue loss with concomitant low/null infection but high comorbidity could suggest using a non-cross-linked BP. The higher resistance to protease enzyme action and to mechanical stress of cross-linked BP suggest using them in situation of high infection and/or big defects. As counterpart, however even in presence of a high grade infection with a low grade tissue loss could be suggested to place a non-cross-linked BP.

Conclusion

The present score represents the first combination of scientific knowledge and clinical expertise that gives some indications about the kind of BP to use. However no definitive recommendations could be given in complicated abdominal wall reconstructive surgery. The lack of definitive evidence-based data and the high costs of the BP suggest to cautiously evaluate each single case.

Competing interests
All authors declare no conflict of interest.

Authors' contributions
All authors participated to the meeting in Bergamo in order to elaborate the decisional model on biological prosthesis use in abdominal surgery, proposed in this article. FeCo and LA drafted the manuscript All authors read and approved the final manuscript.

Author details
[1]General and Emergency Surgery Department, Ospedali Riuniti, Bergamo, Italy. [2]General Surgery Department, Adria Hospital, Rovigo, Italy. [3]General Surgery Department, Cotugno Hospital-CTO, Naples, Italy. [4]General and Emergency Surgery Department, Ospedale Maggiore, Parma, Italy. [5]General Surgery Department, Ospedale Centrale, Bolzano, Italy. [6]General Surgery Department, La Sapienza Univesity Hospital, Rome, Italy. [7]General Surgery Department, New Sant'Agostino Hospital, Modena, Italy. [8]General Surgery Department, Conegliano Hospital, Treviso, Italy. [9]General Surgery Department, Macerata Hospital, Macerata, Italy. [10]Endocrine, Digestive and Emergency Surgery Department, Aldo Moro University Hospital, Bari, Italy.

References

1. Rutkow IM: **Surgical procedure in the United States. Then (1983) and now (1994).** *Arch Surg* 1997, **132**(9):983–990.
2. Engelsman AF, van der Mei H, Ploeg RJ, Busscher HJ: **The phenomenon of infection in abdominal wall reconstruction.** *Biomaterials* 2007, **28**(14):2314–2327.
3. Ansaloni L, Catena F, Coccolini F, Negro P, Campanelli G, Miserez M: **New "biological" meshes: the need for a register, The EHS Registry for Biological Prostheses: call for participating European surgeons.** *Hernia* 2009, **13**(1):103–108.
4. Uscher FC: **Hernia repair with marlex mesh. An analysis of 514 cases.** *Arch Surg* 1962, **84**:325–328.
5. Breuing K, Butler CE, Ferzoco S, Franz M, Hultman CS, Kilbridge JF, Rosen M, Silverman RP, Vargo D: **Incisional ventral hernias: review of the literature and recommendations regarding the grading and technique of repair.** *Surgery* 2010, **148**(3):544–558.
6. Smart NJ, Bloor S: **Durability of biologic implants for use in hernia repair: a review.** *Surg Innov* 2012, **19**(3):221–229.
7. Ansaloni L, Catena F, Coccolini F, Fini M, Gazzotti F, Giardino R, Pinna AD: **Peritoneal adhesions to prosthetic materials: an experimental comparative study of treated and untreated polypropylene meshes placed in the abdominal cavity.** *J Laparoendosc Adv Surg Tech A* 2009, **19**(3):369–374.
8. Deeken CR, Melman L, Jenkins ED, Greco SC, Frisella MM, Matthews BD: **Histologic and biomechanical evaluation of crosslinked and non-crosslinked biologic meshes in a porcine model of ventral incisional hernia repair.** *J Am Coll Surg* 2011, **212**(5):880–888.
9. Catena F, Ansaloni L, D'Alessandro L, Pinna A: **Adverse effects of porcine small intestine submucosa (SIS) implants in experimental ventral hernia repair.** *Surg Endosc* 2007, **21**(4):690.
10. Ansaloni L, Catena F, Coccolini F, Gazzotti F, D'Alessandro L, Pinna AD: **Inguinal hernia repair with porcine small intestine submucosa: 3-year follow-up results of a randomized controlled trial of Lichtenstein's repair with polypropylene mesh versus Surgisis Inguinal Hernia Matrix.** *Am J Surg* 2009, **198**(3):303–312.
11. de Castro Brás LE, Shurey S, Sibbons PD: **Evaluation of crosslinked and non-crosslinked biologic prostheses for abdominal hernia repair.** *Hernia* 2012, **16**(1):77–89.
12. Sipe JD: **Tissue engineering and reparative medicine.** *Ann N Y Acad Sci* 2002, **961**:1–9.
13. Burns NK, Jaffari MV, Rios CN, Mathur AB, Butler CE: **Noncross- linked porcine acellular dermal matrices for abdominal wall reconstruction.** *Plast Reconstr Surg* 2010, **125**(1):167–176.
14. Kaleya RN: **Evaluation of implant/host tissue interactions following intraperitoneal implantation of porcine dermal collagen prosthesis in the rat.** *Hernia* 2005, **9**(3):269–276.
15. Jenkins E, Melman L, Deeken CR, Greco SC, Frisella MM RN, Matthews BD: **Biomechanical and histologic evaluation of fenestrated and nonfenestrated biologic mesh in a porcine model of ventral hernia repair.** *J Am Coll Surg* 2011, **212**:327–339.
16. Smart NJ, Marshall M, Daniels IR: **Biological meshes: a review of their use in abdominal wall hernia repairs.** *Surgeon* 2012, **10**(3):159–171.
17. Alaedeen DI, Lipman J, Medalie D, Rosen MJ: **The single staged approach to the surgical management of abdominal wall hernias in contaminated fields.** *Hernia* 2007, **11**(1):41–45.
18. Jin J, Rosen MJ, Blatnik J, McGee MF, Williams CP, Marks J, Ponsky J: **Use of acellular dermal matrix for complicated ventral hernia repair: does technique affect outcomes?** *J Am Coll Surg* 2007, **205**(5):654–660.
19. Candage R, Jones K, Luchette FA, Sinacore JM, Vandevender D, Reed RL 2nd: **Use of human acellular dermal matrix for hernia repair: friend or foe?** *Surgery* 2008, **144**(4):703–709.
20. Butler CE: **The role of bioprosthetics in abdominal wall reconstruction.** *Clin Plast Surg* 2006, **33**(2):199–211.
21. Ferrara R, Imperiale S, Polato R, Frena A, Martin F: **Impianto di protesi biologica di collagene di derma porcino per laparocele complesso: caso clinico.** *Osp Ital Chir* 2008, **14**(4):451–454.

11

A case of a traumatic chyle leak following an acute thoracic spine injury: successful resolution with strict dietary manipulation

Andrea M Pakula[1*†], Wendy Phillips[2†] and Ruby A Skinner[1†]

Abstract

Background: Chylothorax is a rare form of pleural effusion that can be associated with both traumatic and non-traumatic causes. Thoracic duct ligation is often the treatment of choice in postsurgical patients; however the optimal treatment of this disease process after traumatic injury remains unclear [1]. We present a rare case of a thoracic duct injury secondary to a blunt thoracic spine fracture and subluxation which was successfully treated non-operatively.

Case Presentation: A 51 year old male presented as a tier one trauma code due to an automobile versus bicycle collision. His examination and radiographic work-up revealed fractures and a subluxation at the third and fourth thoracic spine levels resulting in paraplegia. He also sustained bilateral hemothoraces secondary to multiple rib fractures. Drainage of the left hemothorax led to the diagnosis of a traumatic chylothorax. The thoracic spine fractures were addressed with surgical stabilization and the chylothorax was successfully treated with drainage and dietary manipulation.

Conclusions: This unusual and complex blunt thoracic duct injury required a multidisciplinary approach. Although the spine injury required surgical fixation, successful resolution of the chyle leak was achieved without surgical intervention.

Introduction

The majority of reported cases of chylothorax are due to malignancy (50%) specifically non-Hodgkin's lymphoma. Chylothorax due to traumatic thoracic injuries including iatrogenic post surgical injuries comprise approximately twenty-five percent of cases. Other iatrogenic complications primarily related to central access catheters make up the remaining twenty-five percent [2,3]. This disease process, if not properly recognized and treated can lead to profound respiratory, nutritional and immunological dysfunction resulting in significant patient morbidity and mortality. The available treatment modalities include conservative management with drainage and strict dietary regulation or more invasive approaches namely thoracic duct ligation [4,5].

* Correspondence: APakula333@aol.com
† Contributed equally
[1]Department of Surgery, Division of Trauma and Surgical Critical Care, Kern Medical Center, Bakersfield, California
Full list of author information is available at the end of the article

Case Presentation

The patient is a 51 year old male who was struck by an automobile at 35 miles per hour while riding a bicycle. There was loss of consciousness in the field and he arrived to our level II trauma center in full spine precautions, as a tier one trauma code. His primary survey was intact and his initial vital signs were; BP 115/80, HR 84, RR 30, O2 saturation 89% on room air which improved to 98% on a non-rebreather mask at 100%. Pertinent findings on secondary survey revealed bilateral chest wall tenderness to palpation, diminished breath sounds bilaterally, upper thoracic spine tenderness to palpation, a complete loss of motor function in his lower extremities, a loss of sensory function below the level of T4 and a Glascow Coma Scale (GCS) of 15. His American Spine Injury Association Motor Score was 50. He also had a loss of his cremasteric reflex, and bulbar cavernous reflex, and had no sacral tone.

While observing strict spine precautions, the patient had chest and pelvis x-rays taken, and was then transported for computed tomography scans of the head, cervical spine and torso. Positive findings from these studies revealed multiple bilateral rib fractures with associated hemothoraces (Figure 1). He also sustained fractures and subluxation at the third and fourth thoracic levels (Figure 2). The patient was started on spinal dose steroids and strict spine precautions were maintained for anticipated surgical stabilization. Bilateral chest tube thoracostomies were placed for the hemothoraces and a arterial blood gas was then obtained which documented adequate oxygenation and ventilation given this patient's significant pulmonary injury; (pH 7.33 pCO_2 42 PaO2 91 HCO3 21, O_2 saturation 97 BD-4, 2 liters nasal cannula).

The initial drainage from the left chest tube was 500 milliliters (ml) of blood and on his second hospital day it was noted that the chest tube output was 400 ml of milky white fluid suspicious for chyle. Biochemical analysis of the pleural fluid revealed triglycerides of 287 milligrams/decilitre (mg/dL), total protein of 2600 mg/dL, and LDH of 2823 units/L. These results confirmed a diagnosis of chylothorax.

Due to the complexity of the case, a multidisciplinary team approach was taken to develop the appropriate treatment regimen for this patient. The decision to attempt treatment of the chyle leak with dietary manipulation was agreed upon and the patient was started on a very-low-fat oral diet consisting of mainly fresh fruits, vegetables and whole grains. The patient was also given a semi-elemental formula, Peptamen AF, 1 can with each meal which provided additional kilocalories, protein, and medium chain triglyceride (MCT) oil in order to facilitate wound healing. Two scoops of protein powder (beneprotein) were added to each meal as well. The patient was also started on octreotide, 200 mcg subcutaneous every 8 hours to aid in the reduction of lymph production.

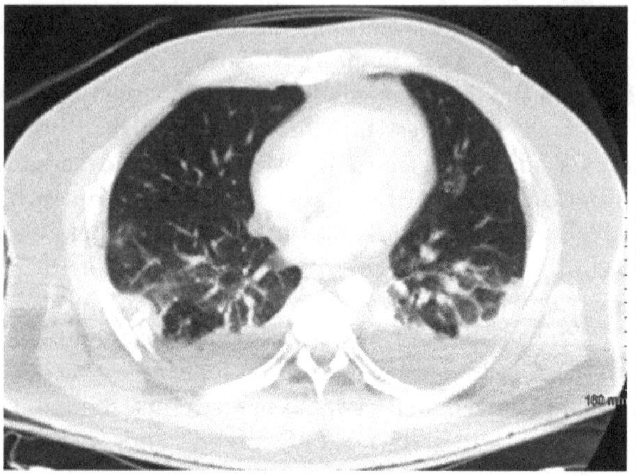

Figure 1 CT scan of the chest illustrates bilateral pleural effusions.

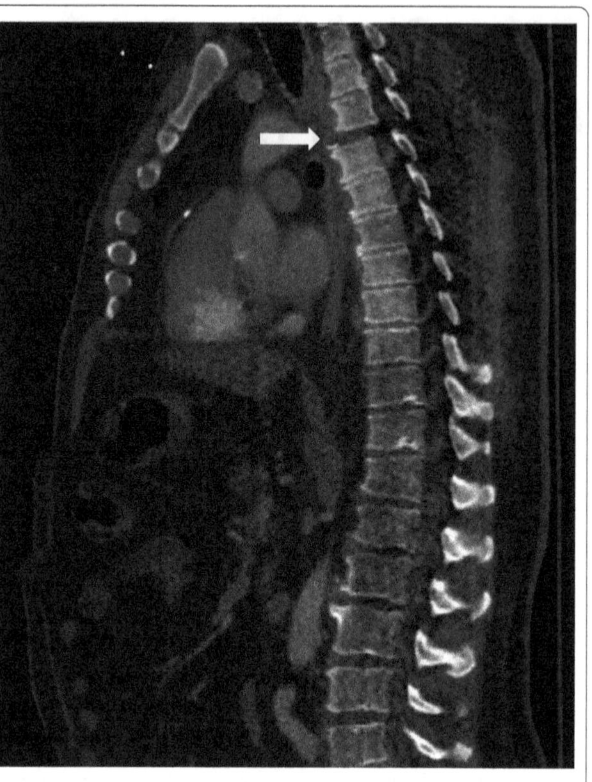

Figure 2 Lateral CT scan of thoracic spine demonstrates T3/4 fracture dislocation (white arrow).

The patient tolerated the diet well and these measures led to a dramatic decrease in the chest tube output to less than 100 ml/day of serous fluid by the time he had operative repair and stabilization of his thoracic spine on hospital day seven. After the surgical procedure there was a transient increase in output from the chest tube to 200 ml per day which declined to 35 ml on hospital day 14. The chest tube was then removed without consequence, he was then started on a regular diet and follow up chest x-rays did not reveal any recurrent pleural effusions. The patient was discharged to an inpatient rehabilitation facility and was seen approximately two months after his injury in our clinic. He still had complete motor paralysis of the lower extremities with a T2 sensory loss. His upper extremity function remained unchanged from admission with his motor function intact. His pulmonary status remained stable as he had no ongoing acute pulmonary issues and saturated 98-100% on room air.

Discussion

Chylous pleural effusion is most commonly caused by malignancy, accounting for more than 50% of cases. Lymphoma is the most common malignant cause, representing about 60% of all cases, with the non-Hodgkins variant being the most prevalent. Traumatic injuries to the upper abdomen and chest including those sustained during surgery are the second leading cause of chylothorax, accounting for approximately 25% of cases.

The first traumatic injury to the thoracic duct was described in 1875 and the first thoracic duct ligation was performed in 1948 [6]. The traumatic causes of injury to the duct vary widely, and the most common blunt mechanism producing injury is related to sudden hyperextension of the spine with rupture of the duct just above the diaphragm [4,7-9]. Sudden stretching over the vertebral bodies for any reason may tear the duct, but this usually occurs in the setting of a thoracic duct previously affected by disease [4,8]. Episodes of vomiting or a violent bout of coughing resulting in shearing of the lymphatic conduit along the crux of the right diaphragm has been reported as well [9]. Penetrating injuries, from a gunshot or stab wound, are less common and usually associated with severe damage to nearby structures.

The pertinent anatomy involved in the development of a chylothorax begins with the cysterna chyli, which is a confluence of lymphatics located in the retroperitoneum, just to the right of the posteromedial aorta at the level of the renal arteries. The thoracic duct ascends from this level and enters the chest through the aortic hiatus into the right hemithorax. The duct crosses over to the left chest at the fourth and fifth thoracic levels and enters the neck anterior to the left subclavian artery to join the venous system at the junction of the left subclavian vein and left internal jugular vein [10,11,13]. Knowledge of this anatomy should alert the physician to the possibility of a thoracic duct injury with thoracic spine fractures or any associated upper abdomen or chest injury involving this trajectory.

As in this case, the diagnosis of a chyle leak was supported by a pleural fluid triglyceride level greater than 110 mg/dL. A pleural fluid triglyceride concentration less than 50 mg/dL excludes a chylothorax. An intermediate level between 50 and 110 mg/dL should be followed by lipoprotein analysis to inspect the pleural fluid for chylomicrons or cholesterol crystals. The presence of chylomicrons and the absence of cholesterol crystals confirm a chyle leak. In addition, a ratio of pleural fluid cholesterol to triglyceride of less than 1 is also diagnostic [11,12].

Although most cases of traumatic chylothorax can be managed non-operatively, the need for surgical intervention in the subset of patients with associated thoracic fractures is higher and approaches 50 percent [5,11]. Indications for surgical intervention include an excessive leak for greater than five days, which for adults is > 500 ml/day and for children > 10 ml/kg/day or > 100 ml/day for each year of age. Any volume of output for greater than 14 days would indicate failure of conservative therapy and the need for surgical intervention as well [10].

Conservative treatment of chylothorax begins with prompt drainage via tube thoracostomy and dietary manipulation. The goal of dietary manipulation is to dramatically decrease lymph production since sixty percent of the dietary fat is absorbed by the lymphatic system, and approximately 1500 to 2000 ml of lymph is produced daily. This can be accomplished by completely bypassing the lymphatic circulation with Total Parenteral Nutrition (TPN), or by strict dietary manipulation based on a very low fat diet. We chose the latter to avoid some of the known infectious complications associated with TPN, especially in this high risk patient with multi-system trauma. With either approach, volume status, electrolyte abnormalities and nutritional parameters of the patient should be followed closely and aggressive replacement of nutritional losses of fat soluble vitamins and proteins should be carried out [10,14,15].

A diet strategy to limit chyle production involves avoidance of long chain triglycerides (LCTs). Medium chain triglycerides (MCTs), however, are absorbed directly into the portal circulation without stimulating lymphatic flow, so inclusion of these MCTs in the diet can help to increase caloric intake for healing [11]. These dietary changes as in our case were accomplished by a strict low fat diet supplemented with extra protein powder and MCT oil. Elemental peptide-based enteric formulas with less than 3% LCTs and MCTs added are also ideal supplements, as they have been shown to reduce the quantity and duration of chyle output. Though there is no consensus on the definitive duration of this nutritional management, the literature supports that these dietary measures be continued for approximately two weeks [10-12]. In general, once the chyle leak is resolved, then a regular diet may be resumed. In complicated cases, however, it may be advisable to ensure leak resolution with a provocative high-fat meal before removing a drainage tube.

Finally, there are anecdotal data supporting the use of octreotide to promote decreased lymphatic production. The mechanism is based on the reduction of gastrointestinal secretions and sphlancnic blood flow associated with octreotide, thus decreasing lymphatic production. The drug can be given as a continuous infusion or bolus injections [16,17].

Conclusions

Although rare, traumatic chylothorax can be a difficult entity to manage especially in a patient with additional traumatic injuries. This case reflects a successful approach to the management of a traumatic chyle leak, using drainage and strict dietary changes, which precluded the need for surgical intervention.

Consent

Written informed consent was obtained from the patient for publication of this case report and accompanying images. A copy of the written consent is available for review by the Editor-in-Chief of this journal.

Author details
[1]Department of Surgery, Division of Trauma and Surgical Critical Care, Kern Medical Center, Bakersfield, California. [2]Department of Nutrition and Dietary Services, Kern Medical Center, Bakersfield, California.

Authors' contributions
All authors contributed to researching, editing and writing the article. All authors read and approved the final manuscript.

Competing interests
The authors declare that they have no competing interests.

References

1. Maldonado F: **Medical and surgical management of chylothorax and associated outcomes.** *Am J Med Sci* 2010, **339(4)**:314-318.
2. Doerr CH, Allen MS, Nichols FC, Ryu JH: **Etiology of Chylothorax in 203 patients.** *Mayo Clinic Proc* 2005, **80(7)**:867-870.
3. Fogli L, Gorini P, Belcastro S: **Conservative management of traumatic chylothorax: a case report.** *Intens Care Med* 1993, **19(3)**:176-177.
4. Valentine V, Raffin T: **The management of chylothorax.** *Chest* 1992, **102**:586-591.
5. Paul S: **Surgical management of chylothorax.** *Thorac Cardiovasc Surg* 2009, **57(4)**:226-228.
6. Browse NL, Allen DR, Wilson NM: **Management of chylothorax.** *Br J Surg* 1997, **84(12)**:1711-1716.
7. Wright P, Gardner A: **Traumatic chylothorax: A case after dislocation of the thoracic spine.** *J Bone Joint Surg* 1952, **34B**:64-67.
8. Brook M, Dupree D: **Bilateral traumatic chylothorax.** *Bilateral traumatic chylothorax* 1988, **17**:69-72.
9. Biet AB, Connolly NK: **Traumatic chylothorax; a report of a case and a survey of literature.** *Br J Surg* 1951, **39**:564-568.
10. Spain DA: **The A.S.P.E.N. Nutrition Support Core Curriculum: A Case-Based Approach–The Adult Patient.** *American Society of Parenteral and Enteral Nutrition* 2007, 477-487.
11. Mason JF: **Chylothorax.** In *Murray and Nadel's Textbook of Respiratory Medicine.* 5 edition. Edited by: Murray JF, Nadel JA. Philadelphia: Saunders; 2010:1764-1792.
12. Staats BA, Ellefson RD, Budahn LL, Dines DE, Prakash UB, Offord UK: **The lipoprotein profile of chylous and nonchylous pleural effusions.** *Mayo Clin Proc* 1980, **55**:700-704.
13. Miller JJ: **Anatomy of the thoracic duct & chylothorax.** In *General Thoracic Surgery.* 6 edition. Edited by: Shields T, Loccicero J, Ponn R, et al. Philadelphia: Lippincott, Williams 2005:879-888.
14. Sahn SA: **Pleural effusions of extra vascular origin.** *Clin of Chest Med* 2006, 285-308.
15. Apostolakis E: **Traumatic chylothorax following blunt trauma: two conservatively treated cases.** *J Card Surg* 2009, **24(2)**:220-2.
16. Barili F: **Administration of octreotide for management of postoperative high-flow chylothorax.** *Ann Vasc Surg* 2007, **21(1)**:90-92.
17. Miura K: **Treatment of a persistent postoperative chylothorax with octreotide.** *Kyobu Geka* 2009, **62(10)**:885-887.

12

An acute care surgery service expedites the treatment of emergency colorectal cancer

Ram Venkatesh Anantha[1], Muriel Brackstone[1], Neil Parry[1,2,3] and Ken Leslie[1,4*]

Abstract

Introduction: Emergency colorectal cancer (CRC) is a complex disease that requires multidisciplinary approaches for management. However, it is unclear whether acute care surgery (ACS) services can expedite the workup and treatment of complex surgical diseases such as emergency CRC. We sought to assess the impact of an Acute Care and Emergency Surgery Service (ACCESS) on wait-times for inpatient colonoscopy and surgical resection among emergency CRC patients.

Methods: This retrospective case–control study was conducted at a tertiary-care, university-affiliated, cancer centre in London, Ontario, Canada. All patients aged 18 or older who presented to the emergency department with a recent (within 48 hours) diagnosis of CRC, or were diagnosed with CRC after admission, were included in the study. Patients were either in the pre-ACCESS (July 1, 2007-June 31, 2010) or post-ACCESS (July 1, 2010-June 30, 2012) groups. A third group of emergency CRC patients treated at an adjacent cancer centre that lacked ACCESS (non-ACCESS) was evaluated separately. The primary outcome was time from admission to colonoscopy and surgery.

Results: A total of 149 patients (47 pre-ACCESS, 37 post-ACCESS, and 65 non-ACCESS) were identified. Only 19% (n = 9) of pre-ACCESS patients underwent inpatient colonoscopy, compared to 38% (n = 14) in the post-ACCESS group (p = 0.023). Additionally, 100% of patients in the post-ACCESS era underwent inpatient colonoscopy and surgery during the same admission, compared to only 44% of pre-ACCESS patients (p = 0.006). Median wait-times for inpatient colonoscopy (2.0 and 1.8 days for pre- and post-ACCESS groups respectively, p = 0.08) and surgical resection (1.6 and 2.3 days for pre- and post-ACCESS groups respectively, p = 0.40) were similar.

Conclusions: Patients admitted to ACCESS underwent more inpatient colonoscopies and were more likely to have definitive surgery on that admission. ACS services can facilitate the workup and management of complex surgical diseases such as emergency CRC without delaying treatment.

Keywords: Colorectal/anal neoplasia, Colonoscopy, Acute care surgery, Health outcomes

Introduction

Colorectal cancer (CRC) is the third most commonly diagnosed cancer in the world, and one of the leading causes of cancer-related mortality [1]. Approximately fifteen to thirty percent of CRCs present as a surgical emergency, with the most common causes being obstruction, perforation, or bleeding [2,3]. Patients with emergency CRC may also present with metabolic, cardiovascular, infectious, or respiratory emergencies that significantly increase mortality [4]. Emergency surgery for CRC has been associated with poorer outcomes compared to elective surgery [2,3,5,6], and the increased morbidity and mortality of emergency CRC surgery places a significant clinical and financial burden on the hospital and the healthcare system [7-9].

Limitations in operating room (OR) resources may also hinder the expedited delivery of care for emergency patients [10,11]. Traditionally, on-call surgeons would either cancel their elective caseload to accommodate emergency surgeries, or delay operating on the emergency patient

* Correspondence: ken.leslie@lhsc.on.ca
[1]Division of General Surgery, Department of Surgery, Schulich School of Medicine and Dentistry, Western University, London, Ontario, Canada
[4]London Health Sciences Centre, Victoria Hospital, Room E2-217, 800 Commissioners Road East, London, Ontario N6A 5 W9, Canada
Full list of author information is available at the end of the article

until they had elective OR time [12-14]. To mitigate this issue, acute care surgery (ACS) services have been widely adopted as a cost-effective model for delivering emergency surgical care [12-14]. ACS teams provide around-the-clock coverage to manage patients with all types of general surgical emergencies [14]. They have been shown to significantly reduce wait-times for urgent and emergent operations [15-18], expedite the efficient disposition of patients from the emergency room [15-18], and reduce hospital costs [11,16] without compromising patient care or safety [19].

However, the management of diseases which are commonly encountered by ACS services do not usually require long-term surveillance for disease recurrence [16,20]. The acute care of emergency CRC patients therefore presents a relatively more complex challenge as it requires the coordination of multiple specialties, including gastroenterologists, surgeons, and oncologists (medical and/or radiation) [2,3,5,8]. While ACS services in the United States are typically staffed by subspecialty trauma and acute care surgeons [19,20], many Canadian ACS teams are run by surgeons who also routinely perform cancer operations as part of their elective practices [14,21]. We, therefore, sought to assess whether the implementation of the Acute Care and Emergency Surgery Service (ACCESS) at our institution would expedite the surgical treatment of emergency CRC patients. Rather than assess the surgical management of emergency CRC *per se*, we elected to focus our study on the delivery of care for these patients.

Methods

Ethics approval for this study was obtained through the Western University Research and Ethics Board (REB Number 102988). This study was conducted at the London Health Sciences Centre (LHSC), a tertiary-care hospital system with two university-affiliated institutions serving a metropolitan population of approximately 450,000. Additionally, the two centres receive referrals from 33 regional hospitals from 7 counties, covering a catchment area of 3 million [22]. Both hospitals within LHSC perform a high volume of colorectal cancer surgeries: University Hospital (UH), which lacks an ACS service (non-ACCESS), and Victoria Hospital (VH), where ACCESS was implemented in July 2010. The two sites function relatively independently, with no crossover of surgical consultants or gastroenterologists. At VH, all surgeons who participate in ACCESS also perform colorectal cancer operations as part of their elective practices.

We retrospectively reviewed adult (over 18 years old) patients who were admitted to LHSC after presenting to the Emergency Room (ER), and diagnosed with CRC. We compared patients whose care took place at VH between July 1, 2007 and June 30, 2010 (pre-ACCESS), and from July 1, 2010 to June 30, 2012 (post-ACCESS) as well as those treated at UH (non- ACCESS) from July 1, 2007 to June 30, 2012. The patients' primary presenting complaints, reasons for admission, time to inpatient colonoscopy, and time to operative treatment were recorded. We assessed wait-times for inpatient endoscopy services (which are performed by gastroenterologists in both hospitals at LHSC) as a surrogate for examining the coordination of multiple specialties in the care of emergency CRC. We also reviewed characteristics of the malignancy such as the stage and tumour location, as well as patient outcomes, including disease-free and overall survival. Patients who underwent urgent diagnostic colonoscopy because of symptoms that suggested the presence of colon cancer (rectal bleeding, symptoms of obstruction, anemia, and weight loss) were considered to have had an inpatient colonoscopy if they were admitted for treatment within 48 hours of their colonoscopy. If patients were admitted to hospital more than 48 hours after their colonoscopy, they were considered to have had an outpatient colonoscopy. Because many of these patients had their colonoscopy at peripheral hospitals, or private endoscopy clinics outside of LHSC, we were unable to accurately ascertain the timing of their outpatient colonoscopy.

We excluded appendiceal neoplasms, carcinoid tumours, and goblet cell cancers since their management differs from the treatment of adenocarcinoma. We also excluded patients who had a previous history of CRC or inflammatory bowel disease as they undergo surveillance colonoscopy more frequently than the general population [23]. We also excluded patients who underwent colonic stenting, because of a lack of data pertaining to the placement of stents during the study period, and because of a lack of consensus regarding the use of stents in emergency CRC patients who are otherwise amenable to surgery [24,25].

Statistical analysis was performed using Graphpad Prism (Graphpad, La Jolla, California). Survival curves were compared by the Kaplan-Meier method. Continuous variables were compared between groups by Kruskal-Wallis one-way ANOVA with post hoc comparison between pre- and post-ACCESS groups by Dunn's test [26]. Discontinuous variables were compared using Pearson chi-squared test. P values less than 0.05 were considered statistically significant.

Results

We identified a total of 149 patients in our study: 47 (32%) were treated in the pre-ACCESS era; 37 (25%) patients were treated in the post-ACCESS era; and 65 (44%) patients were treated in the non-ACCESS hospital. There were no differences in the distribution of symptoms that led patients to present to the Emergency Department ($p = 0.98$): pain (70% of patients), altered bowel habits (54% of patients), and symptoms of obstruction (50% of patients) were the most frequently reported reasons for presenting to the emergency department (Table 1). Twenty two percent of patients (34 patients) presented with overt bleeding.

Seventy eight patients (52%) underwent colonoscopy: 31 patients (48%) were in the non-ACCESS group; 28 patients (60%) were in the pre-ACCESS group; and 19 patients (51%) were in the post-ACCESS group (Table 1). There were no statistical differences between the three groups for symptoms necessitating colonoscopy (p = 0.91), location of the malignancy (p = 0.49), or pathological stage (Table 1; p = 0.15). However, we observed a significant difference in the distribution of inpatient and outpatient colonoscopies between the pre- and post-ACCESS groups. In the pre-ACCESS group, 9 patients (19%) had an inpatient colonoscopy while 19 patients (40%) had an outpatient colonoscopy; in contrast, 14 post-ACCESS patients (38%) had an inpatient colonoscopy compared to only 5 patients (14%) who had an outpatient colonoscopy (p = 0.02).

We also observed a significant difference between the pre- and post-ACCESS groups with respect to the timing of surgical treatment following inpatient colonoscopy (Table 2). In the pre-ACCESS group, five out of 9 patients undergoing inpatient colonoscopy (56%) were discharged and underwent surgery during a separate admission: three patients were diagnosed with CRC after an admission for rectal bleeding, stabilized with blood transfusions, and underwent elective surgery within a week of being discharged from their initial admission, due to a lack of emergency OR time. Two additional patients were discharged following inpatient colonoscopy, and underwent coronary angiograms for optimization of their cardiovascular status and reduction of their perioperative morbidity.

Table 1 Comparison of clinical characteristics among non-ACCESS, pre-ACCESS, and post-ACCESS groups at LHSC

Clinical characteristics	Non-ACCESS	Pre-ACCESS	Post-ACCESS	P value
Number of patients, n	65	47	37	-
Reason for presentation to hospital, n(%):				0.98
Change in bowel movements	40 (62)	26 (55)	14 (38)	
Rectal Bleeding	15 (23)	12 (26)	7 (19)	
Anemia	14 (22)	7 (15)	8 (22)	
Obstruction	37 (57)	22 (47)	15 (41)	
Pain	49 (75)	33 (70)	23 (62)	
Colonoscopy, n(%):				0.02
Prior outpatient colonoscopy	15 (23)	19 (40)	5 (14)	
Inpatient colonoscopy	16 (25)	9 (19)	14 (38)	
Indications for colonoscopy, n(%):				0.91
Change in bowel movements	15 (23)	5 (11)	15 (40)	
Rectal bleeding	13 (20)	7 (15)	11 (30)	
Anemia	14 (22)	6 (13)	7 (19)	
Obstruction	9 (14)	4 (8)	11 (30)	
Pain	17 (26)	9 (19)	15 (40)	
Location of malignancy, n(%):				0.49
Rectal	6 (9)	7 (15)	1 (3)	
Sigmoid and rectosigmoid	15 (23)	17 (36)	11 (30)	
Descending	6 (9)	4 (8)	3 (8)	
Transverse	7 (11)	4 (8)	3 (8)	
Ascending	31 (48)	15 (32)	19 (51)	
Stage, n(%):				0.15
0/I	3 (5)	5 (11)	4 (11)	
II	25 (38)	10 (21)	18 (49)	
III	25 (38)	20 (42)	11 (30)	
IV	10 (15)	9 (19)	4 (11)	
Unknown	2 (3)	4 (8)	0 (0)	

P values are shown for comparisons between pre- and post-ACCESS groups.

Table 2 Comparison of outcomes between non-ACCESS, pre-ACCESS, and post-ACCESS groups at LHSC

Characteristics	Non-ACCESS (*n* = 65)	Pre-ACCESS (*n* = 47)	Post-ACCESS (*n* = 37)	P Value
Inpatient colonoscopy and surgery performed on same or separate admission, n(%):				0.006
Same admission	13 (20)	4 (8)	14 (38)	
Separate admission	3 (5)	5 (11)	0 (0)	
Median time from admission to inpatient colonoscopy, d (IQR[1])	3.5 (2.4-6.9)	2 (0.9-3.6)	1.8 (1.3-3.1)	0.08
Median time from colonoscopy to OR, d (IQR[1]):	3.1 (0.3-8.5)	2.8 (1.0-4.0)	2.1 (1.2-2.5)	0.34
Same admission for colonoscopy and surgery	3.0 (0.14-3.6)	1.8 (0.3-4.0)	2.1 (1.2-2.5)	0.86
Separate admissions for colonoscopy and surgery	11.1 (9.0-12)	3.6 (2.8-11)	0 (0)	0.004
Median time from admission to OR, d (IQR[1]):	2.5 (0.93-45)	1.6 (0.8-4.6)	2.3 (1.1-4.6)	0.40
Without colonoscopy	1.4 (0.8-4.2)	1.6 (0.8-4.4)	1.5 (0.7-2.8)	0.89
With colonoscopy	6.6 (4.7-11.5)	4.4 (2.7-4.8)	4.5 (3.5-5.3)	0.87
Type of operation performed, n(%):				0.96
Primary anastomosis	49 (75)	35 (74)	27 (73)	
Ostomy	16 (25)	12 (26)	10 (27)	
Median length of stay, d (IQR[1])	13.5 (8.8-19.2)	10.0 (6–17.2)	12 (8.5-18.5)	0.16
Status as of September 2012:				0.31
Disease-free	28 (43)	19 (40)	26 (70)	
Alive with disease	11 (17)	2 (5)	6 (16)	
Died of disease	18 (28)	19 (40)	3 (8)	
Died of other causes	8 (12)	7 (15)	2 (6)	

P values are shown for comparisons between pre- and post-ACCESS groups.
[1]IQR: Inter-quartile range (25%-75%).

In contrast, 100% of patients in the post-ACCESS group had their surgery during the same admission as their colonoscopy (p = 0.006). In the non-ACCESS group, three patients (19%) were discharged following inpatient colonoscopy for rectal bleeding and were operated in separate admissions within one to two weeks after their initial admission.

Median wait-times from admission to inpatient colonoscopy were similar among the three groups (Table 2). Additionally, there were no differences in median wait-times from inpatient colonoscopy to surgery, if both were performed during the same admission (p = 0.86). When the inpatient colonoscopy and surgery were performed on separate admissions, however, we observed a significant difference in wait-times between the pre- and post-ACCESS groups (3.6 and 0 days respectively, p = 0.004). We did not observe any differences in hospital stay (p = 0.16), overall survival, or disease-free survival between the three groups of patients (Table 2).

Discussion

The emergency presentation of CRC may be considered an extreme expression of the waiting time paradox where the outcomes are poor but the "waiting time" is very short [27]. Although many factors may contribute to the increased morbidity and mortality of emergency CRC patients compared to their elective counterparts [4,28-30], the presentation of these patients at night or on weekends to centres with reduced clinical services after-hours has been implicated as a potential contributor to mortality [28]. In this study, we demonstrate that an ACS service which provides around-the-clock emergency general surgery coverage expedites the in-hospital workup and treatment of emergency CRC patients within a single admission.

To date, many studies of ACS services have focussed on the delivery of care for patients presenting with acute appendicitis and cholecystitis, the two most frequently encountered diseases in acute care surgery [14-16,31]. Following an operation for these conditions, patients typically have a short hospital stay and limited outpatient follow-up. Emergency CRC therefore represents a more complex disease in the context of an ACS service, because its management requires the coordination of multiple aspects of care (diagnosis, workup, and treatment) provided by different medical and surgical specialties. Since most inpatient colonoscopies are performed by gastroenterologists at LHSC, we assessed inpatient endoscopy wait-times as a surrogate for the multidisciplinary coordination of care among emergency CRC patients. While a significant proportion of pre-ACCESS patients had received a colonoscopy as an outpatient, the implementation of ACCESS enabled a majority of emergency CRC patients to undergo inpatient colonoscopy after admission to hospital, and facilitated the performance of their surgery during the same admission. In contrast, more than half of all pre-ACCESS patients were discharged after their colonoscopy due to the lack of emergency operative time, and readmitted at a later date for elective surgery, with significantly increased wait-times as a consequence. Therefore, ACS services such as ACCESS may represent a model of high-value care [9,32], wherein the availability of dedicated ACS hospital beds and nursing staff, as well as the concentration of multiple procedures and operations within a single admission, facilitates the workup and treatment of emergency surgical patients in a timely and cost-effective manner [11,12,19,31].

Similar to other studies, 50% of patients presented with obstruction, while 22% presented with overt bleeding [6,33]. Interestingly, we did not observe the preponderance towards higher stages that previous studies have shown among patients with emergency CRC [29,30,34]. Among our population, only 15% of patients had distant metastases, compared to 25% in a retrospective study and 37% in a large prospective analysis [30,34]. Although select patients with metastatic CRC may benefit from a concurrent resection of the primary malignancy and liver metastases [35], coordination with a hepatobiliary surgeon may be challenging in emergency CRC due to time constraints. Moreover, the limited sample size in our study precludes an evaluation of outcomes, which may be resolved by a multi-centre analysis of emergency CRC patients operated by ACS services.

In our study of emergency CRC patients, 52% were diagnosed by colonoscopy, which is slightly higher than other studies [36]. Concerns about the median wait-times for inpatient endoscopy in emergency CRC patients mirror the concerns for outpatients with CRC [37]. While we observed a trend toward reduced wait-times for inpatient colonoscopy in the post-ACCESS group, future cost-benefit analyses are necessary to determine the ideal balance for allocating endoscopy resources towards outpatient and inpatient procedures within the constraints of a publicly-funded healthcare system [38].

In the absence of an ACS service with dedicated OR time, access to emergency OR resources may be affected by a multitude of factors, including competing surgical specialty access, consultant practice patterns, and the availability of anesthesiologists and other OR support staff [10,11,13,14,39]. The overall hospital length of stay was similar among the three groups, and comparable to other studies [33]. While we did not observe differences in patient outcomes, long-term follow-up of a large number of patients will be necessary to identify differences between groups. However, given that the biology of CRC tumours among emergency patients may be more aggressive and invasive compared to non-emergency or elective CRC patients [29], the expedited treatment of patients within a single admission, as demonstrated by our study, may play a role in improving clinical outcomes for emergency CRC.

As with the implementation of any new surgical service, the organization of ACCESS underwent subtle changes throughout the study period in order to optimize the utilization of operative resources. While we observed a longer, but statistically insignificant, wait-time between colonoscopy and surgery for post-ACCESS patients, a large prospective multi-centre analysis of institutions with ACS services may help identify more emergency CRC patients, determine their outcomes in and out of hospital, and highlight any potential inefficiency in the setup of ACS services with respect to wait-times for colonoscopies and surgeries.

There are several limitations in this study. Although endoscopy can be used to provide symptomatic relief for patients (including decompressing an acutely obstructed colon [40,41] or halting gastrointestinal bleeding), it was beyond the scope of our study to examine whether the colonoscopies were performed with therapeutic intent. Additionally, none of the patients in our study underwent colonic stenting. While its use as a bridge to elective surgery remains controversial in patients presenting with emergency CRC [24,25], future prospective cohort studies of all emergency CRC patients (surgical and non-surgical) are needed to assess the value of colonic stenting in this population. Additionally, we did not consider whether the surgeries were performed with curative or palliative intent, because it may not have been clearly evident at the time of the operation. Since pathology information—a necessity prior to referral to our regional cancer centre— was usually not available during the patients' hospital stay, patients would be typically sent home and provided a referral to the cancer centre by the operating surgeon's office once the pathology results were provided. Therefore, information regarding referral to adjunct services was not available for our study population.

Our study focuses on access to colonoscopic diagnosis of emergency CRC as a surrogate for multidisciplinary care. However, referral to other subspecialty services may potentially confound our analysis, especially if procedures are needed to optimize patients prior to surgery, such as placement of inferior vena cava filters (as prophylaxis to prevent pulmonary emboli), or performance of angiograms to diagnose and treat cardiovascular disease. We were also unable to obtain information regarding the number and timing of outpatient colonoscopies in our study population, because the procedures were often performed in community hospitals or private endoscopy clinics outside of our institution. This data would provide a true reflection of overall wait-times for surgical resection among emergency CRC patients, and could be addressed by a prospective analysis. While it is possible that patients who underwent colonoscopy may have presented to a peripheral facility for management of their emergency CRC (thereby underestimating estimates of the study population overall), we believe this is unlikely in most cases because these patients are typically transferred to LHSC, which serves as the regional cancer centre, for surgical management.

In conclusion, we demonstrate that the implementation of ACCESS expedites the treatment of emergency colorectal cancer patients by combining the diagnosis, workup, and surgical treatment within a single admission without delaying treatment. This study adds to the growing body of evidence that ACS programs effectively deliver surgical care, and can also potentially improve the quality of delivered care for patients who require more complex care. Although the availability of colonoscopy resources for emergency CRC patients is only one of many equally valid outcomes for CRC, our experience demonstrates that the reorganization of resources can significantly improve access to emergency colonoscopies for a vulnerable population. Future multi-centre studies examining the impact of ACS services on emergency cancer care are needed to demonstrate differences in clinical outcomes among this population.

Competing interest

The authors do not declare any actual or potential conflicts of interest.

Authors' contributions

RVA designed the study, collected the data, performed the data analysis and drafted the manuscript. NP and KL helped to design the study. MB, NP, and KL provided critical revisions of the manuscript for important intellectual content. All authors approved the final version of the manuscript.

Acknowledgements

The authors would like to thank Ms. Lisa Creasor (Health Records, London Health Sciences Centre) and Ms. Frances Whiston (Clinical Research Unit, London Regional Cancer Program, London Health Sciences Centre). RVA is supported by the Royal College of Physicians and Surgeons of Canada (RCPSC) Clinician-Investigator Program, the Canadian Institutes of Health Research (CIHR) Canada Graduate Scholarship, and the Ontario Graduate Scholarship (Ontario Ministry of Education).

Author details

[1]Division of General Surgery, Department of Surgery, Schulich School of Medicine and Dentistry, Western University, London, Ontario, Canada. [2]Division of Critical Care, Department of Medicine, Schulich School of Medicine and Dentistry, Western University, London, Ontario, Canada. [3]Trauma Program, London Health Sciences Centre, London, Ontario, Canada. [4]London Health Sciences Centre, Victoria Hospital, Room E2-217, 800 Commissioners Road East, London, Ontario N6A 5 W9, Canada.

References

1. Quinten C, Martinelli F, Coens C, Sprangers MA, Ringash J, Gotay C, Bjordal K, Greimel E, Reeve BB, Maringwa J, Ediebah DE, Zikos E, King MT, Osoba D, Taphoorn MJ, Flechtner H, Schmucker-Von Koch J, Weis J, Bottomley A: **A global analysis of multitrial data investigating quality of life and symptoms as prognostic factors for survival in different tumor sites.** *Cancer* 2013, **120**:302–311.
2. Rabeneck L, Paszat LF, Li C: **Risk factors for obstruction, perforation, or emergency admission at presentation in patients with colorectal cancer: a population-based study.** *Am J Gastroenterol* 2006, **101**:1098–1103.
3. Scott NA, Jeacock J, Kingston RD: **Risk factors in patients presenting as an emergency with colorectal cancer.** *Br J Surg* 1995, **82**:321–323.
4. Lewis MA, Hendrickson AW, Moynihan TJ: **Oncologic emergencies: Pathophysiology, presentation, diagnosis, and treatment.** *CA Cancer J Clin* 2011: Epub ahead of print.
5. McGillicuddy EA, Schuster KM, Davis KA, Longo WE: **Factors predicting morbidity and mortality in emergency colorectal procedures in elderly patients.** *Arch Surg* 2009, **144**:1157–1162.
6. McArdle CS, Hole DJ: **Emergency presentation of colorectal cancer is associated with poor 5-year survival.** *Br J Surg* 2004, **91**:605–609.
7. Kelly M, Sharp L, Dwane F, Kelleher T, Comber H: **Factors predicting hospital length-of-stay and readmission after colorectal resection: a population-based study of elective and emergency admissions.** *BMC Health Serv Res* 2012, **12**:77.
8. Shah NA, Halverson J, Madhavan S: **Burden of emergency and non-emergency colorectal cancer surgeries in West Virginia and the USA.** *J Gastrointest Cancer* 2013, **44**:46–53.
9. Stukel TA, Fisher ES, Alter DA, Guttmann A, Ko DT, Fung K, Wodchis WP, Baxter NN, Earle CC, Lee DS: **Association of hospital spending intensity with mortality and readmission rates in Ontario hospitals.** *JAMA* 2012, **307**:1037–1045.
10. Von Conrady DH: **The acute surgical unit: improving emergency care.** *ANZ J Surg* 2010, **80**:933–936.
11. Ciesla DJ, Cha JY, Smith JS 3rd, Llerena LE, Smith DJ: **Implementation of an acute care surgery service at an academic trauma center.** *Am J Surg* 2011, **202**:779–785. discussion 785–776.
12. Hameed SB: **General surgery 2.0: the emergence of acute care surgery in Canada.** *Can J Surg* 2010, **53**:79–83.
13. Ball CG: **Acute care surgery: a new strategy for the general surgery patients left behind.** *Can J Surg* 2010, **53**:84–85.
14. Anantha RVPN, Vogt KN, Jain V, Crawford S, Leslie K: **The Implementation of an Acute Care Emergency Surgical Service: A Cost Analysis from the Surgeon's Perspective.** *Can J Surg* 2014: (doi:10.1503/cjs.001213).
15. Britt RC, Weireter LJ, Britt LD: **Initial implementation of an acute care surgery model: implications for timeliness of care.** *J Am Coll Surg* 2009, **209**:421–424.
16. Cubas RF, Gomez NR, Rodriguez S, Wanis M, Sivanandam A, Garberoglio CA: **Outcomes in the management of appendicitis and cholecystitis in the setting of a new acute care surgery service model: impact on timing and cost.** *J Am Coll Surg* 2012, **215**:715–721.
17. Gandy RC, Truskett PG, Wong SW, Smith S, Bennett MH, Parasyn AD: **Outcomes of appendicectomy in an acute care surgery model.** *Med J Aust* 2010, **193**:281–284.
18. Geere SL, Aseervatham R, Grieve D: **Outcomes of appendicectomy in an acute care surgery model.** *Med J Aust* 2011, **194**:373–374.
19. Schuster KM, McGillicuddy EA, Maung AA, Kaplan LJ, Davis KA: **Can acute care surgeons perform emergency colorectal procedures with good outcomes?** *J Trauma* 2011, **71**:94–100.
20. Britt RB: **Impact of acute care surgery on biliary disease.** *J Am Coll Surg* 2010, **210**:595–599.
21. Johner AM, Merchant S, Aslani N, Planting A, Ball CG, Widder S, Pagliarello G, Parry NG, Klassen D, Hameed SM, Canadian Association of General Surgery Committee on Acute Surgery and Critical Care: **Acute general surgery in Canada: a survey of current handover practices.** *Can J Surg* 2013, **56**:E24–E28.
22. **Census Profile - Population Centre.** http://www12.statcan.gc.ca/census-recensement/2011/dp-pd/prof/details/page.cfm?Lang=E&Geo1=POPC&Code1=0480&Geo2=PR&Code2=35&Data=Count&SearchText=London&SearchType=Begins&SearchPR=01&B1=All&Custom=&TABID=1.
23. Baumgart DC, Sandborn WJ: **Inflammatory bowel disease: clinical aspects and established and evolving therapies.** *Lancet* 2007, **369**:1641–1657.
24. Sagar J: **Colorectal stents for the management of malignant colonic obstructions.** *Cochrane Database Syst Rev* 2011, **11**:CD007378.
25. van Hooft JE, Bemelman WA, Oldenburg B, Marinelli AW, Holzik MF, Grubben MJ, Sprangers MA, Dijkgraaf MG, Fockens P, Collaborative Dutch Stent-In study g: **Colonic stenting versus emergency surgery for acute left-sided malignant colonic obstruction: a multicentre randomised trial.** *Lancet Oncol* 2011, **12**:344–352.

26. Dunn OJ: **Multiple contrasts using rank sums.** *Technometrics* 1964, **5:**241–252.
27. Torring ML, Frydenberg M, Hansen RP, Olesen F, Hamilton W, Vedsted P: **Time to diagnosis and mortality in colorectal cancer: a cohort study in primary care.** *Br J Cancer* 2011, **104:**934–940.
28. McPhail S, Elliss-Brookes L, Shelton J, Ives A, Greenslade M, Vernon S, Morris EJ, Richards M: **Emergency presentation of cancer and short-term mortality.** *Br J Cancer* 2013, **109:**2027–2034.
29. Ghazi S, Berg E, Lindblom A, Lindforss U, Low-Risk Colorectal Cancer Study G: **Clinicopathological analysis of colorectal cancer: a comparison between emergency and elective surgical cases.** *World J Surg Oncol* 2013, **11:**133.
30. Wong SK, Jalaludin BB, Morgan MJ, Berthelsen AS, Morgan A, Gatenby AH, Fulham SB: **Tumor pathology and long-term survival in emergency colorectal cancer.** *Dis Colon Rectum* 2008, **51:**223–230.
31. Earley AS, Pryor JP, Kim PK, Hedrick JH, Kurichi JE, Minogue AC, Sonnad SS, Reilly PM, Schwab CW: **An acute care surgery model improves outcomes in patients with appendicitis.** *Ann Surg* 2006, **244:**498–504.
32. Porter ME: **What is value in health care?** *N Engl J Med* 2010, **363:**2477–2481.
33. Coco C, Verbo A, Manno A, Mattana C, Covino M, Pedretti G, Petito L, Rizzo G, Picciocchi A: **Impact of emergency surgery in the outcome of rectal and left colon carcinoma.** *World J Surg* 2005, **29:**1458–1464.
34. Anderson JH, Hole D, McArdle CS: **Elective versus emergency surgery for patients with colorectal cancer.** *Br J Surg* 1992, **79:**706–709.
35. Carpizo DR, Are C, Jarnagin W, Dematteo R, Fong Y, Gonen M, Blumgart L, D'Angelica M: **Liver resection for metastatic colorectal cancer in patients with concurrent extrahepatic disease: results in 127 patients treated at a single center.** *Ann Surg Oncol* 2009, **16:**2138–2146.
36. Bass G, Fleming C, Conneely J, Martin Z, Mealy K: **Emergency first presentation of colorectal cancer predicts significantly poorer outcomes: a review of 356 consecutive Irish patients.** *Dis Colon Rectum* 2009, **52:**678–684.
37. Sey MS, Gregor J, Adams P, Khanna N, Vinden C, Driman D, Chande N: **Wait times for diagnostic colonoscopy among outpatients with colorectal cancer: a comparison with Canadian Association of Gastroenterology targets.** *Can J Gastroenterol* 2012, **26:**894–896.
38. Yong E, Zenkova O, Saibil F, Cohen LB, Rhodes K, Rabeneck L: **Efficiency of an endoscopy suite in a teaching hospital: delays, prolonged procedures, and hospital waiting times.** *Gastrointest Endosc* 2006, **64:**760–764.
39. Parasyn AT: **Acute-care surgical service: a change in culture.** *ANZ J Surg* 2009, **79:**12–18.
40. Soto S, Lopez-Roses L, Gonzalez-Ramirez A, Lancho A, Santos A, Olivencia P: **Endoscopic treatment of acute colorectal obstruction with self-expandable metallic stents: experience in a community hospital.** *Surg Endosc* 2006, **20:**1072–1076.
41. Morino M, Bertello A, Garbarini A, Rozzio G, Repici A: **Malignant colonic obstruction managed by endoscopic stent decompression followed by laparoscopic resections.** *Surg Endosc* 2002, **16:**1483–1487.

13

Extra-curricular supervised training at an academic hospital: is 200 hours the threshold for medical students to perform well in an emergency room?

Phillipe Abreu-Reis[1,4*†], Guilherme Czelusniak Oliveira[1,4†], Arthur Curtarelli de Oliveira[3,4†], Hammad Sadique[5], Adonis Nasr[2,4†], Flávio Daniel Saavedra Tomasich[2,4†]

Abstract

Introduction: Due to high number of jobs in Emergency Medicine (EM) and the lack of specialist to work in this field, recent graduates work in the emergency room straight after medical school. Additional courses on EM are available through Academic Leagues. This organizations offer lectures and supervised extra-curricular practical activities in their teaching university-affiliated hospital. The objectives of the present study are to assess the influence of hours undertaken in the extra-curricular practical activities on the performance and confidence of students in carrying out the different procedures in the emergency department, and on their own perception of how well they did. Also, to assess the influence the practical activities have on student´s future choice of specialty.

Methods: A Cross-sectional study conducted by collecting data through a questionnaire. 102 eligible individuals were included and divided into two groups according to the number of extra-curricular hours performed (Group 1- up to 200 hours and Group 2- over 200 hours).

Results: Students in Group 2 (over 200 hours) had a greater number of procedures performed on all variables evaluated, in particular, initial patient care (mean 363.8 vs.136.905 in Group 1 - p = 0.001), Simple Sutures (mean of 96.2 vs 33.980 respectively) (p = 0.00003). To determine patient follow-up by the student, the number of initial patient care was correlated with number of discharge procedures performed (in Group 1, 49.6% of patients were not followed up and discharged by the same students who first talked to them in the hospital. While in Group 2, this value becomes 29.4 % - values for Group 1 - p = 0.011 and Group 2 - p = 0.117). Regarding the influence of the practical extra-curricular activities, 76.5% of the total reported that it had influenced their choice of future specialty.

Conclusions: The aptitude, confidence and skill of students are closely linked to the practice time (number of training hours served). Two hundred hours appeared to be a relatively significant time for the student to demonstrate good conduct and ability. Practical extra-curricular activities had the ability to influence the future choice of specialty, either positively or negatively.

* Correspondence: phillipeareis@gmail.com
† Contributed equally
[1]Federal University of Parana, Curitiba, Brazil
Full list of author information is available at the end of the article

Introduction

Emergency Medicine (EM) is a fascinating area to most medical students. However in developing countries like Brazil, EM is not considered a specialty. Consequently EM is taught to medical students as part of their core curriculum inside rotations, but no emergency dedicated residency training exists (like in other parts of the world), leaving gaps in medical training in these countries. Due to high number of jobs in EM and the lack of specialist to work in this field, recent graduates in developing countries sometimes work in the emergency room straight after medical school and have to either acquire knowledge by experience only or take additional courses during their graduation. Examples of additional courses in EM include the ATLS (Advanced Trauma Life Support), Trauma academic weeks, conferences and lectures. A more feasible alternative for countries like Brazil has been the formation of extra-curricular groups linked to both academic and non-academic hospitals where students are taught by qualified teachers, and thus complement their learning in specific areas such as EM [1-4]. In Brazil, these groups are known as "Academic leagues."

Academic Leagues offer lectures and supervised extra-curricular practical activities in their teaching university-affiliated hospital and form part of an overall parallel curriculum. The name Academic Leagues come from medical students creating these activities in order to acquire theoretic and practical experience [1,2]. This parallel curriculum has become essential for medical students in Brazil due to the gaps in Medical School core teaching and the amount of learning and training medical students need to be competent clinicians. Tavares et al. showed that 82.5% of medical students of a Brazilian University actively take part in the "Parallel curriculum", spending on average 8.2 hours per week [2]. Furthermore, a similar study in the Brazilian state of Alagoas demonstrated that by the third year of medical school, 98.4% of the students are involved in some form of extracurricular activity [3] and for 12.5% of them, these activities lasted for more than 12 hours per week [3].

Extra-curricular activities in non-teaching hospitals without University affiliation may influence career choices as well. A study of medical students involved in extra-curricular activities in Critical Care Medicine in the city of Salvador, Brazil, concluded that the students' in a career in Critical Care rose from 32% to 65% the establishment of an Academic League in this field [1]. Extra-curricular activities also boost good social work practice [3], providing valuable experience in dealing with death, suffering and feelings of powerlessness [4].

Some authors dispute the importance of the Academic Leagues in the training of medical students. Despite their potential benefits, these authors warn of the possible risk of premature specialization and too much practical work without being accompanied by theoretical knowledge, which can skew medical training [5].

The Hospital do Trabalhador in the city of Curitiba, Brazil, is a well-established Level I Trauma Center. It has the only emergency department in the city that utilizes an "open door system" (where the citizen can seek assistance directly) without referral by other hospitals or physicians. The Emergency Room of the Hospital do Trabalhador admitted 63,057 patients in 2010 and performed approximately 1,500 surgeries per month [6]. This public hospital is covered exclusively by the Brazilian Unified Health System (SUS). The hospital offers residency programs in general surgery and orthopedics/trauma. The hospital currently has 140 medical students in a supervised extra-curricular program. For this program, medical students are divided into teams that work according to a pre-established system of shifts. Medical students are selected for this extra-curricular program by examination. In order to be eligible for the exam, students must be in at least their fourth year and be regular students of one of the 4 medical schools in the region. The range of activities that can be undertaken in this extra-curricular program is broad and includes trauma, orthopedics and general surgery. The minimum number of hours required to complete the program is 250 hours (and the maximum allowed is 500 hours) over a maximum period of 12 months. The objective of this supervised program is to expose the student to everyday situations in trauma, teach how to diagnose and treat these diseases as well as help in decisions about their future specialty. The objectives of the present study are to assess the influence of hours undertaken in the extra-curricular practical activities on the performance and confidence of students in carrying out the different procedures in the emergency department, and on their own perception of how well they did. Also, we aim to assess the influence that the clerkship has on the student´s future choice of specialty.

Methods

A Cross-sectional study conducted by collecting data through a questionnaire developed by the research group consisting of three parts. The first part recorded general information about the student i.e. name, semester, university, etc. The second part recorded an estimated number of procedures performed routinely in surgical emergency department. The student was also asked to evaluate themselves on how confident they were, how much their previous training contributed to their ability, how helpful supervision was (by residents and the attendings) and to record a score on a scale of 0-10 for each of these fields. The third part recorded how much the clerkship influenced their future career choice by closed (yes/no) questions.

The inclusion criteria of the study were all students who were studying medicine and participated in the surgical emergency medicine clerkship of the Hospital do Trabalhador in the second half of 2011.

The exclusion criteria of the study were all students who did not attend the annual meeting or who refused to complete the questionnaire.

If one (or more) of the three sections of the questionnaire had incomplete fields, that section(s) was removed but the remaining data was still included in the statistical analysis.

The students were divided into two groups: the first contained the students with less than 200 hours on duty in the emergency room and the second group contained those that had 200 hours or more on duty. Data was tabulated in spreadsheet format and analyzed using SPSS 19 software IBM. We used the non-paired non-parametric t-test.

Data was collected during the Annual General Meeting (AGM) of students at the Hospital do Trabalhador.

Results

Of the 140 students in the emergency clerkship, 38 did not meet the inclusion criteria and were excluded, leading to a total of 102 questionnaires eligible for analysis. These 102 subjects were divided into two groups, Group 1 (with less than 200 hours of training in the clerkship = 71 students) and Group 2 (those with 200 or more hours of training in the clerkship = 31 student) and were analyzed against each other in each of the objectives mentioned above.

When comparing the number of patients: Group 2 students took care of an average 363.8 initial evaluations, whilst Group 1 students took care of an average of 136.9, giving an absolute difference of 226.9 patients, corresponding to an increase of 167.5 % by Group 2. The comparison between the two groups was statistically significant (p = 0.001075). (Table 1)

Under the guidance and supervision of ED doctors, medical students have the ability to request imaging to those patients requiring further investigation. Students are then requested to follow-up the results afterwards, with the attending physician. Evaluation of the student radiographs revealed that Group 1 students requested an average of 152.6 radiographs while Group 2 students requested an average of 335.500 radiographs, an absolute increase of 182.8 examinations which represents a 119.7% increase for Group 2. When comparing the numbers of radiographs requested with the numbers of radiographs followed up with the attending/radiologist, Group 1 had an average of 44.8 radiographs followed up and Group 2 had an average of 167.4 followed up/evaluated (giving a difference of 122.6 – an increase of 273.8%). (p = 0.000128 for Group 1)(p = 0.012034 for Group 2). (Figure 1)

The results comparing the orthopedic immobilization procedures were divided into plastered and non-plastered. Regarding non-plaster immobilizations, it was observed that students in the Group 1 on average performed 19.3 procedures and Group 2 students performed on average 63.5 procedures (resulting in an increase of 44.2 immobilizations for Group 2, that represents a 229% increase – p value = 0.0053). In addition to this, for plaster immobilizations, Group 1 students on average performed 32.8 procedures compared to an average of 102.1 procedures by Group 2. This represents an increase of 69.3 procedures (211.2% more plaster immobilization) for Group 2 (p = 0, 00029). (Table 1)

We also collected data of surgical procedures such as sutures of skin lacerations, with a simple separated or a Donatti stitch. Once again, under supervision of ED doctors, students are able to perform these procedures. Group 1 students averaged 33.9 single stitch sutures, while Group 2 students averaged 96.2 of the same procedure (a difference of 183.7% of procedures, p = 0.000032). Regarding Donatti stitches, Group 1 students

Table 1 Number of procedures versus number of hours of extra-curricular supervised activities.

Number of Procedures	< 200h	> 200h	p value
History Takings in Initial Patient Care	136.905	363.800	0.001075
Non-cast immobilizations	19.360	63.577	0.005303793
Cast immobilizations	32.811	102.160	0.000295235
Simple sutures	33.980	96.200	0.000032826369841
Donatti sutures	5.283	12.214	0.019836
Trauma Resuscitation Room visits	2.804	21.036	0.000045965

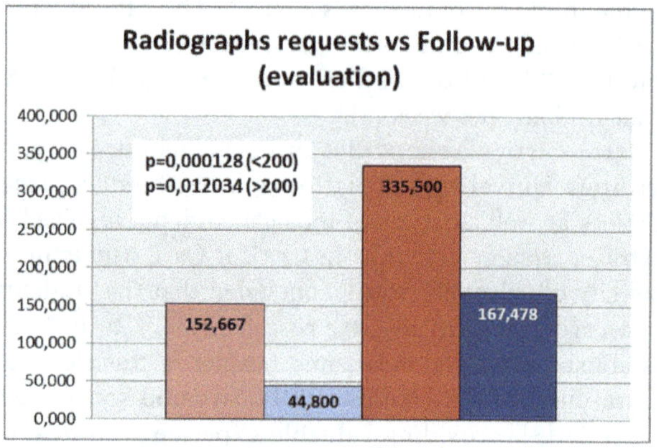

Figure 1 Number of Radiographs Requests vs number of Radiographs evaluation/follow-up. Rose: Group 1 requests. Light-Blue: Group 1 evaluations/follow-ups. Red: Group 2 requests. Dark-Blue: Group 2 evaluations/follow-ups.

reported having done an average of 5.2 sutures, while in Group 2 the recorded average was 12.2, with a difference of 7 procedures (131% more for Group 2). (Table 1)

Students have an established role in the Emergency Department, but sometimes their help is needed for trauma patients in the resuscitation room. The student on duty estimated the number of supervised visits to the trauma resuscitation room. Group 1 showed a mean of 2.8 visits, compared with a mean of 21 visits in Group 2 (an increase of 650.2% for the Group 2, p = 0.000045). (Table 1)

In order to achieve the clerkship objectives, it is important for the students to participate in all parts of patient care, from the patient admission in the ED to the management (discharge, admission to hospital floor, admission to ICU, admission to mini-unit, etc). However, these objectives are not required. Consequently, the study found that while students from Group 1 aided in discharging the patient, 69.1 times on average, Group 2 performed the same task 256.7 times (a 271.5% increase for Group 2). In addition, correlation with the numbers of histories taken revealed that in Group 1, 49.6% of patients whose history had been taken were not followed up and discharged by the same student. In comparison to Group 2, this percentage decreases to 29.4% (p = 0.011 for Group 1, p = 0.117 for Group 2). Concerning the number of supervised prescriptions, Group 1 students wrote 56.7 prescriptions at discharge, and Group 2 students wrote 232.4 (309.9% more). (Figure 2)

Finally, students were asked about their intention to pursue a surgical career. The vast majority of students (70.6%) said they want to be surgeons, 21.6% said they have no interest in surgical careers and the remainder (7.8%) did not answer the question. Also, when asked if the participation in this clerkship influenced their choice, we found that in 41.6% of cases, the clerkship had a positive influence, 7.8% had a negative influence and 35.3% reported it did not influence their decision. However, 15.7% declined to answer the question. (Figure 3) (Figure 4)

Discussion

There are only a few studies in the field of extra-curricular academic learning activities, probably because of the methodological difficulty in this form of study. [7,8] However, the rising incidence of students seeking alternative ways to learn medicine and increase their knowledge and skills makes it an extremely important issue that needs to be addressed.

Data collected reflects a major difference between the two groups of students. There are many reasons why students withdraw from the clerkship before they accomplish enough hours to fulfill the requirements for a proper certificate. Personal issues, excessive workload, the increasing service demand, night shifts, lack of sympathy of the health care providers may all be suggested as causes for abandoning the clerkship. However, those students who go on to complete the 200 hours appear to be well ahead in knowledge, skill and medical maturity.

Students in Group 2 outperformed students in Group 1 countless times over. This observation can be explained by the greater length of stay in the clerkship, so that the student is able to repeat over and over again whatever is needed to get used to it.

Furthermore, Group 2 requested 119.7% more radiographs than the Group 1 did. This number seems to be higher only because of their greater length of stay in the service, probably having no direct connection with the quality of their request or need for patient evaluation. However, when we interpret this with the number of supervised evaluations and follow up of the radiographs that the students performed, Group 2 did it almost four

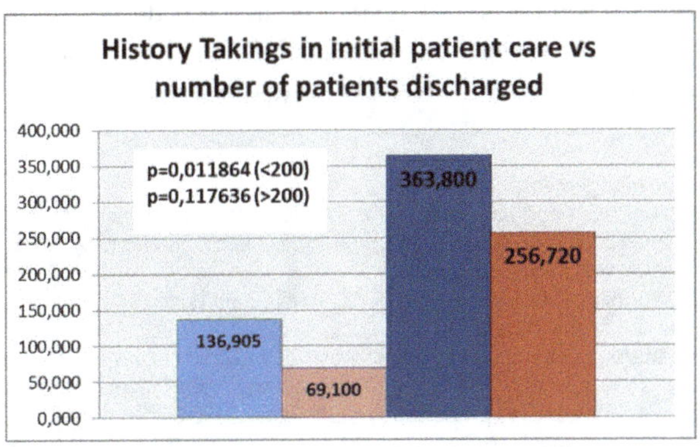

Figure 2 Number histories takings in initial patient care vs number of patients discharged. Rose: Group 1 patient discharged. Light-Blue: Group 1 histories taken. Red: Group 2 patient discharged. Dark-Blue: Group 2 histories taken.

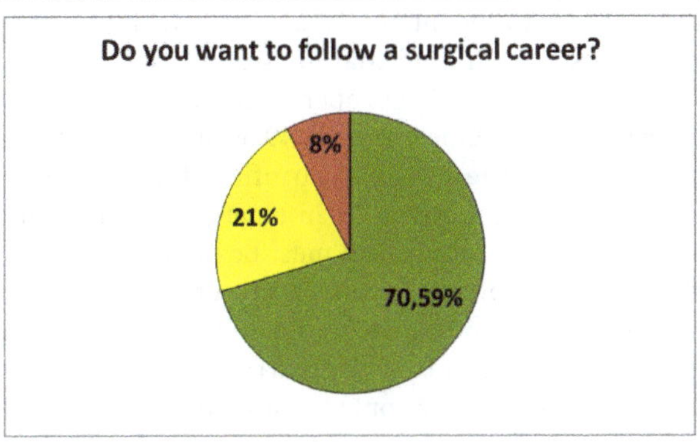

Figure 3 Percentage of Students that want to follow a surgical career. Yellow: No. Red: Not Answered. Green: Yes.

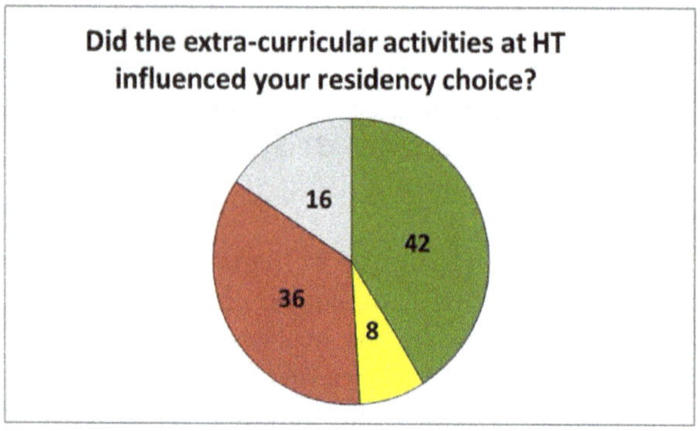

Figure 4 The supervised extra-curricular practical activity influence in their Decision. Green: Yes, Positive. Yellow: Yes, Negative. Red: No. Grey: Not Answered.

times more than Group 1 (273.8%). This seems to be related to better learning, and may even be a sign of maturity, as students begin to understand their own educational process. It is necessary for them to help in every steps of patient care to get the best picture in a better perspective of the entire process.

Also, the number of immobilization and sutures are directly proportional to the student's number of hours in the clerkship. Although it can be assumed that the more a procedure is performed the better the student's skill is, it has been proved that self-evaluation is not reliable as a good method to assess abilities [7]. Rather, objective assessment should be applied.

Considering all fields, Group 2 made significantly more of the following procedures: 229% more plaster immobilizations, 211.2% more non-plaster immobilizations, 183.7% more single stitch sutures, 131% more Donatti stitch sutures and 650.2% more Resuscitation Room patient care, which reflect their experience and knowledge for future practice.

We can also observe that students in Group 2 discharged 187.6 times more patients than the ones in Group 2, what can also be explained by more hours in the clerkship. However, if we correlate the number of history taking with the number discharge orientation given to patients, we will find that in Group 2 only 29.4% of patients did not receive proper instructions and follow up, whereas this number rises to 49.6% in the Group 1.

Considering the possible harmful effects of having medical students working in an emergency department alone, all activities developed must be under supervision, what help their practical training process that will never be achieved only by books.[5,9] Nevertheless, replacing curricular activities by extra-curricular ones shall be always discouraged. Not only but also, many Universities unfortunately do not offer a good enough plan of activities for their medical students, making regular lectures not a priority in their schedules (an issue that shall be addressed in a different paper).

Despite the better quality of medical care that can be offered by dedicated doctors compared to medical students, in Brazilian busy public emergency rooms most of the time it is impossible to dedicate the appropriate time on consultations to each patient (what may be the reality in most of the countries worldwide). Then, a team of committed medical students can be extremely helpful on patient care.

Even being non-licensed not-fully-trained, if properly supervised, they can play an important role in this environment. Tutors must be always aware of eventual medical errors that if not promptly approached will be under their legal responsibility as well as a threat to patients' safety.

Since it is a surgical clerkship, it is expected that the vast majority of students aim to follow a surgical career beforehand (70.6%). However, data concerning the influence of the extra-curricular activity in their decision should be analyzed carefully. Most of the students that do not have interest on a surgical career and find the practical activities a bad influence for them may abandon it before its completion (500 hours), or even before 200 hours, and would not participate in the present study.

Conclusions

Our data suggests that 200 hours seems to be a suitable threshold in medical students' learning surgical manual dexterity in an Emergency Department clerkship, even in the absence of objective parameters to further evaluate this theory. Last but not least, maturity and quality of medical care significantly improved proportional to the number of hours served in the ED clerkship. Therefore the practice of leaving before 200 hours should be actively discouraged.

Further comparative studies with objective criteria to evaluate students and residents' manual dexterity and their own perception of their abilities should be performed in order to assess our initial findings.

Acknowledgements

We thank Iwan Augusto Collaço, MD, PhD, TCBC, for his substantial academic contributions in the field of Trauma, and for his efforts by which this study was made possible.

We also thank Kenneth Stahl, MD, FACS, for his contribution with the discussion of this study.

This article has been published as part of *World Journal of Emergency Surgery* Volume 7 Supplement 1, 2012: Proceedings of the World Trauma Congress 2012. The full contents of the supplement are available online at http://www.wjes.org/supplements/7/S1.

Author details

[1]Federal University of Parana, Curitiba, Brazil. [2]Department of Surgery, Federal University of Parana, Curitiba, Brazil. [3]University Positivo, Curitiba, Brazil.

[4]Hospital do Trabalhador, State Health Department, Parana, Brazil. [5]University of Birmingham, UK.

Authors' contributions

PGTAR conceived the study idea, conducted the study design, writing and applying questionnaires, data analysis and contributed writing the manuscript and translation into English. GCO contributed applying questionnaires, helped with the data analysis and to write the manuscript. ACO participated applying questionnaires, data analysis and writing the manuscript. HS participated in the design of the study, performed the data analysis and discussion, and writing the manuscript and translation into English. AN participated in the design of the study, performed the data analysis, coordination and helped to draft the manuscript. FDST participated in the design of the study, performed the data analysis, coordination and helped to draft the manuscript. All authors read and approved the final manuscript.

Competing interests

No competing interests declared.

References

1. Nascimento DT, Dias MA, Mota RS, Barberino L, Durães L, Santos PAJ: **Avaliação dos estágios extracurriculares de medicina em unidade de terapia intensiva adulto.** *Rev Bras Ter Intensiva* 2008, **20(4)**:355-361.
2. Tavares AP, Ferreira RA, França EB, Fonseca CA Jr, Lopes GC, Dantas GT, Cardoso SAV: **O "Currículo Paralelo" dos estudantes de medicina da Universidade Federal de Minas Gerais.** *Rev Bras Edu Med* 2007, **31(3)**:254-265.
3. Tavares CHF, Maia JA, Muniz MCH, Malta MV, Magalhães BRC, Thomaz ACP: **O Currículo Paralelo dos Estudantes da Terceira Série do Curso Médico da Universidade Federal de Alagoas.** *Rev Bras Educ Med* 2007, **31(3)**:245-253.
4. Vieira EM, Barbieri CLA, Vilela DB, Ianhez E Jr, Tomé FS, Woida FM, Martinez GL, Vicente LM, Gava NF, Lira PG, Brandão TO, Mendonça TN: **O que eles fazem depoisa da aula? As atividades extracurriculares dos alunos de ciências médicas da FMRP-USP.** *Rev Fac Med Rib Preto* 2004, **37**:84-90.
5. Torres AR, Oliveira GM, Yamamoto FM, Lima MCP: **Ligas Acadêmicas e formação médica: contribuições e desafios.** *Rev Interface Com Sau Edu* 2008, **12(27)**:713-20.
6. Governo do Estado do Parana: **Dados públicos de atendimento do hospital do Trabalhador.** [http://www.hospitaldotrabalhador.saude.pr.gov.br/].
7. Kruger J, Dunning D: **Unskilled and unaware of it: how difficulties in recognizing one's own incompetence lead to inflated self-assessments.** *J Pers Soc Psychol* 1999, **77(6)**:1121-34.
8. Pego-Fernandes PM, Mariani AW: **Medical teaching beyond graduation: undergraduate study groups.** *São Paulo Med J* 2010, **128(5)**:257-8.
9. Block EF, Lottenberg L, Flint L, Jakobsen J, Liebnitzky D: **Use of human patient simulator for the advenced trauma life support course.** *Am Surg* 2002, **68(7)**:648-51.

14

Reexpansion pulmonary edema following a posttraumatic pneumothorax

Mark Malota[1*], Markus C Kowarik[2], Barbara Bechtold[3] and Reinhard Kopp[1]

Abstract

The reexpansion pulmonary edema is a rare, but life threatening complication of a pneumothorax. Early recognition and a fast symptom orientated therapy are necessary for a good outcome. Several cases after non traumatic pneumothoraces are reported. We describe a patient who presented with a post-traumatic right pneumothorax. After the insertion of a chest tube he developed a reexpansion pulmonary edema, which had to be treated by an intubation.

Additionally, a review of the literature regarding case reports of reexpansion pulmonary edema is presented.

Keywords: reexpansion pulmonary edema, acute pulmonary failure, posttraumatic pneumothorax, chest tube

Background

Cases of posttraumatic or spontaneous pneumothorax are usually treated by the insertion of a chest tube. A rare, potentially life-threatening complication of pneumothorax drainage is the pulmonary reexpansion edema. Usually it occurs after non traumatic pneumothoraces. Early recognition and a fast symptom orientated therapy of pulmonary reexpansion edema are necessary for a good outcome. Here we present a case of the development of a reexpansion pulmonary edema after a traumatic pneumothorax

Case Presentation

A 21-year-old male, sportive patient was admitted to our surgical emergency department after he had been involved in a traffic accident. As the unbelted driver of a car, he crashed frontally against another car with approximately 50 km/h.

On first sight he was complaining of jabbing pain in the right hemothorax and in the sternal region, thoracic constriction and a considerable dyspnoea. Apart from that, he had signs of a beginning cold: since two days he had a cough and suffered from an acute rhinitis. The patient was an occasional smoker but did not have any history of pulmonary or other diseases.

The asthenic man (weight 62 kg, size 179 cm) was orientated and had no neurological deficit with stable vital parameters. Some small superficial wounds and haematoma in the lower part of the sternum and the right hemithorax could be found. Furthermore a discrete cyanosis of the lips was seen. On auscultation, the patient was found to have no respiratory murmur and hyperresonant percussion on the right side, with the left lung completely normal.

Using a chest x-ray, we saw a pneumothorax on the right with a subtotal lung collapse (Figure 1).

Under insufflation of 4 l O1/2/min, the arterial blood gas showed signs of a respiratory partial insufficiency: the pO^2 was 50 mmHg and pCO^2 43 mmHg. Apart from a leucocytosis of 17, 9 mg/dl, the blood examination was without pathological findings.

Based on the diagnosis of a posttraumatic pneumothorax we immediately performed the insertion of a chest tube in Buelau technique located in the 5th ICR, proximal axillary line under local anaesthesia, and connected it to a 3-chamber chest drain system with suction of 20 cm water column. The pre-treatment time took approximately twenty minutes.

The pulmonary condition of the patient ameliorated (pO^2 72 mmHg, pCO^2 38 mmHg), both lungs were

* Correspondence: markmalota@hotmail.com
[1]Krankenhaus München Harlaching, Departement of Surgery, Munich, Germany
Full list of author information is available at the end of the article

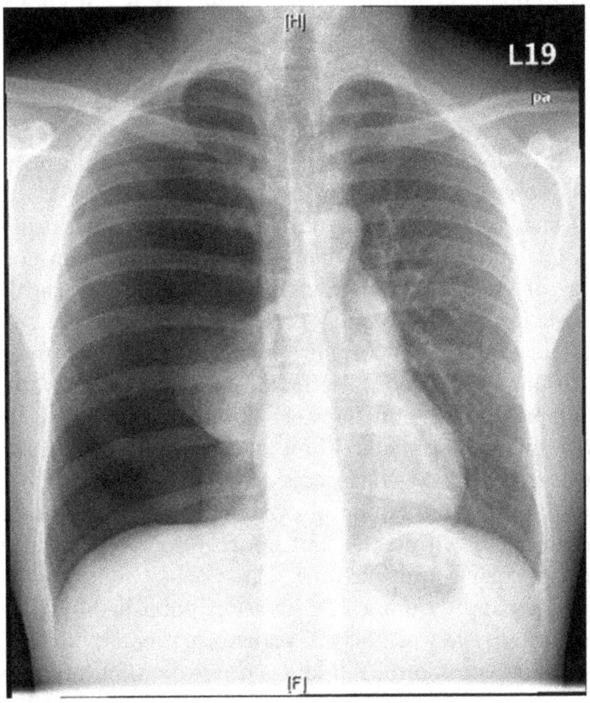

Figure 1 The first chest x-ray. We find a pneumothorax on the right with a subtotal lung collapse.

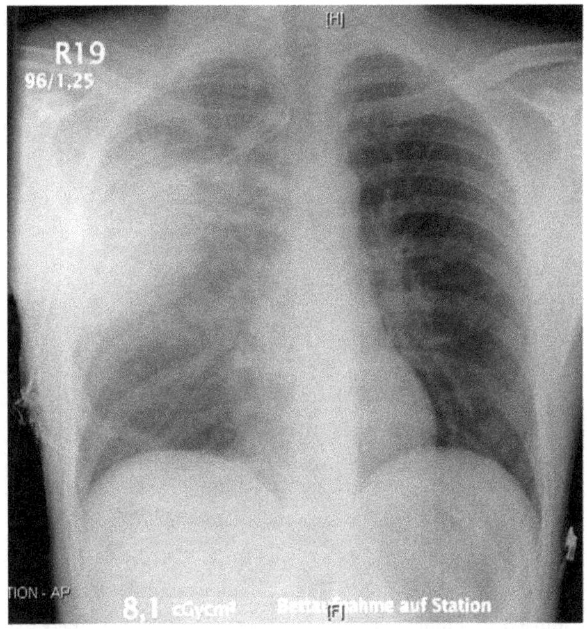

Figure 2 The second chest x-ray with the thoracic drain. The lung is correctly expanded. There is a suspect shadow along the lateral right chest wall.

ventilated and SpO1/2 increased ten minutes after the intervention up to 99%. Because of a moderate analgesic and sedative medication, we kept the patient for further monitoring in our anaesthetic recovery room. Here the patient reported only light pain at the entrance of the drainage, without having any dyspnoea.

Two hours later, the patient's condition rapidly worsened. He was pale, sweating, tachypnoic and complained of increasing chest pain with dyspnoea. In spite of 10 l/min O1/2, the SpO1/2 was only 82% with a heart rate of 122/min and a decreasing blood pressure. Checking the arterial blood gas, the pO^2 was 61 mmHg and pCO^2 58 mmHg, indicating now a global respiratory failure

Immediately a chest x-ray was taken (Figure 2). Although the lung seemed expanded correctly, there was a suspect shadow along the chest wall, where the tube was entering. Because of the suspicion of a haematoma of the thoracic wall, we checked the haemoglobin, which was stable at 14 g/dl. Furthermore there was no blood in the tube. Meanwhile the patient's condition got worse progressively, so that we decided to initiate an intubation to be able to improve the oxygenation using mechanical respiration. At the inspection of the pharynx, an immense amount of suppuration was blocking the upper respiratory tract. Finally 350 ml of putrid mucos were sucked off, whereupon a tracheal intubation could be performed. Now the mechanical ventilation of the patient was easy to handle and in the following twenty minutes another 300 ml mucos were removed.

After that, we did a CT scan of the thorax, which surprisingly showed a marked ipsilateral lung edema, designated as a reexpansion pulmonary edema. Furthermore a small edema was seen on the contralateral side, however without any other pathological findings concerning the lung or the complete rib cage (Figure 3).

The patient was rapidly stabilized under automatic continuous positive airway pressure respiration (CPAP) and short-term therapy with Noradrenaline and Furosemid. After transferring the patient to our intensive care unit, the respiratory and haemodynamic situation remained stable.

Under a calculated antimicrobiotic therapy with Piperacilin and Sulbactam the respiratory condition quickly improved and the patient could be extubated after 48 hours. Chest tubes could be removed soon and the patient was released from hospital on the 4th post OP day with normally expanded lung.

Discussion

"Reexpansion pulmonary edema" (RPE) has been described as a rare, life threatening complication in the treatment of lung atelectasis, pleural effusions or spontaneous pneumothorax with a mortality up to 20% [1].

Pinault in Paris was the first to describe the clinical situation in 1853 after the drainage of 3 l pleural

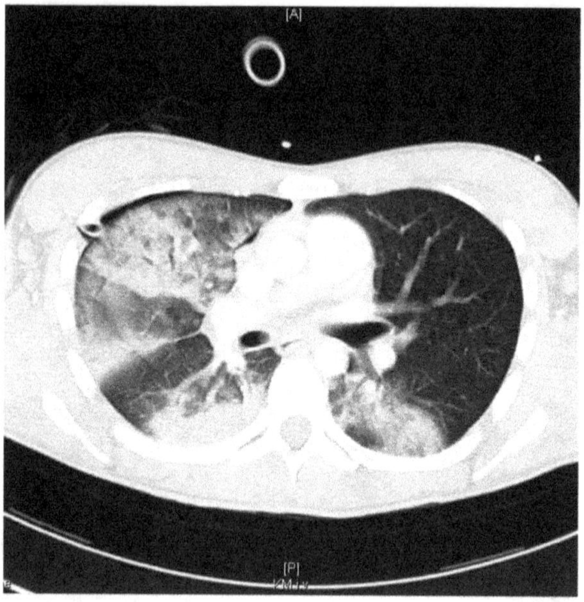

Figure 3 CT findings of the lung edema. A bilateral lung edema can be seen in the CT of the chest.

effusion [2]. The first report of a RPE after treatment for a totally collapsed lung because of pneumothorax was published in 1958 by Carlson [3]. In the following years, there were several cases reporting on the occurrence of RPE after spontaneous pneumothorax, the resection of a mediastinal tumor, thoracoscopy, or talc pleurodesis [3-5].

Mahfood et al reviewed all reported cases from 1958 to 1987 with 47 cases of RPE. Here the clinical disorders occur from almost free of complaints to foydurant processes with lethal ending. A rapid onset of dyspnoea is the cardinal symptom, followed by cough and hypotension. Risk factors seem to be age (the younger the patient, the higher the risk), female sex, degree of lung collapse, a pneumothorax existing more than 24 hours, a reexpansion of the lung in less than ten minutes, using a suction system and - in cases of a pleural effusion - an evacuation volume of more than 2000 ml [1].

RPE can occur as well after talc pleurodesis. In a retrospective study of 614 patients, 12 patients developed transient interstitial opacities on the chest x-ray, indicating a RPE [4].

In one case report, RPE occurred after left thoracoscopic resection of a mediastinal tumor. Here, the lung had been preoperatively compressed by the tumor and one-lung ventilation was used [5].

Fujino et al reported an intraoperative RPE during a video assisted thoracoscopy, where high-frequency jet ventilation was used to reexpand the lung, which had collapsed 23 days before [6]. All cases had in common that the duration of the lung collapse was at least 12 hours.

Although the precise incidence of RPE is not known, it is generally considered to be very low. A series of 320 cases of spontaneous pneumothorax was published by Rozenman et al in 1996 with 3 cases of RPE [7]. In another case series of a combined total of 775 cases with patients treated for spontaneous pneumothorax was no reported case of RPE [8,9].

Usually, most of the reported cases were described as an ipsilateral RPE, but there are few patients with contra- or even bilateral edema, which seem to raise the mortality. Her and Mandy published 3 cases with a contralateral RPE after a right upper lobectomy for cancer, a drainage of a pleural effusion and an intraoperative collapse during non thoracic surgery. In all cases, the RPE in the contralateral lung occurred faster and more severe than in the collapsed side [10].

Appraising the temporal dynamic, the first symptoms often occur within the first hour up to 24 hours after the re-expansion of the lung [7].

As we know from a 22 case series published by Gleeson, who reviewed the CT scans of patients with RPE, the most common CT findings of reexpansion pulmonary edema include ipsilateral ground-glass opacities, septal thickening, foci of consolidation and areas of atelectasis [11].

The aetiology depends on multiple factors; however the pathophysiological process has not yet been completely explored. From several animal experiments it could be seen, that a chronic lung collapse causes a thickening of the capillary endothelium by the release of MCP1 (monocyte chemoattractant protein 1), Leukotriene B4 and IL-8 (Interleukin 8). On reexpansion of the lung, the microvessels are suddenly stretched, which harms their endothelium. Thereby the capillary permeability is increased and a loss of alveolar surfactant can be observed. Thus the perivascular pressure of the microvessels decreases, which leads to further endothelial damage. In addition to that, it could be demonstrated, that oxidases are induced, which leads to apoptosis of alveolar and endothelial cells [12,13].

The treatment for RPE is symptomatic. Apart from monitoring the patient's vital parameters, invasive respiration with a high positive end-expiratory pressure may be necessary to reexpand the collapsed alveoli. Supportively anti-inflammatory drugs and diuretics should be given [14].

Conclusion

Although the RPE is a rare complication after the treatment of a pneumothorax, the physician should be aware of the severity of this disease pattern and always keep it in mind. Furthermore he should be aware of the fact that it can as well occur after a traumatic pneumothorax.

Consent

Written informed consent was obtained from the patient for publication of this Case report and any accompanying images. A copy of the written consent is available for review by the Editor-in-Chief of this journal.

Author details

[1]Krankenhaus München Harlaching, Departement of Surgery, Munich, Germany. [2]Klinikum Rechts der Isar, Munich, Germany. [3]Krankenhaus München Harlaching, Departement of Anaesthesiology, Munich, Germany.

Authors' contributions

MM drafted the manuscript. MCK made substantial revisions. BB searched the literature and the findings. RK had given final approval of the version to be published. All authors read and approved the final manuscript.

Competing interests

The authors declare that they have no competing interests.

References

1. Mahfood S, Hix WR, Aaron BL: **Reexpansion pulmonary edema.** *Ann Thorac Surg* 1998, **45**:340-345.
2. Pinault H: **Considérations cliniques sur la thoracentèse.**, 1853 [doctoral thesis]. Paris.
3. Carlson RI, Classen KL, Gollan F: **Pulmonary edema following the rapid expansion of a totally collapsed lung due to pneumothorax: A clinical and experimental study.** *Surg Forum* 1958, **9**:367-371.
4. de Campos JRM, Vargas FS, Werebe EDC: **Thoracoscopy talc poudrage.** *Chest* 2001, **119**:801-806.
5. Matsumiya N, Dohi S, Kimura T, Naito H: **Reexpansion pulmonary edema after mediastenal tumor removal.** *Anesth Analg* 1991, **73**:646-8.
6. Fujino S, Tezuka N, Inoue N, *et al*: **Reexpansion pulmonary edema due to high-frequency jet ventilation: Report of a case.** *Surg Today* 2000, **30**:1110-1111.
7. Rozenman J, Yellin A, Simansky DA, Shiner RJ: **Re-expansion pulmonary oedema following spontaneous pneumothorax.** *Respir Med* 1996, **90(4)**:235-8.
8. Mills M, Balsch BF: **Spontaneous pneumothorax: A series of 400 cases.** *Ann Thorac Surg* 1965, **122**:286-297.
9. Brooks JW: **Open thoracotomy in the management of spontaneous pneumothorax.** *Ann Surg* 1973, **177**:798-805.
10. Her C, Mandy S: **Acute respiratory distress syndrome of the contralateral lung after reexpansion pulmonary edema of a collapsed lung.** *J Clin Anesth* 2004, **16**:244-250.
11. Gleeson T, Thiessen R, Müller N: **Reexpansion pulmonary edema: computed tomography findings in 22 patients.** *J Thorac Imaging* 2011, **26(1)**:36-41.
12. Nakamura H, Ishizaka A, Sawafuji M, *et al*: **Elevated levels of interleukin-8 and leukotriene B4 in pulmonary edema fluid of a patient with reexpansion pulmonary edema.** *Am J Respir Crit Care Med* 1994, **149**:1037-1040.
13. Wright RM, Ginger LA, Kosila N: **Mononuclear phagocyte xanthine oxidoreductase contributes to cytokine-induced acute lung injury.** *Am J Respir Cell Mol Biol* 2004, **30**:479-490.
14. Cho SR, Lee JS, Kim MS: **New treatment method for reexpansion pulmonary edema: Differential lung ventilation.** *Ann Thorac Surg* 2005, **80**:1933-1934.

15

Bariatric emergencies: current evidence and strategies of management

Abdulzahra Hussain[1,2*] and Shamsi EL-Hasani[1]

Abstract

Background: The demand for bariatric surgery is increasing and the postoperative complications are seen more frequently. The aim of this paper is to review the current outcomes of bariatric surgery emergencies and to formulate a pathway of safe management.

Methods: The PubMed and Google search for English literatures relevant to emergencies of bariatric surgery was made, 6358 articles were found and 90 papers were selected based on relevance, power of the study, recent papers and laparoscopic workload. The pooled data was collected from these articles that were addressing the complications and emergency treatment of bariatric patients. 830,998 patients were included in this review.

Results: Bariatric emergencies were increasingly seen in the Accident and Emergency departments, the serious outcomes were reported following complex operations like gastric bypass but also after gastric band and the causes were technical errors, suboptimal evaluation, failure of effective communication with bariatric teams who performed the initial operation, patients factors, and delay in the presentation. The mortality ranged from 0.14%-2.2% and increased for revisional surgery to 6.5% ($p = 0.002$). Inspite of this, mortality following bariatric surgery is still less than that of control group of obese patients (p = value 0.01).

Conclusions: Most mortality and catastrophic outcomes following bariatric surgery are preventable. The awareness of bariatric emergencies and its effective management are the gold standards for best outcomes. An algorithm is suggested and needs further evaluation.

Keywords: Laparoscopic roux en-Y gastric bypass, Laparoscopic sleeve gastrectomy, Laparoscopic adjustable gastric band, Stomal ulceration

Introduction

Definitions

Bariatric surgery: Relating to the treatment of obesity. Origin: Greek bar (os) weight (cf. baro-) + –iatrics (http://dictionary.reference.com/browse/bariatrics).

British Obesity and Metabolic Surgery Society BOMSS defined it as: Surgeons involved in obesity management (www.bomss.org.uk).

Metabolic surgery: The procedures for weight loss, whether designated as restrictive, restrictive/malabsorptive, malabsorptive, and others, or neuro-hormonal, all fall under the definition as the operative manipulation of a normal organ or organ system to achieve a biological result for a potential health gain [1].

Current indications for bariatric surgery

The National Institute for health and Clinical Excellence (NICE) UK guidelines and the American Gastroenterological Association (AGA) recommend bariatric surgery as a treatment option for adults with a Body Mass Index (BMI) 40–50, or those with BMI > 35-40 and one or more severe obesity-related medical complication (e.g., hypertension, heart failure, or sleep apnea) if they have been unable to achieve or maintain weight loss with conventional therapy, have acceptable operative risks, and are able to comply with long-term treatment and follow-up [2,3]. The updates of these indications are going to be published in the Endocrine Practice 2013; the most updated version of guidelines sponsored by American Association of Clinical

* Correspondence: azahrahussain@yahoo.coml
[1]Minimal access and bariatric unit, King's College Hospital NHS Foundation Trust, Princess Royal University Hospital, Orpington, London BR6 8ND, UK
[2]Honorary Senior Lecturer at King's College Medical School, London, UK

Endocrinologists (AACE), The Obesity Society (TOS), and American Society for Metabolic & Bariatric Surgery (ASMBS).

Types of operations: Different types of operations including gastric balloon, gastric plication and different types of intestinal bypasses are practiced but the most popular are: Gastric bypass, Sleeve gastrectomy, Gastric band, Bilio-pancreatic diversion+/–Duodenal switch.

Background

Bariatric and metabolic surgery to treat obesity and type 2 diabetes has promising results of cure rather than improvement [4], Level of evidence (L2+), such outcome is not without risks due to a limited physiological reserve, thus patients can easily deteriorate when complications occur. Modern technology and minimal access experience have contributed to the current quality and safety of bariatric operations but unfortunately mortality is still reported in the literature and especially after complex procedures such as duodenal switch and bilio-pancreatic diversion and to a less extent after gastric bypass [5,6], (L2+). The Swedish Obese Subject Study has shown clear benefits of Bariatric Surgery (BS) in terms of reduced mortality and weight loss compared to control group of conventional therapy [7]. Such benefits can be improved by reducing the mortality of emergencies of BS.

The AACE, TOS and ASMBS updated document of guidelines is referring to 6 recommendations concerning acute presentations of the bariatric patients, stressing the admission and surgical approach if medical treatment is not effective for malnutrition, gastrointestinal complications, strictures and revisional surgery [8], (variable levels). Currently there are no comprehensive guidelines for managing the acute presentations of BS and the on-call general surgical and anaesthetic/critical care teams are increasingly facing such clinical scenarios with no standard plan of management.

To address the problem of morbidity and mortality, it is important to predict which patient is going to develop complications after BS and one way of doing so is by using certain indices; like the Elixhauser index [9], (L2+).

Recent study of more than 44,000 patients from the United States of America (USA) showed independent predictors associated with significantly increased mortality included age >45 years, male gender, a body mass index (BMI) of 50 kg/m or higher, open bariatric procedures, diabetes, functional status of total dependency before surgery, prior coronary intervention, dyspnea at preoperative evaluation, more than 10% unintentional weight loss in 6 months, and bleeding disorder [10,11], (L2+). Intensive care unit admission for bariatric patients has increased owing to revisional surgeries [12], (L2+), and the trend has changed from elective to an emergency admission.

The Accident & Emergency (A&E) doctors, the on-call surgical teams and sometimes the on-call medical team are initially seeing and managing bariatric patients for different presentations [13] (L2+), one of the reasons of poor outcomes of these patients is primary failure of recognition of the problem [14], (L2++). Hence, there is a definite need for clear pathways to reduce the incidents of delaying investigations, initiating appropriate treatment and start effective communication with bariatric and critical care teams [15], (L2+), [16,17], (L2++). The aim of this document is to study the current evidence and to highlight the initial management plan for emergencies of BS and streamlining a timely and safe management pathway.

Materials and methods

The PubMed and Google engines were searched for English literatures relevant to the acute presentations and management of bariatric emergencies. The search words were bariatric emergencies, management of acute bariatric patients, acute abdomen in obesity and metabolic surgery; post bariatric complications, nutritional complications following bariatric and metabolic surgery. Two independent authors selected the studies. 6358 articles were found. The abstracts of these articles were filtered and 90 papers were selected for this review. The pooled data from selected studies were further analysed. Heterogeneity was obvious. A review was undertaken to assess the evidence in each of 7 common complications (bleeding, leak, obstruction, stomal ulceration, pulmonary embolism and respiratory complication, blood sugar disturbances and nutritional disturbances) that were seen in the A&E department and required an urgent and safe approach.

Scottish Intercollegiate Guidelines Network (SIGN) grading of evidence was adopted (see Table 1). The heterogeneity among the studies because of the different causes of morbidity and mortality after different types of BS for different categories of patients and different surgical teams and centres, has made a robust meta-analysis or systematic review almost impossible. The reference followed by the level of evidence (L) was used for citation.

Results

The pooled data of 830,998 patients were included in this study. The evidence was variable in strength [4 guidelines, one meta-analysis, 10 Randomised Controlled Trials (RCTs), 2 comparative studies, 4 prospective cohorts, 20 reviews, 48 retrospective observational studies and 9 case series (in rare complications only)]. Majority of the current body of knowledge was reported by retrospective and observational studies (see Figure 1). 80% of the presented evidence was published

Table 1 Level of evidence

Levels of Evidence (Scottish Intercollegiate Guidelines Network, SIGN)	
1++	High quality meta-analyses, systematic reviews of RCTs, or RCTs with a very low risk of bias
1+	Well conducted meta-analyses, systematic reviews, or RCTs with a low risk of bias
1-	Meta-analyses, systematic reviews, or RCTs with a high risk of bias
2++	High quality systematic reviews of case control or cohort studies
	High quality case control or cohort studies with a very low risk of confounding or bias and a high probability that the relationship is causal
2+	Well conducted case control or cohort studies with a low risk of confounding or bias and a moderate probability that the relationship is causal
2-	Case control or cohort studies with a high risk of confounding or bias and a significant risk that the relationship is not causal
3	Non-analytic studies, eg case reports, case series
4	Expert opinion

in the last 5 years. Catastrophic and avoidable mortality and severe disabling morbidities were still seen in the current bariatric practice, complex multifactor aetiology was reported and included low degree of awareness among the admitting teams, unavailability of bariatric services at the admitting hospitals, failure of communication with the bariatric team who performed the initial operation, technical errors and delay in the presentation and referral by general practitioners, and personal factors. The outcomes of each of research areas were reported under each of the following headings. As a result a conclusion algorithm was suggested (see Figures 2, 3 and 4).

Bleeding

Bleeding complications could follow any operation and bariatric surgery is not an exempt. Luckily, relatively rare, following gastric bypass it was around 0.94% [18], (L2+), but it could reach 4.4% [19], (L2+). A systematic review concluded a higher rate in laparoscopic Roux en-Y Gastric bypass (LRYGB) versus open one [20], (L2+). Bleeding following Adjustable Gastric Band (LAGB) was extremely rare and could be related to organ injury or band erosions [21], (L3), [22], (L2+). Bleeding following LRYGB, sleeve gastrectomy and bilio-pancreatic diversion could be intralumenal or extralumenal types. Early bleeding (within 30 days of operation) was more common than late bleeding. The presentation was variable and diverse from low haemoglobin to fainting and un-stability, heamatemesis, malena and fresh blood per rectum were another forms [23], (L3), small bowel obstruction may be the initial presentation of bleeding and can occur in 0.5% of patients [24], (L2+), [25], (L2++).

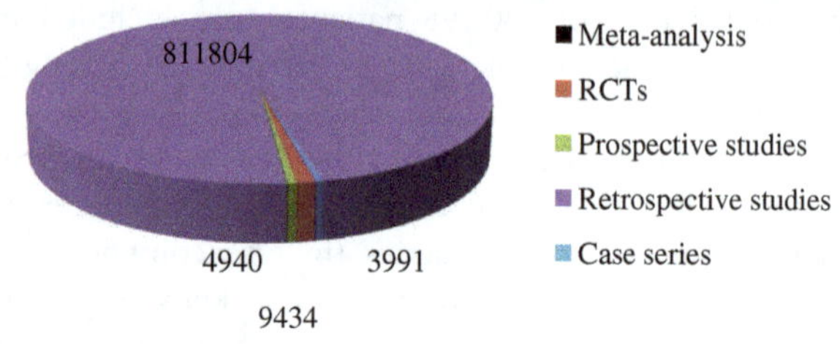

Figure 1 Weight of the studies.

The underlying causes of bleeding could be due to patient factors such as bleeding tendencies, anti-coagulations, infection, ulceration or surgeon factors of poor surgical or haemostatic technique, while the type and the length of the operation is reflected by the degree of complexity (the more complex and prolong procedure, the more the incidence of bleeding) [26], (L2++). LRYGB caused more bleeding complication [27], (L2++), which can be related to the type of stapler. A meta-analysis showed linear stapler was associated with less bleeding [28], (L1+), and enforcement of staple line after Laparoscopic Sleeve Gastrectomy (SG) could reduce bleeding significantly (odd ratio was 0.559) [29], (L2++).

NICE guideline of acute upper gastrointestinal bleeding management was an excellent reference [30], (variable levels). However, some specific measures may help to control the bleeding in this particular group of patients [31], (L2+), [32], (L3). This was largely related to the type of the procedure and whether the bleeding was intra or extra luminal. Intra-lumenal bleeding especially at the gastro-jejunostomy (G-J) can be controlled with the aid of endoscopic therapy [33], (L2++). Jejuno-jenunostomy (J-J) intra lumenal bleeding site may be difficult to reach with good visualization by the endoscopy and majority of unstable patients were candidates of laparoscopic or laparotomy exploration of the anastomosis and controlling of bleeder(s). Extra-lumenal bleeding in stable patient can be treated conservatively. Unstable cases were managed by laparoscopic or laparotomy exploration [18], (L2+), with the use of clips, diathermy, suturing of bleeding points if the cause was staple line or more aggressive approach of splenectomy if the source was uncontrollable splenic bleed due to organ injury. Mesenteric, port site bleeder and other intra peritoneal bleeders can be controlled accordingly. As some of the patients would need blood transfusion for the bleeding, this raised the question of safety of bariatric surgery in 0.5% of American patients who refused transfusion for religious or personal causes. Safety was concluded for these patients, provided other measures have been used to manage the bleeding [34], (L2+).

Leak

Leak was a major killer and an enemy to the success of BS, it can follow procedures where anastomosis is

A.Gastric bypass B.Gastric band C.Sleeve gastrectomy D.Gastric balloon E.Biliopancreatic diversion & duodenal switch F.Gastric plication	1.Obstruction 2.Bleeding 3.Leak (acute abdomen) 4.Sepsis 5.Wounds complications 6.Metabolic acidosis and blood sugar abnormalities 7.Thiamine and other nutritional deficiencies 8.Respiratory complications (Pulmonary embolism, Atelectasis, Pneumonia)	1.full blood count, renal & liver functions, coagulation and blood sugar (thiamine,Vit C, Vit A, B12, Calcium and other rare elements when nutritional deficiencies are suspected) 2.Chest X-Ray 3.Abdominal X-Ray 4.Arterial blood gas 5.CT scanning depends on the case	1.Nil by mouth 2.IV Fluids (Hartman/or Normal saline when low sodium) 3.Antibiotics (Augmentin+ metronidazole) in suspicion of sepsis or wound infection 4.Omeprazole 40 mgs iv when upper GI bleed or ulcer. 5.Urinary catheter in unwell patient, sepsis and acute abdomen 6.Don't put NG until check ing with the bariatric team. 7.Don't give iv glucose to any bariatric patients unless hypoglycaemia 8.Moniter observations *9.Involve on call surgical & bariatric teams early*

Figure 2 Acute presentations of bariatric surgeries and initial accident & emergency management.

Gastric band adjustment problems	1.Obstructive (dysphagia) No pain. 2.Vomiting & pregnancy. 3.The above presentations should be differentiated from slippage and acute gastric ischemia.	1.Full blood count, renal & liver function, coagulation and blood sugar. 2.Stable patient needs no investigations.	1.Nil by mouth 2.IV Fluids (Hartman /or Normal saline when low sodium). 3.Stable patient can be managed by deflation of the band & discharged. 4.The band should be deflated during pregnancy. *5.Involve on call surgical & bariatric teams early*

Figure 3 Acute presentations and management of gastric band adjustment problems.

A.Gastric bypass B.Gastric band C.Sleeve gastrectomy D.Gastric balloon E.Biliopancreatic diversion & duodenal switch F.Gastric plication	1.Recurrent or chronic abdominal pain (more than 3 months) 2.Occasional vomiting 3.Dysphagia Other than table (1) presentations	1.Full blood count, renal, liver function, coagulation and blood sugar 2.Chest X-Ray 3.Abdominal X-Ray 4.Blood gas 5.CT scanning depends on the case	1.Depends on the initial diagnosis 2.Prepare for surgery or endoscopy until prove otherwise 3.Conservative management if initial assessment and investigations show no abdominal catastrophe 4.*Involve on call surgical & bariatric teams early*

Figure 4 **Presentations and initial management of chronic or subacute post bariatric surgery complications which are seen in emergency department.**

undertaken like gastric bypass, the incidence of which could reach 1.4% [35], (L2+). It can also follow laparoscopic Sleeve Gastrectomy (SG) or organ injury during LAGB insertion. Sepsis was reported as a major cause of death and this was largely due to diagnosed or undiagnosed leak [36], (L2+). After gastric bypass, a large study of 226,452 patients showed factors associated with higher risk of gastro-intestinal tract (GIT) leak were open gastric bypass, congestive heart failure, chronic renal failure, age older than 50 years, Medicare payer, male sex and chronic lung disease [37], (L2+). Routine use of per-operative endoscopy during LRYGB was associated with low leak (0.2%) and stricture (1.1%) rates [38], (L2+) while the use of drain provided no benefit and the diagnosis of leak was largely clinical, aided by appropriate imaging [39], (L2++). Leak was the most common cause of major morbidity and mortality after LSG [40], (L2+) and was associated with mortality rate of 4.5% [41], (L3).

Although reinforcement of sleeve line was thought to reduce the leak incidence [29], (L2++), a recent meta-analysis has failed to confirm that, but concluded the use of bougie larger than 40 FR was reducing the leak rate [42], (L2+), this may refer to the stenosis of the sleeve as a predisposing factor for leak in the LSG patients. The initial management of the leaks was that of peritonitis, some additional steps and tips depended on the type of operation. The choice of conservative or emergency exploration was dictated by the overall assessment of the patient. In a stable patient, the use of covered stent was effective [43], (L3). Emergency management was composed of drainage, control of sepsis, antibiotics, nutritional support [44], and intensive care management (L2++). If no response to the conservative treatment or deterioration, laparoscopy and/or laparotomy were suggested [45], (L3).

Obstruction

Obstruction following bariatric surgery can be serious and GIT ischemia should be ruled out early in the course of presentation, late diagnosis and intervention could be disastrous [35], (L2+). Four types of internal hernia were seen following gastric bypass; Mesenteric, and mesojejunal, Petersons and jejuno-jejunal herniae are identified [46,47], (L2+), [48], (L2++). Obstruction could be due to a mechanical problem or technical error at the anastomosis or from banded gastric bypass operation [49], (L3). G-J stricture was another cause of obstruction and the incidence could reach 27% [50], (L2++). However, recent series reported much lower incidence of less than 1% [51], (L2+). J-J obstruction was reported and its incidence was much less that G-J stricture at 0.001%, the causes of which were different; technical error or clot obstruction [52,53], (L2+). Gastric band obstruction (a common complication) can be easily managed by deflation of the band. More serious slippage with gastric strangulation should be excluded in any case with dysphagia [54], (L2++). The initial assessment is outlined in the algorithm. The main question to the surgeon is: does this patient have gastrointestinal ischemia or not? Clinical presentation, Computerized Tomography (CT) scan, arterial blood gasses will help to direct the course of management.

Stomal ulceration (SU)

This was an unusual complication following LRYGB. Early series reported high incidence of 12.5% [55], (L2+), however later studies showed much lower incidence of refractory SU of 0.1% [56], (L2+). Early experience showed SU was the result of acid production in the bypassed stomach in the presence of a gastrogastric fistula, could happen in 20% of patients [57], (L2+), however wider experience indicated that SU was caused by possible ischemia, narrow G-J stoma, smoking, medications including steroid and Non Steroidal Anti-Inflammatory Drugs (NSAID), H Pylori infection, foreign bodies at the base of ulcer [58], (L3), [59,60], (L2+).

Prophylactic short course of proton pump inhibitor PPI has reduced the incidence of SU [61], (L2+). The PPI may works in presence of Helicobacter Pylori infection. There are other studies that contradict these findings. The presentation of SU was variable, but ranged from epigastric pain to dysphagia, vomiting and obstruction. However, 28% were asymptomatic [62], (L2++).

Avoidance of the above risk factors should reduce the incidence of the SU. The management of established case was ranging from PPI and cytoprotective scrulfate, endoscopic and radiological dilatation of associated stricture and revisional surgery [63,64], (L2+).

Pulmonary embolism and respiratory complications

Pulmonary embolism was rare after bariatric surgery; the weighted incidence was 0.5% [65], (L1+). The analysis of mortality of 13,871 patients in Italy after bariatric surgery showed 11.8% were due to respiratory failure including pulmonary embolism [66], (L2+). Not only LRYGB, but also LAGB was associated with major respiratory complications of aspiration pneumonia, atelectasis, exacerbation of asthma and empyema and lung abscess [67], (L2+). Prediction of patients who are likely to develop respiratory complication and prevention was the corner stone in reducing this kind of complications. Congestive heart failure and stroke were the greatest preoperative risk factors for pneumonia. Previous percutaneous coronary intervention, dyspnoea at rest, bleeding disorder, age, chronic obstructive pulmonary disease, and type of surgery, smoking, diabetes mellitus, anesthesia time and increasing weight were predisposing to respiratory complications [68], (L2+). Age, waist circumference, systolic blood pressure, and witnessed sleep apnea episodes were important risk factors in patient with sleep apnoea, thus preoperative optimization was necessary to reduce respiratory morbidity [69], (L2+). The main task for admitting and managing teams was to exclude abdominal catastrophe. When that's done; the respiratory complications management was following the same concept of treatment of individual complication. Please see the algorithm (Figures 2, 3 and 4).

Blood sugar disturbance

The American Diabetes Association (ADA) has defined the cure of diabetes following bariatric surgery as a return to normal measures of glucose metabolism (haemoglobin) HbA1c below 6 per cent, fasting glucose less than 5·6 mmol/l at least 1 year after bariatric surgery without hypoglycaemic medication [70], (L2+). All bariatric surgeries were influencing blood sugar level and improving insulin sensitivity and decreasing HgbA1c [71], (L2++), this effect was especially associated with more complex type such as gastric bypass, ileal or jejunal bypass and duodenal switch or bilio-pancreatic diversion [72,73], (L2++, [74], (L3). Hypotheses of the mechanisms were ranged from beta cell expansion to altered beta cell function as well as non-beta cell factors [75], (L2+). Post-prandial hyper insulinemic hypoglycemia associated with nesidioblastosis may be related to the changes in Glucagon Like Peptide (GLP-1) and other gut hormones [76], (L2++). The cases of hypoglycaemia and acidosis were seen in A&E department and can be successfully managed by joint care with the medical and endocrinology teams. Low carbohydrate diets may be effective in treating post-gastric bypass hyperinsulinemic hypoglycemia [77], (L3). Blood sugar disturbance and acidosis was also presented following LAGB and special association with early pregnancy was noticed. Deflation of the band will resolve the problem.

Nutritional disturbances

Hypovitaminosis D and secondary hyperparathyroidism were associated with morbid obesity and therefore calcium deficiencies and acute hypocalcemia syndromes were reported following BS [78], (L2++), especially in patients who had thyroidectomy before [79], (L2++). 25-hydroxyvitamin D was the most commonly observed deficiency after SG & LRYGB [80], (L2++) while the major macronutrient deficiency after bariatric surgery was protein malnutrition [81], (L2++). A number of gastrointestinal or extra-gastrointestinal symptoms had raised the suspicion of malabsorption or dumping syndromes. Although it was rare for these patients to present acutely, physicians who care for patients after bariatric surgery need to be familiar with common postoperative syndromes that result from specific nutrient deficiencies [82,83], (L2++). Fat soluble vitamines and minerals abnormalities were reported following metabolic and bariatric surgery, the most common: vitamin B12, folate, zinc, thiamin, copper, vitamin A, and vitamin E deficiencies [84,85], (L2++), [86], (L1+), [87], (L2+), [88], (L2++). Water-soluble vitamins deficiency such as vitamin C (Scurvey) was extremely rare [89], (L3). Acute Wernicke's encephalopathy secondary to thiamine and B12 deficiencies can induce permanent damage despite aggressive replacement therapy [90], (L3).

Acute presentation of these clinical syndromes was rare but great index of suspicion by General Practitioners (GPs) and bariatric teams is expected and needed for early diagnosis and effective treatment. In any acute presentation of the nutritional syndromes, acute surgical catastrophe has to be excluded first, then a multidisciplinary team approach of collaboration of admitting surgeon or physician, endocrinologist and gastroenterologist would resolve the problem. Acute psychiatric and neurological bariatric emergencies such as Wernicke's encephalopathy would entail involvement of neuro-psychiatric teams.

Algorithm of management of acute presentations after bariatric surgery

Based on the evidence from 90 papers including 830,998 patients an algorithm was suggested (Figures 2, 3 and 4).

This pathway is helping to initiate a correct management plan and to provide a standardised care for these critical patients. This algorithm is expected to induce hot discussions among surgeons, emergency physicians and endocrinologists, as there are no comprehensive guidelines of management. The current evidence of more than 800,000 patients is supporting the pathway and the conclusions of this article. The algorithm is in its initial stage and it needs independent assessment by further research.

Limitations of the study

1. The opinions and conclusions of this review were based on the assessing pool data of the outcomes following bariatric operations. The presented evidence was variable in strength as in any meta-analysis or systematic review studies. Most recent studies were included. 80% studies were published in or after 2008. This supports the current evidence of how to manage this special group of patients.
2. The evidence was concluded from the most common operations; i.e. LRYGB, SG & LAGB. Referral to other operations like bilio-pancreatic diversion or duodenal switch was made on specific issues.
3. Great heterogeneity was found among the studies and a systematic review or meta-analysis looking at 7 complications following different bariatric operations, surgical teams and experience, type of patients, co-morbidities, period of follow up was considered impossible.
4. Studies selection: the abstracts of 6358 studies were assessed, only 90 studies were selected. Studies were excluded when they were small (less than 5 subjects, except in case of very rare complications like Scurvy following BS), not relevant to the research subjects. Some of the studies were not included because they were published before laparoscopic era or they were open bariatric studies. Also bariatric studies, which were published in other languages, were not searched and not included. This indicates a certain degree of selection bias. However, efforts were made to include the most powerful and robust study where possible.
5. Algorithm tables for management pathway is based on the evidence from these papers, majority of which were published in the last 3 years (2010–2013). It provides general management route and by no means represents a pathway for managing every case. Every patient has to be taken as an individual case.
6. Level of majority of evidence was L2+ (except in some areas), and this has to be taken in consideration when applying evidence in clinical practice. Surgeons, medical colleagues and emergency physicians practices and experience in dealing with bariatric patients have been evolving and the current view in this paper may help towards formulating guidelines to improve the standards of care these patients currently receiving, and avoid the preventable mortality and severe morbidity that unfortunately happening.

Conclusions

Preventable serious complications can follow bariatric surgery, the effective management of which is depending on the awareness and early diagnosis of the acute surgical or medical cause. Effective communication with the bariatric team is essential to initiate an early and active management plan. Catastrophic outcomes are still reported and an algorithm of actions is proposed to prevent or reduce these incidents and mortality associated with bariatric emergencies.

Competing interests

Dr AH and Dr SE have no conflicts of interest or financial ties to disclose.

Author's contribution

Dr AH designed the study, drafted the manuscript, critically appraised the paper and approved the final version. Dr SE contributed to the design and concept of the study, critically reviewed and approved the final version.

Disclosure

The authors confirm no conflict of interest and no financial interest or ties of any kind in relation to this paper.

References

1. Buchwald H, Oien DM: **Metabolic/bariatric surgery Worldwide 2008.** *Obes Surg* 2009, **12**:1605–1611.
2. Obesity, NICE Clinical Guideline: *Obesity: the prevention, identification, assessment and management of overweight and obesity in adults and children.* 2006. http://www.nice.org.uk/guidance/date of access 20/11/2012.
3. American Gastroenterological Association: **American Gastroenterology Association medical position statement on obesity.** *Gastroenterology* 2002, **123**:879–881.
4. Hussain A, Mahmood H, EL-Hasani S: **Can gastric bypass surgery provide a lifelong solution for diabetes mellitus?** *Can J Surg* 2009, **52**:E269–E275.
5. Cossu ML, Meloni GB, Alagna S, Tilocca PL, Pilo L, Profili S, Noya G: **Emergency surgical conditions after biliopancreatic diversion.** *Obes Surg* 2007, **5**:637–641.

6. Zhang N, Maffei A, Cerabona T, Pahuja A, Omana J, Kaul A: **Reduction in obesity-related comorbidities: is gastric bypass better than sleeve gastrectomy?** *Surg Endosc* 2013, **27**:1273–1280.
7. Sjöström L, Narbro K, Sjöström CD, Karason K, Larsson B, Wedel H, Lystig T, Sullivan M, Bouchard C, Carlsson B, Bengtsson C, Dahlgren S, Gummesson A, Jacobson P, Karlsson J, Lindroos AK, Lönroth H, Näslund I, Olbers T, Stenlöf K, Torgerson J, Agren G, Carlsson LM: **Effects of bariatric surgery on mortality in Swedish obese subjects.** *N Engl J Med* 2007, **357**:741–752.
8. Mechanick JI, Youdim A, Jones DB, Garvey T, Hurley D, McMahon M, Heinberg L, Kushner R, Adams T, Shikora S, Dixon J, Brethauer S: **Clinical practice guidelines for the perioperative nutritional, metabolic, and nonsurgical support of the bariatric surgery patient —2013 update: cosponsored by American Association of Clinical Endocrinologists, The Obesity Society, and American Society for Meta bolic & Bariatric Surgery.** *Endocr Pract* 2013 doi:10.4158/EP12437.GL.
9. Shin JH, Worni M, Castleberry AW, Pietrobon R, Omotosho PA, Silberberg M, Østbye T: **The application of comorbidity indices to predict early postoperative outcomes after laparoscopic Roux-en-Y gastric bypass: a nationwide comparative analysis of over 70,000 cases.** *Obes Surg* 2013, **23**:638–649.
10. Fernández-Esparrach G, Córdova H, Bordas JM, Gómez-Molins I, Ginès A, Pellisé M, Sendino O, González-Suárez B, Cárdenas A, Balderramo D, Lacy AM, Delgado S: **Llach J [Endoscopic management of the complications of bariatric surgery. Experience of more than 400 interventions].** *Gastroenterol Hepatol* 2011, **34**:131–136.
11. Khan MA, Grinberg R, Johnson S, Afthinos JN, Gibbs KE: **Perioperative risk factors for 30-day mortality after bariatric surgery: is functional status important?** *Surg Endosc* 2013, **27**:1772–1777.
12. Cendán JC, Abu-aouf D, Gabrielli A, Caruso LJ, Rout WR, Hocking MP, Layon AJ: **Utilization of intensive care resources in bariatric surgery.** *Obes Surg* 2005, **9**:1247–1251.
13. Gonzalez-Sánchez JA, Corujo-Vázquez O, Sahai-Hernández M: **Bariatric surgery patients: reasons to visit emergency department after surgery.** *Bol Asoc Med P R* 2007, **4**:279–8.
14. Campanile FC, Boru CE, Rizzello M, Puzziello A, Copaescu C, Cavallaro G, Silecchia G: **Acute complications after laparoscopic bariatric procedures: update for the general surgeon.** *Langenbecks Arch Surg* 2013, **398**:669–686.
15. Kirshtein B, Lantsberg L, Mizrahi S, Avinoach E: **Bariatric emergencies for non-bariatric surgeons: complications of laparoscopic gastric banding.** *Obes Surg* 2010, **11**:1468–1478.
16. Monkhouse SJ, Morgan JD, Norton SA: **Complications of bariatric surgery: presentation and emergency management–a review.** *Ann R Coll Surg Engl* 2009, **94**:280–286.
17. Car Peterko A, Kirac I, Gaurina A, Diklić D, Bekavac-Bešlin M: **Diagnosis and management of acute and early complications of/after bariatric surgery.** *Dig Dis* 2012, **30**:178–181.
18. Heneghan HM, Meron-Eldar S, Yenumula P, Rogula T, Brethauer SA, Schauer PR: **Incidence and management of bleeding complications after gastric bypass surgery in the morbidly obese.** *Surg Obes Relat Dis* 2012, **6**:729–735.
19. Mehran A, Szomstein S, Zundel N, Rosenthal R: **Management of acute bleeding after laparoscopic Roux-en-Y gastric bypass.** *Obes Surg* 2003, **13**:842–847.
20. Podnos YD, Jimenez JCWilson SE, Stevens CM, Nguyen NT: **Complications after laparoscopic gastric bypass: a review of 3464 cases.** *Arch Surg* 2003, **138**:957–961.
21. Torab FC, Hefny AF, Taha M, Abou-Rebyeh H, Abu-Zidan FM: **Delayed life-threatening upper gastrointestinal bleeding as a complication of laparoscopic adjustable gastric banding: case report and review of the literature.** *Asian J Surg* 2012, **35**:127–130.
22. Rao AD, Ramalingam G: **Exsanguinating hemorrhage following gastric erosion after laparoscopic adjustable gastric banding.** *Obes Surg* 2006, **16**:1675–1678.
23. Rabl C, Peeva S, Prado K, James AW, Rogers SJ, Posselt A, Campos GM: **Early and late abdominal bleeding after Roux-en-Y gastric bypass: sources and tailored therapeutic strategies.** *Obes Surg* 2011, **21**:413–420.
24. Mala T, Søvik TT, Schou CF, Kristinsson J: **Blood clot obstruction of the jejunojejunostomy after laparoscopic gastric bypass.** *Surg Obes Relat Dis* 2012, **9**:234–237.
25. Boru C, Silecchia G: **Bariatric emergencies: what the general surgeon should know.** *Chirurgia (Bucur)* 2010, **105**:455–464.
26. Nandipati K, Lin E, Husain F, Perez S, Srinivasan J, Sweeney JF, Davis SS: **Factors predicting the increased risk for return to the operating room in bariatric patients: a NSQIP database study.** *Surg Endosc* 2013, **27**:1172–1177.
27. Ferreira LE, Song LM, Baron TH: **Management of acute postoperative hemorrhage in the bariatric patient.** *Gastrointest Endosc Clin N Am* 2011, **21**:287–294.
28. Penna M, Markar SR, Venkat-Raman V, Karthikesalingam A, Hashemi M: **Linear-stapled versus circular-stapled laparoscopic gastrojejunal anastomosis in morbid obesity: meta-analysis.** *Surg Laparosc Endosc Percutan Tech* 2012, **22**:95–101.
29. Choi YY, Bae J, Hur KY, Choi D, Kim YJ: **Reinforcing the staple line during laparoscopic sleeve gastrectomy: does it have advantages? A meta-analysis.** *Obes Surg* 2012, **8**:1206–1213.
30. **Acute upper gastrointestinal bleeding Management.** http://www.nice.org.uk/nicemedia/live/13762/59549/59549.pdf. Date of access 20/11/2012.
31. Bakhos C, Alkhoury F, Kyriakides T, Reinhold R, Nadzam G: **Early postoperative hemorrhage after open and laparoscopic roux-en-y gastric bypass.** *Obes Surg* 2009, **2**:153–157.
32. Tang SJ, Rivas H, Tang L, Lara LF, Sreenarasimhaiah J, Rockey DC: **Endoscopic hemostasis using endoclip in early gastrointestinal hemorrhage after gastric bypass surgery.** *Obes Surg* 2007, **9**:1261–1267.
33. Gill RS, Whitlock KA, Mohamed R, Sarkhosh K, Birch DW, Karmali S: **The role of upper gastrointestinal endoscopy in treating postoperative complications in bariatric surgery.** *J Interv Gastroenterol* 2012, **2**:37–41.
34. Kitahama S, Smith MD, Rosencrantz DR, Patterson EJ: **Is bariatric surgery safe in patients who refuse blood transfusion?** *Surg Obes Relat Dis* 2012, **9**:390–394.
35. Edwards MA, Jones DB, Ellsmere J, Grinbaum R, Schneider BE: **Anastomotic leak following antecolic versus retrocolic laparoscopic Roux-en-Y gastric bypass for morbid obesity.** *Obes Surg* 2007, **3**:292–297.
36. Smith MD, Patterson E, Wahed AS, Belle SH, Berk PD, Courcoulas AP, Dakin GF, Flum DR, Machado L, Mitchell JE, Pender J, Pomp A, Pories W, Ramanathan R, Schrope B, Staten M, Ude A, Wolfe BM: **Thirty-day mortality after bariatric surgery: independently adjudicated causes of death in the longitudinal assessment of bariatric surgery.** *Obes Surg* 2011, **21**:1687–1692.
37. Masoomi H, Kim H, Reavis KM, Mills S, Stamos MJ, Nguyen NT: **Analysis of factors predictive of gastrointestinal tract leak in laparoscopic and open gastric bypass.** *Arch Surg* 2011, **146**:1048–1051.
38. Haddad A, Tapazoglou N, Singh K, Averbach A: **Role of intraoperative esophagogastroenteroscopy in minimizing gastrojejunostomy-related morbidity: experience with 2,311 laparoscopic gastric bypasses with linear stapler anastomosis.** *Obes Surg* 2012, **22**:1928–1933.
39. Kavuturu S, Rogers AM, Haluck RS: **Routine drain placement in Roux-en-Y gastric bypass: an expanded retrospective comparative study of 755 patients and review of the literature.** *Obes Surg* 2012, **22**:177–181.
40. Sakran N, Goitein D, Raziel A, Keidar A, Beglaibter N, Grinbaum R, Matter I, Alfici R, Mahajna A, Waksman I, Shimonov M, Assalia A: **Gastric leaks after sleeve gastrectomy: a multicenter experience with 2,834 patients.** *Surg Endosc* 2013, **27**:240–245.
41. Moszkowicz D, Arienzo R, Khettab I, Rahmi G, Zinzindohoué F, Berger A, Chevallier JM: **Sleeve gastrectomy severe complications: is it always a reasonable surgical option?** *Obes Surg* 2013, **23**:1675–1676.
42. Parikh M, Issa R, McCrillis A, Saunders JK, Ude-Welcome A, Gagner M: **Surgical strategies that may decrease leak after laparoscopic sleeve gastrectomy: a systematic review and meta-analysis of 9991 cases.** *Ann Surg* 2013, **257**:231–237.
43. Simon F, Siciliano I, Gillet A, Castel B, Coffin B, Msika S: **Gastric Leak After Laparoscopic Sleeve Gastrectomy: Early Covered Self-Expandable Stent Reduces Healing Time.** *Obes Surg* 2013, **23**:687–692.
44. Morales MP, Miedema BW, Scott JS, de la Torre RA: **Management of postsurgical leaks in the bariatric patient.** *Gastrointest Endosc Clin N Am* 2011, **21**:295–304.
45. de Aretxabala X, Leon J, Wiedmaier G, Turu I, Ovalle C, Maluenda F, Gonzalez C, Humphrey J, Hurtado M, Benavides C: **Gastric leak after sleeve gastrectomy: analysis of its management.** *Obes Surg* 2011, **21**:1232–1237.
46. Kawkabani Marchini A, Denys A, Paroz A, Romy S, Suter M, Desmartines N, Meuli R, Schmidt S: **The four different types of internal hernia occurring after laparascopic Roux-en-Y gastric bypass performed for morbid obesity: are there any multidetector computed tomography (MDCT) features permitting their distinction?** *Obes Surg* 2011, **4**:506–516.

47. De la Cruz-Muñoz N, Cabrera JC, Cuesta M, Hartnett S, Rojas R: **Closure of mesenteric defect can lead to decrease in internal hernias after Roux-en-Y gastric bypass.** *Surg Obes Relat Dis* 2011, **2**:176–180.
48. Bell BJ, Bour ES, Scott JD, Cobb WS, Carbonell AM: **Management of complications after laparoscopic Roux-en-Y gastric bypass.** *Minerva Chir* 2009, **3**:265–276.
49. Campos JM, Evangelista LF, Ferraz AA, Galvao Neto MP, De Moura EG, Sakai P, Ferraz EM: **Treatment of ring slippage after gastric bypass: long-term results after endoscopic dilation with an achalasia balloon (with videos).** *Gastrointest Endosc* 2010, **1**:44–49.
50. Matthews BD, Sing RF, De Legge MH, Ponsky JL, Heniford BT: **Initial results with a stapled gastrojejunostomy for the laparoscopic isolated laparoscopic Roux-en-Y gastric bypass.** *Am J Surg* 2000, **179**:476–481.
51. Brockmeyer JR, Simon TE, Jacob RK, Husain F, Choi Y: **Upper gastrointestinal swallow study following bariatric surgery: institutional review and review of the literature.** *Obes Surg* 2012, **22**:1039–1043.
52. Abasbassi M, Pottel H, Deylgat B, Vansteenkiste F, Van Rooy F, Devriendt D, D'Hondt M: **Small bowel obstruction after antecolic antegastric laparoscopic Roux-en-Y gastric bypass without division of small bowel mesentery: a single-centre, 7-year review.** *Obes Surg* 2011, **21**:1822–1827.
53. Shimizu H, Maia M, Kroh M, Schauer PR, Brethauer SA: **Surgical management of early small bowel obstruction after laparoscopic Roux-en-Y gastric bypass.** *Surg Obes Relat Dis* 2012, **9**:718–724.
54. Egan RJ, Monkhouse SJ, Meredith HE, Bates SE, Morgan JD, Norton SA, Egan RJ, Monkhouse SJ, Meredith HE, Bates SE, Morgan JD, Norton SA: **The Reporting of gastric band slip and related complications; a review of the literature.** *Obes Surg* 2010, **24**:1280–1288.
55. Sanyal AJ, Sugerman HJ, Kellum JM, Engle KM, Wolfe L: **Stomal complications of gastric bypass: incidence and outcome of therapy.** *Am J Gastroenterol* 1992, **9**:1165–1169.
56. Deylgat B, D'Hondt M, Pottel H, Vansteenkiste F, Van Rooy F, Devriendt D: **Indications, safety, and feasibility of conversion of failed bariatric surgery to Roux-en-Y gastric bypass: a retrospective comparative study with primary laparoscopic Roux-en-Y gastric bypass.** *Surg Endosc* 2012, **7**:1997–2002.
57. MacLean L, Rhode B, Nohr C, Katz S: **P McLean.Stomal ulcer after gastric bypass.** *J Am Coll Surg* 1997, **185**:1–7.
58. Frezza EE, Herbert H, Ford R, Wachtel MS: **Endoscopic suture removal at gastrojejunal anastomosis after Roux-en-Y gastric bypass to prevent marginal ulceration.** *Surg Obes Relat Dis* 2007, **3**:619–622.
59. Schirmer B, Erenoglu C, Miller A: **Flexible endoscopy in the management of patients undergoing Roux-en-Y gastric bypass.** *Obes Surg* 2002, **12**:634–638.
60. Capella JF, Capella RF: **Gastro-gastric fistulas and marginal ulcers in gastric bypass procedures for weight reduction.** *Obes Surg* 1999, **9**:22–27.
61. D'Hondt MA, Pottel H, Devriendt D, Van Rooy F, Vansteenkiste F: **Can a short course of prophylactic low-dose proton pump inhibitor therapy prevent stomal ulceration after laparoscopic Roux-en-Y gastric bypass?** *Obes Surg* 2010, **20**:595–599.
62. Csendes A, Burgos AM, Altuve J, Bonacic S: **Incidence of marginal ulcer 1 month and 1 to 2 years after gastric bypass: a prospective consecutive endoscopic evaluation of 442 patients with morbid obesity.** *Obes Surg* 2009, **19**:135–138.
63. Racu C, Mehran A: **Marginal ulcer after Roux-en-Y Gastric Bypass. Pain for the patient Pain for the Surgeon.** *Bariatric Times* 2010, **7**:23–25.
64. Ukleja A, Afonso BB, Pimentel R, Szomstein S, Rosenthal R: **Outcome of endoscopic balloon dilation of strictures after laparoscopic gastric bypass.** *Surg Endosc* 2008, **22**:1746–1750.
65. Becattini C, Agnelli G, Manina G, Noya G, Rondelli F: **Venous thromboembolism after laparoscopic bariatric surgery for morbid obesity: clinical burden and prevention.** *Surg Obes Relat Dis* 2012, **1**:108–115.
66. Morino M, Toppino M, Forestieri P, Angrisani L, Allaix ME, Scopinaro N: **Mortality after bariatric surgery: analysis of 13,871 morbidly obese patients from a national registry.** *Ann Surg* 2007, **6**:1002–1007.
67. Avriel A, Warner E, Avinoach E, Avnon LS, Shteinberg M, Shteinberg D, Heimer D, Yona S, Maimon N: **Major respiratory adverse events after laparascopic gastric banding surgery for morbid obesity.** *Respir Med* 2012, **106**:1192–1198.
68. Gupta PK, Gupta H, Kaushik M, Fang X, Miller WJ, Morrow LE, Armour-Forse R: **Predictors of pulmonary complications after bariatric surgery.** *Surg Obes Relat Dis* 2012, **8**:574–581.
69. Gasa M, Salord N, Fortuna AM, Mayos M, Embid C, Vilarrasa N, Montserrat JM, Monasterio C: **Optimizing screening of severe obstructive sleep apnea in patients undergoing bariatric surgery.** *Surg Obes Relat Dis* 2012, **9**:539–546.
70. Pournaras DJ, Aasheim ET, Søvik TT, Andrews R, Mahon D, Welbourn R, Olbers T, le Roux CW: **Effect of the definition of type II diabetes remission in the evaluation of bariatric surgery for metabolic disorders.** *Br J Surg* 2012, **99**:100–103.
71. Roslin MS, Dudiy Y, Weiskopf J, Damani T, Shah P: **Comparison between RYGB, DS, and VSG effect on glucose homeostasis.** *Obes Surg* 2012, **22**:1281–1286.
72. Reis CE, Alvarez-Leite JI, Bressan J, Alfenas RC: **Role of bariatric-metabolic surgery in the treatment of obese type 2 diabetes with body mass index < 35 kg/m2: a literature review.** *Diabetes Technol Ther* 2012, **14**:365–372.
73. Foster-Schubert KE: **Hypoglycemia complicating bariatric surgery: incidence and mechanisms.** *Curr Opin Endocrinol Diabetes Obes* 2011, **2**:129–133.
74. Ritz P, Vaurs C, Bertrand M, Anduze Y, Guillaume E, Hanaire H: **Usefulness of acarbose and dietary modifications to limit glycemic variability following Roux-en-Y gastric bypass as assessed by continuous glucose monitoring.** *Diabetes Technol Ther* 2012, **8**:736–740.
75. Nannipieri M, Mari A, Anselmino M, Baldi S, Barsotti E, Guarino D, Camastra S, Bellini R, Berta RD, Ferrannini E: **The role of beta-cell function and insulin sensitivity in the remission of type 2 diabetes after gastric bypass surgery.** *J Clin Endocrinol Metab* 2011, **96**:E1372–E1379.
76. Meneghini LF: **Impact of bariatric surgery on type 2 diabetes.** *Cell Biochem Biophys* 2007, **48**:97–102.
77. Bantle JP, Ikramuddin S, Kellogg TA, Buchwald H: **Hyperinsulinemic hypoglycemia developing late after gastric bypass.** *Obes Surg* 2007, **17**:592–594.
78. Miñambres I, Chico A, Pérez A: **Severe Hypocalcemia due to Vitamin D Deficiency after Extended Roux-en-Y Gastric Bypass.** *Journal of Obesity* 2011, **2011**:3.
79. Pietras SM, Holick MF: **Refractory hypocalcemia following near-total thyroidectomy in a patient with a prior roux-en-y gastric bypass.** *Obes Surg* 2009, **19**:524–526.
80. Moizé V, Andreu A, Flores L, Torres F, Ibarzabal A, Delgado S, Lacy A, Rodriguez L, Vidal J: **Long-term dietary intake and nutritional deficiencies following Sleeve gastrectomy or Roux-En-Y gastric bypass in a Mediterranean population.** *J Acad Nutr Diet* 2013, **113**:400–410.
81. Bal BS, Finelli FC, Shope TR, Koch TR: **Nutritional deficiencies after bariatric surgery.** *Nat Rev Endocrinol* 2012, **8**:544–556.
82. Koch TR, Finelli FC: **Postoperative metabolic and nutritional complications of bariatric surgery.** *Gastroenterol Clin North Am* 2010, **39**:109–124.
83. Hammer HF: **Medical complications of bariatric surgery: focus on malabsorption and dumping syndrome.** *Dig Dis* 2012, **30**:182–186.
84. Frantz DJ: **Neurologic complications of bariatric surgery: involvement of central, peripheral, and enteric nervous systems.** *Curr Gastroenterol Rep* 2012, **14**:367–372.
85. Schweitzer DH, Posthuma EF: **Prevention of vitamin and mineral deficiencies after bariatric surgery: evidence and algorithms.** *Obes Surg* 2008, **18**:1485–1488.
86. Aasheim ET, Björkman S, Søvik TT, Engström M, Hanvold SE, Mala T, Olbers T, Bøhmer T: **Vitamin status after bariatric surgery: a randomized study of gastric bypass and duodenal switch.** *Am J Clin Nutr* 2009, **90**:15–22.
87. Granado-Lorencio F, Simal-Antón A, Blanco-Navarro I, González-Dominguez T, Pérez-Sacristán B: **Depletion of serum carotenoid and other fat-soluble vitamin concentrations following obesity surgery.** *Obes Surg* 2011, **21**:1605–1611.
88. Folope V, Coëffier M, Déchelotte P: **Nutritional deficiencies associated with bariatric surgery.** *Gastroenterol Clin Biol* 2007, **31**:369–377.
89. Stolle LB, Heidemann E, Bischoff-Mikkelsen M: **Scurvy is not entirely a historical disease.** *Ugeskr Laeger* 2012, **174**:499–500.
90. Jethava A, Dasanu CA: **Acute Wernicke encephalopathy and sensorineural hearing loss complicating bariatric surgery.** *Conn Med* 2012, **76**:603–605.

16

Sigmoid volvulus in pregnancy and puerperium: a surgical and obstetric catastrophe

Muhammad R Khan* and Sameer ur Rehman

Abstract

Sigmoid volvulus is a rare surgical complication occurring in pregnancy and puerperium. Only 84 cases of sigmoid volvulus in pregnancy have been reported in the English literature so far. We have reviewed the available literature on this subject and present another case recently managed at our institution. The available literature suggests that over the years, there has been an improvement in the maternal and fetal outcome for this critical condition, but delay in presentation and a further delay in diagnosis remain a challenge for the treating physicians. Our patient was a 30-week pregnant lady, who presented late with 6 days history of abdominal pain, distension and absolute constipation. She had evidence of multi-organ dysfunction at presentation due to complicated sigmoid volvulus. She was resuscitated and surgical exploration revealed gangrenous large bowel. Bowel resection with diverting ileostomy was performed, but she succumbed to the septic shock due to late presentation. Acute surgical pathology may be overlooked in pregnant patients due to reluctance in radiological workup and a high index of suspicion is essential for enhanced outcome. There is a need to increase the awareness amongst the obstetricians and general practitioners. Early diagnosis and referral and timely surgical intervention could significantly improve the outcome of this surgical and obstetric catastrophe.

Keywords: Sigmoid volvulus, Pregnancy, Outcome

Background

Sigmoid volvulus in pregnancy is a rare but serious complication associated with a significant maternal and fetal mortality [1]. The fundamental problem of sigmoid volvulus in pregnancy is that of delay in presentation and further delay in diagnosis leading to ischemia of the colon, which requires bowel resection and colostomy as seen in most of the reported cases [2-20]. Timely surgical intervention is essential to reduce maternal and fetal morbidity and mortality [1]. Perforation, peritonitis and sepsis can be the maternal complications if intervention is not done early in the course of the disease. The fetal complications include preterm delivery, intrauterine death and neonatal sepsis. We have reviewed the available literature on this subject and report another case of a 30-week pregnant lady who presented to us with complicated sigmoid volvulus (Table 1). There is a need to increase the awareness amongst the general practitioners and community obstetricians for this potentially life threatening condition. A high index of suspicion and judicious use of modern radiological imaging may help make an early diagnosis and improve the maternal and fetal outcomes.

Case presentation

A 25-year-old pregnant lady, gravida 2 and para 1, presented to the emergency room with 6 days history of lower abdominal pain, abdominal distension, bilious vomiting and constipation. She had no significant past medical or surgical history and her menstrual and antenatal history were uneventful. She was being managed conservatively for these complaints at a local hospital before presenting to us in the emergency. On examination, she was dehydrated, tachycardiac with a heart rate of 136 beats per minute and tachypneic with a respiratory rate of 28 per minute. Her initial blood pressure was 102/69 mmHg and she was drowsy. Her abdomen

* Correspondence: khan.rizwan@aku.edu
Department of Surgery and Medical College, Aga Khan University & Hospital, Stadium Road, Karachi, 74800, Pakistan

Table 1 Reported Cases of Sigmoid Volvulus in Pregnancy and Puerperium

Authors	Year of the study	Number of cases reported	Stage of pregnancy in weeks	Duration of symptoms in days	Status of colon	Treatment offered	Outcome	
							Mother	Fetus
Recent Cases	1978 – 2011	20						
Present case	2011	1	30	6 days	Gangrenous	Total colectomy with proximal ileostomy	Expired	IUD
Kolusari A et al [2]	2009	4	7	1	Gangrenous	Resection of sigmoid colon with primary anastomosis	Healthy	Alive
			31	2	Gangrenous	Resection of sigmoid colon with proximal colostomy	Healthy	IUD
			32	2	Gangrenous	Resection of sigmoid colon with proximal colostomy	Healthy	Alive
			Puerperium	3	Gangrenous	Resection of sigmoid colon with proximal colostomy	Expired	Alive
Vo TM et al [3]	2008	1	28	1	Gangrenous	Resection of sigmoid colon with proximal colostomy	Healthy	Alive
Iwamoto I et al [4]	2007	1	35	3	Perforated	Repair of perforation with proximal colostomy	Expired	IUD
Sascha Dua R et al [5]	2007	1	Puerperium	1	Viable	Laparotomy and sigmoidopexy	Healthy	Alive
Machado NO et al [6]	2006	1	18	1	Viable	Resection of sigmoid colon with primary anastomosis	Healthy	Alive
Alshawi JS [7]	2005	1	28 & 35 (recurrent)	1	Viable	Sigmoidoscopy and decompression followed by elective sigmoid colectomy	Healthy	Alive
De U et al [8]	2005	1	24	3	Gangrenous	Resection of sigmoid colon with proximal colostomy	Healthy	IUD
Joshi MA et al [9]	1999	1	28	2	Gangrenous	Resection of sigmoid colon with proximal colostomy	Healthy	IUD
Lurie S et al [10]	1997	1	Ectopic Pregnancy	2	Viable	Laparotomy and de-torsion of volvulus	Healthy	Ectopic
Lord SA et al [11]	1996	1	36	2	Gangrenous	Resection of sigmoid colon with proximal colostomy	Healthy	Alive
Allen JC [12]	1990	1	28	1	Viable	Sigmoidoscopy and decompression	Healthy	Alive
Keating JP et al [13]	1985	1	34	1	Viable	Resection of sigmoid colon with double barrel colostomy	Healthy	Alive
Hofmeyr GJ et al [14]	1985	2	33	3	Gangrenous	Resection of sigmoid colon with proximal colostomy	Healthy	IUD
			26	3	Gangrenous	Resection of sigmoid colon with proximal colostomy	Expired	IUD
Fraser JL et al [15]	1983	1	32	1	Viable	Laparotomy and de-torsion of volvulus	Healthy	Alive
Fuller JK et al [16]	1978	1	Puerperium	1	Viable	Laparotomy and de-torsion of volvulus	Healthy	Alive
Lazaro EJ et al [17]	1958 – 1969	13						
Harer WB Jr. et al [18]	1944 – 1958	11						
Kohn SG et al [19]	1931 – 1944	12						
Lambert AC [20]	Before 1931	29						

Legend: IUD = Intrauterine Death

was distended and tense, with generalized tenderness and a tympanitic note on percussion. The uterine size was of 30 weeks gestation. Rectal examination revealed no stool and cervical os was closed on per vaginal examination. She was clinically suspected to have peritonitis with evidence of septic shock. She was resuscitated with intravenous fluids and antibiotics.

Plain radiographs of the chest and abdomen showed pneumoperitoneum, a single fetus and a distended gas filled transverse colon. Ultrasound scan of the abdomen revealed moderate amount of free fluid with mobile internal echoes representing bowel content and intra-uterine death of the fetus. Her laboratory workup revealed severe electrolyte imbalance with serum potassium of 6.3 mmol/L (normal 3.5-5) and blood glucose level of 39 mg/dL (normal 80–160). She had evidence of severe metabolic acidosis with serum pH of 7.18 (normal 7.36-7.44), hypoxia with pO2 of 39 mmHg (normal 85–105) and deranged coagulation. The surgical and obstetric teams in the emergency room evaluated the patient. While being resuscitated in the emergency room, the conscious level of the patient dropped further and she was intubated and put on the mechanical ventilator.

With the clinical diagnosis of bowel perforation and peritonitis, the patient was taken up for emergency laparotomy. Intra-operatively findings were of sigmoid volvulus resulting in closed loop obstruction leading to distension and ischemia of whole large bowel. The whole of the colon was dilated, friable, and gangrenous. Multiple perforations were identified in the colon with around 800 ml of feculent material aspirated on opening the abdomen. Whole colon was mobilized & resected and diverting ileostomy with a Hartman's procedure was done. A lower segment caesarean section was done for delivering the dead fetus and modified B-lynch sutures applied to the uterus. Post-operatively, she was continued on broad-spectrum antibiotics and shifted to the intensive care unit. She had an initial period of recovery for a couple of days, but subsequently, her pulmonary function deteriorated with development of pneumonia and adult respiratory distress syndrome. In addition to high ventilator support, she also needed increasing dose of inotropes and eventually expired on the 8th post-operative day due to overwhelming sepsis and organ dysfunction.

Discussion

The incidence of intestinal obstruction in pregnancy ranges from 1 in 1500 to 1 in 66431 deliveries [2]. Intestinal obstruction in pregnancy can be caused by many factors including congenital or postoperative adhesions, volvulus, intussusceptions, hernia and appendicitis [1]. Sigmoid volvulus is the most common cause of bowel obstruction complicating pregnancy, accounting for up to 44 per cent of cases [21]. Pregnancy itself is considered to be the precipitating factor for sigmoid volvulus. The occurrence of sigmoid volvulus in pregnancy is due to displacement, compression and partial obstruction of a redundant or abnormally elongated sigmoid colon by the gravid uterus [18]. This could probably explain the increased incidence of sigmoid volvulus in the third trimester of pregnancy [1]. Despite this higher propensity in the third trimester, there have been reports of this complication developing in the early pregnancy as well as the puerperium [2,5,16,18].

To date, 84 cases of sigmoid volvulus have been reported occurring in the pregnancy and puerperium (Table 1). Lambert [20] reported 29 cases of sigmoid volvulus before 1931, followed by another 12 cases reported by Kohn et al [19] between 1931 and 1944. Subsequently, all the previously reported cases were reviewed by Harer et al [18] in 1958, who reported an additional 11 cases between 1994 and 1958. Later on, Lazaro et al [17] compiled another 13 cases occurring between 1558 and 1969. In this report, we have identified 19 more cases reported till 2009, and include another case managed recently at our institution.

The diagnosis of sigmoid volvulus is suspected when a pregnant female presents with a clinical triad of abdominal pain, distention, and absolute constipation. The average time from the onset of obstructive symptoms until presentation has been reported to be 48 hours [1]. This is largely because pregnancy itself masks the clinical picture since abdominal pain, nausea, and leukocytosis can occur in an otherwise normal course of pregnancy [13]. In our review of recent 20 cases, the mean delay between the onset of symptoms to presentation was 2 days, with a range from few hours to as many as 6 days, as seen in our case. Six patients presented more than 48 hours after the onset of symptoms. Harer et al [18] also noted similar delay in presentation in their review and concluded that such a delay in diagnosis and surgical intervention had a significant impact on the ultimate outcome of the mother and fetus.

The maternal and fetal outcome in sigmoid volvulus has been directly related to the degree of bowel ischemia and subsequent systemic sepsis. In our analysis of recent 20 cases, there were 4 (20 %) maternal and 8 (40 %) fetal deaths, including one ectopic pregnancy. It is important to note that all the maternal deaths occurred in the group of patients where delay in presentation and surgical intervention was more than 2 days. [2,4,14] Similarly, 5 fetal deaths were seen in patients who presented after 48 hours of onset of symptoms, as compared to 2 fetal deaths in patients presenting early in the course of the disease. This observation highlights the fact that high index of clinical suspicion is vital in cases of intestinal obstruction in pregnant patients. This facts needs to be emphasized amongst the general practitioners and community obstetricians primarily responsible for taking care of these patients.

Another important area of concern is the reluctance in the utilization of modern radiological diagnostic tools in pregnant patients. There have always been concerns about the radiation exposure of the fetus during pregnancy. Significant radiation exposure may lead to chromosomal mutations, neurologic abnormalities, mental retardation, and increased risk of childhood leukemia. Cumulating radiation dosage is the primary risk factor for adverse fetal effects, but fetal age at exposure is also important [22-24]. Exposure during the first week of gestation results in highest rates of fetal mortality. The next most sensitive time period is between 10 and 17 weeks of gestation, when central nervous system teratogenesis becomes an important consideration. After this period, the concern shifts from teratogenesis to the risk of childhood hematologic malignancy. It has been recommended that the cumulative radiation dose to the fetus during pregnancy should be less than 5–10 rads [25]. In general, no single diagnostic study exceeds 5 rads of radiation exposure. As an example, the radiation dose to the fetus for a plain abdominal radiograph averages 0.1–0.3 rads, while a CT of the pelvis and abdomen yields up to 5 rads of fetal exposure [26]. In any case, the health and life of the mother takes priority over the concerns for the fetus and judicious use of radiation may help make an early diagnosis with optimal outcome for both the mother and the fetus.

The management of intestinal obstruction and perforation in pregnant women is pretty much similar to that of non-pregnant women. The basis of therapy is early surgical intervention [27]. Surgery should be performed via midline vertical laparotomy. In the third trimester, if sufficient intestinal exposure cannot be obtained due to enlarged uterus, a caesarean section must be carried out [28]. The entire bowel should be examined for other areas of obstruction. Intestinal viability should be assessed cautiously and segmental resection with or without anastomosis is often necessary [27].

Conclusions

Sigmoid volvulus complicating pregnancy is very rare condition with significant maternal and fetal morbidity and mortality. Timely diagnosis mandates high index of clinical suspicion in patients presenting with abdominal pain, distension and absolute constipation. Hesitancy in getting X-rays in view of pregnant situation must be avoided and appropriate management must be defined. Delay in diagnosis and treatment beyond 48 hours results in increased fetal and maternal morbidity and mortality. Review of the available literature emphasizes the importance of early diagnosis and timely intervention to minimize maternal and fetal morbidity and mortality.

Consent

A written informed consent was obtained from the next of kin of the patient for publication of this Case report and any accompanying images. A copy of the written consent is available for review by the Editor-in-Chief of this journal.

Competing interests

The author declares that they have no competing interest.

Authors' contribution

MRK conceived the study. SR collected the data and prepared the initial manuscript. The manuscript was critically reviewed and approved by all the authors.

References

1. Perdue PW, Johnson HW Jr, Stafford PW: **Intestinal obstruction complicating pregnancy.** *Am J Surg* 1992, **164:**384–388.
2. Kolusari A, Kurdoglu M, Adali E, Yildizhan R, Sahin HG, Kotan C: **Sigmoid volvulus in pregnancy and puerperium: a case series.** *Cases Journal* 2009, **2:**9275.
3. Vo TM, Gyaneshwar R, Mayer C: **Concurrent sigmoid volvulus and herniation through broad ligament defect during pregnancy: case report and literature review.** *J Obstet Gynaecol Res* 2008, **34:**658–662.
4. Iwamoto I, Miwa K, Fujino T, Douchi T: **Perforated colon volvulus coiling around the uterus in a pregnant woman with a history of severe constipation.** *J Obstet Gynaecol Res* 2007, **33:**731–733.
5. Sascha Dua R, Rothnie ND, Gray EA: **Sigmoid volvulus in the Puerperium.** *Int J Gynaecol Obstet* 2007, **97:**195.
6. Machado NO, Machado LS: **Sigmoid volvulus complicating pregnancy managed by resection and primary anastomosis; case report with literature review.** *Sultan Qaboos Univ Med J* 2009, **9:**84–88.
7. Alshawi JS: **Recurrent sigmoid volvulus in pregnancy: report of a case and review of the literature.** *Dis Colon Rectum* 2005, **48:**1811–1813.
8. De U, De KK: **Sigmoid volvulus complicating pregnancy.** *Indian J Med Sci* 2005, **59:**317–319.
9. Joshi MA, Balsarkar D, Avasare N, Pradhan C, Pereira G, Subramanyan P, *et al*: **Gangrenous sigmoid colon in a pregnant woman.** *Trop Gastroenterol* 1999, **20:**141–142.
10. Lurie S, Katz Z, Rabinerson D, Simon D: **Sigmoid volvulus after medical management with subsequent operative laparoscopy of unruptured ectopic pregnancy.** *Gynecol Obstet Invest* 1997, **43:**204–205.
11. Lord SA, Boswell WC, Hungerpiller JC: **Sigmoid volvulus in pregnancy.** *Am Surg* 1996, **62:**380–382.
12. Allen JC: **Sigmoid volvulus in pregnancy.** *J R Army Med Corps* 1990, **136:**55–56.
13. Keating JP, Jackson DS: **Sigmoid volvulus in late pregnancy.** *J R Army Med Corps* 1985, **131:**72–74.
14. Hofmeyr GJ, Sonnendecker EW: **Sigmoid volvulus in advanced pregnancy. Report of 2 cases.** *S Afr Med J* 1985, **67:**63–64.
15. Fraser JL, Eckert LA: **Volvulus complicating pregnancy.** *Can Med Assoc J* 1983, **128:**1045–1048.
16. Fuller JK, Larrieu AJ: **Sigmoid volvulus in the young: a case following cesarean section.** *Arch Surg* 1978, **113:**316–317.
17. Lazaro EJ, Das PB, Abraham PV: **Volvulus of the sigmoid colon complicating pregnancy.** *Obstet Gynecol* 1969, **33:**553–557.
18. Harer WB Jr, Harer WB Sr: **Volvulus complicating pregnancy and puerperium; report of three cases and review of literature.** *Obstet Gynecol* 1958, **12:**399–406.
19. Kohen SG, Briele HA, Douglas LH: **Volvulus in pregnancy.** *Am J Obst & Gynec* 1944, **48:**398.
20. Lambert AC: *Paris thesis.*: ; 1931.
21. Ballantyne GH, Brandner MD, Beart RW Jr, Ilstrup DM: **Volvulus of the colon.** *Incidence and mortality. Ann Surg* 1985, **202:**83–92.
22. Kennedy A: **Assessment of acute abdominal pain in the pregnant patient.** *Semin Ultrasound CT MR* 2000, **21:**64–77.
23. Toppenberg KS, Hill DA, Miller DP: **Safety of radiographic imaging during pregnancy.** *Am Fam Physician* 1999, **59:**1813–1818.
24. Timins JK: **Radiation during pregnancy.** *N J Med* 2001, **98:**29–33.
25. Karam PA: **Determining and reporting fetal radiation exposure from diagnostic radiation.** *Health Phys* 2000, **79:**S85–S90.
26. Chen MM, Coakley FV, Kaimal A, Laros RK Jr: **Guidelines for computed tomography and magnetic resonance imaging use during pregnancy and lactation.** *Obstet Gynecol* 2008, **112:**333–340.
27. Allen JR, Helling TS, Langenfeld M: **Intraabdominal surgery during pregnancy.** *Am J Surg* 1989, **158:**567–569.

17

Can we respect the principles of oncologic resection in an emergency surgery to treat colon cancer?

Frederico Teixeira, Eduardo Hiroshi Akaishi, Adriano Zuardi Ushinohama, Tiago Cypriano Dutra, Sérgio Dias do Couto Netto*, Edivaldo Massazo Utiyama, Celso Oliveira Bernini and Samir Rasslan

Abstract

Patients with colorectal cancer admitted to the emergency room are generally at more advanced stage of the disease and are usually submitted to a resection with curative intent in a smaller scale. In such scenario, one of the aspects to be considered is whether the principles of oncologic resection are observed when those patients diagnosed with colon cancer are treated with surgery. We selected 87 patients with adenocarcinoma of colon and/ or upper rectum submitted to an emergency surgical resection. The major variables reviewed retrospectively were: the extent of resection performed, the number of dissected regional lymph nodes and the overall survival rate. Intestinal obstruction was observed in 67 patients (77%) while perforation was found in 20 patients (23%). Seven (8%) specimens had circumferential compromised margins, all found in patients with T4 tumors combine with poor clinical status. The number of dissected regional lymph nodes was greater than, or equal to, 12 in 71% of patients. While the average days of stay in the ICU was 5.7 days, the median was 3 days. The morbidity and peri-operative mortality stood at 33.6% and 20%, respectively. The outcome of an emergency surgery of colorectal cancer observed in this study was similar to those found in the literature. The principles of oncologic resection were respected when considering and analyzing the extent of the resection, the surgical margins and the number of dissected lymph nodes.

Keywords: Colorectal Cancer, Emergency Surgery, Colorectal emercency surgery

Introduction

The Colorectal Cancer (CC) is the third most frequent type of malignancy and the second cause of death by cancer in men and women [1]. It is a common disease in the world, with approximately 850,000 annual new cases and 500,000 deaths annually [2].

According to 2009 statistics from the U.S., 106,100 new cases of colon cancer and 40,870 new cases of rectum cancer are estimated to emerge every year, with about 49,920 deaths in the U.S. [3]. In Brazil, according to the National Cancer Institute (INC) numbers from 2009, 12,490 new annual cases of CC were likely to be found in men and 14,500 new cases in women. The statiscs show an estimated risk of 13 new cases in every 100,000 men and 15 per 100,000 women [4].

Despite preventive measures and early detection, from 6% to 30% of patients have symptoms or late complications related to the disease, requiring an emergency intervention [5-7].

Patients with colorectal cancer admitted to an emergency room are at a more advanced stage of the disease and are submitted to resection with curative intent in a smaller scale. A bowel obstruction also increases the risk of perforation and is accompanied by elevated rates of potential local recurrence.

Colorectal cancer surgical intervention performed to address an acute obstruction is associated with a mortality of 15% to 20% and a morbidity of 40% to 50%, which are significantly higher than in an elective situation [8-12]. These elevated rates of morbidity and mortality are generally related to apparence of the CC in its more complicated forms: obstruction, intestinal necrosis, perforation, diffuse or localized peritonitis; also aggravated

* Correspondence: sergiodcnetto@gmail.com
Division of Clinical Surgery III, Department of Surgery, São Paulo University School of Medicine, São Paulo, Brazil

by others diseases which some of these patients already have.

Considering such circumstances, one of the aspects to be considered is whether the principles of oncologic resection are observed when patients with colon cancer are subjected to an emergency surgical treatment.

Objectives

This study aims to examine whether the principles of cancer surgery could be observed in the operations performed in patients who had been admitted in the emergency room, with a previous diagnosis of CC, with the presence of intestinal obstruction or perforation. The extent of resection, the microscopic analysis of resected surgical margins and number of regional lymph nodes were observed in this study.

As a secondary objective, the analysis aims to describe the demographic characteristics of the population observed, complications related to surgical treatment and the long-term survival of those patients.

The study selected 87 patients from all people admitted in the Emergency Room Service. The persons who were chosen had been diagnosed with adenocarcinoma of colon and/or upper rectum and were submitted to a surgical resection.

Patients with a diagnosis other than the adenocarcinoma of the colon, primary tumor in the middle or lower rectum, or not submitted to colectomy were excluded.

We have retrospectively reviewed data on age, race, sex, presence of comorbidities and status classification of risk factors according to the criteria set by the American Society of Anesthesiologists (ASA) (Table 1).

Certain variables specifically related to the malignancy under analysis, which have been considered were: complications of the cancer disease in the clinical presentation (obstruction or perforation), site of primary tumor in the large intestine, staging with the TNM system of the American Joint Committee on Cancer (AJCC), and histological type, according to its degree of cellular differentiation.

Certain variables related to the colectomy were also analyzed and they were: the extent of resection performed, the number of dissected regional lymph nodes and the final outcome of the resection, considering the presence or absence of residual disease. The study also examined the percentage of patients who underwent primary anastomosis versus those who underwent resection with stoma procedures.

Postoperative complications were divided into local and systemic. The number of days of hospitalization in the ICU and the overall survival rate were also observed.

Table 1 Demographics and risk factor stratification of the population

Average age (years)	60 (24–89)
Race (white/all)	71/87
Systemic hypertension	34/87
Diabetes mellitus	6/87
Chronic pulmonary obstructive disease	1/87
ASA	
I	39/87 (45%)
II	38/87 (44%)
III	8/87 (9%)
IV	2/87 (2%)

Results

Review of medical record data (Table 2) revealed a predominance of sigmoid and right colon cancer. Intestinal obstruction was observed in 67 patients (77%) while perforation was found in 20 patients (23%). Bleeding was never observed in these cases.

Primary anastomosis was performed in 48 patients (55%), while the remainder (45%) resections were performed with stoma procedures.

The extent of the resections performed, the number of primary anastomotic dehiscence and the anatomical site of the colon resection are shown in Table 3. In the right colon, 89% patients were submitted to primary anastomosis and 12% developed anastomotic dehiscence. In the left colon, primary anastomosis was performed in 27% of the cases and no dehiscence was observed. In the sigmoid colon and upper rectum, only five primary anastomosis were performed (16.6%) and no further complications were observed.

Seven (8%) specimens of surgical resection had circumferential compromised margins. Those patients had bulky T4 tumors - four with tumors in the upper rectum and three with tumors located in the right colon. Four of these patients had bowel perforation presented as a primary symptom. Multivisceral *en bloc* resection was precluded due to poor clinical status of the patients.

Histological analysis of the degree of cellular differentiation of the resected specimens revealed well differentiated tumors in 63 patients (72%), moderately differentiated adenocarcinoma in 15 (17%) and poorly

Table 2 Site of the primary tumor according to the colonic anatomic division

Localization	N	%
Right colon	37	42,6
Transverse colon	5	5,8
Left colon	14	16
Sigmoid	27	31
Upper rectum	4	4,6

Table 3 Extent of colon resection performed, number of primary anastomosis and number of dehiscences in the population studied

Right colectomy	Anastomosis	33	Dehiscence	4 (12%)
	Colostomy	4		
Left colectomy	Anastomosis	3	Dehiscence	0
	Colostomy	8		
Sigmoidectomy	Anastomosis	5	Dehiscence	0
	Colostomy	25		
Transversectomy	Anastomosis	2	Dehiscence	1 (50%)
	Colostomy	2		
Total colectomy	Anastomosis	5	Dehiscence	0

differentiated adenocarcinoma in nine of the patients (11%).

The number of regional lymph nodes which were dissected was greater than or equal to 12 in 71% of patients undergoing resection of the tumor, with a mean of 4.02 metastatic lymph nodes (median of 1).

Table 4 shows the rates of major postoperative complications in the group of selected patients. There was dehiscence in 10.4% of the anastomosis, evisceration in 2.2% of patients and other infectious complications, such as septic shock (5.7% of the patients) and infected wound (6.8%). The rates of overall survival, according to pathological staging at three and five years, are shown in Tables 5 and 6 and the Kaplan-Meyer curve (probability of survival) is demonstrated in Figure 1.

The average days of stay in the ICU was 5.7 days, with a median of three days, while the morbidity and perioperative mortality (30 days after surgery) were 33.6% and 20%, respectively.

Discussion

A review of the literature shows colon cancer patients admitted to the emergence room present more frequently a bowel obstruction (8% to 60% of cases) [13,14], followed by perforation (2% to 22% of cases) [15-17] and bleeding. In our study, 77% of patients had intestinal obstruction while the remainder presented a perforation. Almost half (42.6%) of our patients had right colon cancer and 36% of patients had sigmoid or upper rectum cancer.

The emergency operation is usually associated with higher rates of morbidity, mortality and worse prognosis when compared to an elective surgery. Both overall survival rate and percentage of survival specifically related to cancer are lower in patients with CC operated on an emergency situation. When compared with elective surgery patients, those diagnosed with obstructive colorectal cancer submitted to an emergency surgery have a two-fold higher risk of dying as a result of their disease, despite the attempt of a curative operation [18]. Smothers et al., in 2003, published the first case–control study of patients who were operated on because of an emergency related to colorectal cancer (Table 7). The results showed an emergency colectomy as an independent negative prognostic factor in terms of morbidity and mortality related to the surgery. In their series, the authors have found a morbidity and mortality related to emergency operation of 64% and 34%, respectively [19]. Tobaruela et al., (Table 7) in a review of 51 patients operated on for obstruction or perforation, found a morbidity and mortality of 41% and 15% respectively. The overall survival was 15% in 62 months [20]. Ascanelli et al., in 2003, found 27% of morbidity and 12% of mortality in 118 patients submitted to emergency surgery [21].

In our series of 87 patients, we also observed increased rates of morbidity and mortality: 33.6% and 20% respectively (Table 7).

Table 4 Number and percentage of local and systemic complications of the population submitted to the emergency operation

Complications	n	%
Anastomotic dehiscence	5	10,4
Evisceration	2	2,2
Infected wound	6	6,8
Septic shock	5	5,7
Pneumonia	3	5,7
Colostomy complications	2	5,1

Table 5 Number of patients operated on emergency in accordance with anatomical and pathological TNM staging of AJCC/UICC 6th edition

Stage	N	%
I	1	1,1
IIa	11	12,7
IIb	4	4,6
IIIa	4	4,6
IIIb	17	19,6
IIIc	12	13,8
IV	38	43,6

Table 6 Overall survival at three and five years according to AJCC/UICC 6th ed

Stage	Overall survival at three years	Overall survival at five years
I	100,0%	0%
II	50,0%	21%
III	9%	9%
IV	10%	10%

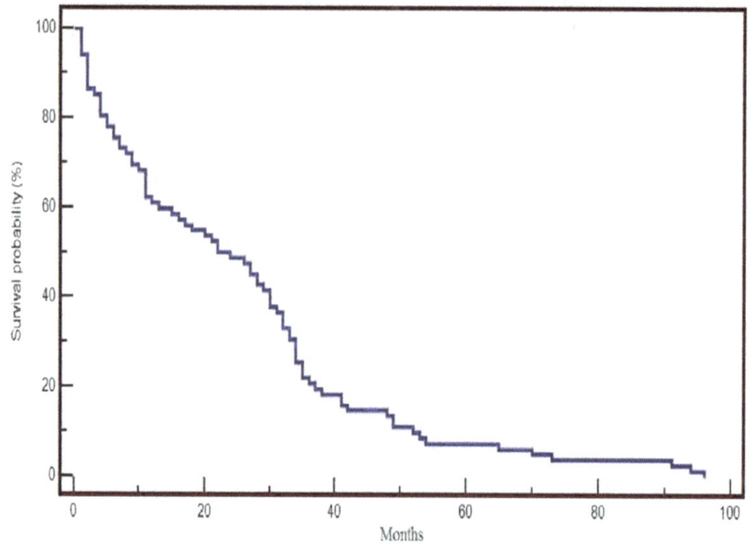

Figure 1

A peculiarity in this study was the higher-than-reported rate of dehiscence in right colectomy (12%) [22]. The right colectomy with primary anastomosis in an emergency intervention is considered to have lower rate of anastomotic complications, although Candelária et al. have also shown significant rate of anastomotic dehiscence in his series [23]. Another relevant aspect in the treatment of CC in an emergency, a primary objective of this study, concerns the feasibility of the appropriate oncologic resection with curative intent. Oncologic principles have been established in accordance with practical parameters which include: (1) extent of resection and negative surgical margins, (2) en bloc resection of contiguous tissue attached to the primary tumor, (3) lymph node dissection of at least 12 regional lymph nodes examined by pathologists [24,25]. It is unclear if the oncologic principles of surgery can be, in fact, implemented in the scenario of emergency operations, although it can be seen a small number of publications demonstrating the efforts to follow these principles in patients with a complicated form of colon cancer [12-30]. Recently, it was suggested that the principles of oncologic resection for CC operated on an emergency can be met, also achieving results related to the long-term survival [31]. Some clinical and surgical aspects are considered when choosing an oncologic resection in the emergency setting: the fear of causing further physiological deterioration in a critical patient; the possibility of extending the resection and the time spent in surgery; the difficulty of making an appropriate lymph node dissection; the struggle to manipulate and mobilize the distended colon; and the potential severe contamination and inflammation of the peritoneal cavity in cases involving bowel perforation are factors adversely affecting the choice of an oncologic resection.

Table 7 Morbidity and mortality: Literature analysis

Authors	Series	Morbidity	Peroperative mortality
Tobaruela et al. [20]	51	41%	14%
Smothers et al. [19]	29	64%	34%
Ascanelli et al. [21]	118	27,1%	11,9%
Current Series	87	33,6%	20%

It has been suggested a surgery for CC performed by specialized surgeon has a significant impact on survival [32]. Surgeons who attend the emergency setting have variable degrees of specialization. However, the majority of them are less specialized and they may perform a resection intended only to address the urgency of the situation without respecting oncologic principles.

The first criterion considered in our study concerns the extent of resection and the pathological status of the surgical margins. In general, clear margins can be obtained even in an emergency situation. With about 5 cm to 10 cm of margins, the epiploic and paracolics lymph nodes can be removed and the risk of anastomotic recurrence minimized. In the group studied, 92% of patients had R0 resection. Although the achievement of clear margins is technically simple for colectomies, the study observed 8% of positive microscopic margins, all in T4 tumors, which could be related to the impossibility of *en bloc* multivisceral resection, since these patients might have presented poor clinical conditions. The second criterion examined was the number of dissected regional lymph nodes, which has prognostic and therapeutic implications. The resection of all metastatic lymph nodes also defines an R0 resection and a sample of at least 12 lymph nodes is needed to secure appropriate accuracy. In this series, 71% of patients had at least 12 regional lymph nodes dissected. The absolute number of lymph nodes dissected may be influenced by the extent of the resection and was higher in patients undergoing total or subtotal colectomy.

Conclusion

The study shows the outcome of an emergency surgery of colorectal cancer was similar to those found in the literature. It was possible to respect the principles of oncologic resection, as regards the extent of resection, surgical margins and lymph node dissection. The morbidity and mortality were higher, however, the different rates were attributed to further complications of the disease and the clinical condition of some of the patients than to the fact those patients had undergone a left colectomy and sigmoidectomy. In the group of patients submitted to right colectomy, we have observed a higher rate of dehiscence of the ileo-transverse anastomosis, superior to the percentage reported in the literature. It has been possible to respect the oncologic principles of resection in the emergency surgery for colorectal cancer.

Competing interests

The authors declare that they have no competing interests.

Authors' contributions

All authors FJRT Jr, EHA, AZU, TCD, SDCN, EMU, COB, and SR read and approved the final manuscript.

References

1. Jemal A, Siegel R, Ward E, Murray T, Xu J, Thun MJ. Cancer statistics, 2007. CA Cancer J Clin. 2007;57:43–66.
2. Ries LAG, Eisner MP. SEER Cancer Statistics Review, 1973–1997. Bethesda, MD: National Cancer Institute; 2000.
3. Risk Factor on Colon Cancer Treatment. 2016. Available at: www.cancer.gov/cancertopics/pdq/treatment/colon/HealthProfessional#_8_toc . Acessed at Jan, 16 th, 2015.
4. Epidemiologia em Cancer Colorretal. Available at: http://www2.inca.gov.br/wps/wcm/connect/tiposdecancer/site/home/colorretal+. Acessed at January, 16th, 2015.
5. Ponz de Leon M, Sassatelli R, Scalmati A, Di Gregorio C, Fante R, Zanguieri G. Descriptive epidemiology of colorectal câncer in Italy: the 6 year experience of a specialized registry. Eur J Cancer. 1993;29(3):367–71.
6. Phang PT, MacFarlane JK, Taylor RH, Chiefetz R, Davis N, Hay J. Effect of emergent presentation on outcome from rectal cancer management. Am J Surg. 2003;185:450–4.
7. Scott NA, Jeacock J, Kingston RD. Risk factors in patients presenting as an emergency with colorectal cancer. Br J Surg. 1995;82:321–3.
8. Letiman IM, Sullivan JD, Brams D, De Cosse JJ. Multivariate analysis of morbity and mortality from the initial surgical management of obstructing carcinoma of the colon. Surg Gynecol Obstet. 1992;174:513–8.
9. Tekkis PP, Kinsman R, Thompson MR, Statamakis JD. The Association of Coloproctology of Great Britain and Ireland study of large bowel obstruction caused by colorectal cancer. Ann Surg. 2004;240:76–81.
10. Fielding LP, Wells BW. Survival after primary and after staged resection for large bowel obstrucion caused by cancer. Br J Surg. 1974;61:16–8.
11. Runkel NS, Schlag P, Schwarz V, Herfarth C. Outcome after emergency surgery for cancer of the large intestine. Br J Surg. 1991;78:183–8.
12. Runkel NS, Hinz U, Lehnert T, Buhr HJ, Herfarth C. Improved outcome after emergency surgery for cancer of the large intestine. Br J Surg. 1998;85:1260–5.
13. Kronborg O, Backer O, Sprechler M. Acute obstruction in cancer of the colon and rectum. Dis Colon Rectum. 1975;18(1):22.
14. Stower M, Hard CJ. The results of 1115 patients with colorectal cancer treated over an 8-year period in a single hospital. Eur J Surg Oncol. 1985;11(2):119–23.
15. Carraro P, Segala M, Orlotti C, Tiberio G. Outcome of large-bowel perforation in patients with colorectal cancer. Dis Colon Rectum. 1998;41(11):1421–6.
16. Mandava N, Kumar S, Plzzi WF, Aprille IJ. Perforated colorectal carcinomas. Am J Surg. 1996;172(3):236–8.
17. Alcobendas F, Jorba R, Poves I, Busquets J, Engel A, Jaurrieta E. Perforated colonic cancer. Evolution and prognosis. Rev Esp Enferm Dig. 2000;92(5):326–33.
18. McArdle CS, Mc Millan D, Hole DJ. The impact of blood loss, obstruction and perforation on survival in patients undergoing curative resection for colon cancer. Br J Surg. 2006;93:383–8.
19. Smothers L, Hynan L, Fleming J, Turnage R, Simmang C, Anthony T. Emergency surgery for colon carcinoma. Dis Colon Rectum. 2003;46(1):24–30.
20. Tobaruela E, Camuñas J, Navascúes JM E –, Díez M, Ratia T, Martin A, et al. Medical factors in the morbidity and mortality associated with emergency colorectal cancer surgery. Rev Esp Enferm Dig. 1997;89(1):13–22.
21. Ascanelli A, Navarra G, Tonini G, Feo C, Zerbinati A, Pozza E, et al. Early and late outcome after surgery for colorectal cancer: elective versus emergency surgery. Tumori. 2003;89(1):36–41.
22. Wyrzycovski A, Feliciano DV, George TA, Tremblay LN, Rozycki GS, Murphy TW, et al. Emergent right hemicolectomies. Am Surg. 2005;71(8):653–6. discussion 656–7.
23. Candelaria P, Rasslan S, Soldá SC, Parreira JG. Right hemicolectomy for nontraumatic surgical emergencies. Int Surg. 2005;90(4):231–5.
24. Nelson H, Petrelli N, Carlin A, Couture J, Fleshman J, Guilhem J. Guidelines 2000 for Colon and Rectal Cancer Surgery. J Natl Canc Inst. 2001;93:No. 8.
25. Chang GJ, Rodriguez-Bigas MA, Skibber JM, Moyer VA. Lymph node evaluation and survival after curative resection of colon cancer: systematic review. J Natl Canc Inst. 2007;99(6):433–41.
26. Kruscheswisk M, Runkel N, Buhr HJ. Radical resection in obstructing colorectal carcinomas. Int J Colorectal Dis. 1998;13(5–6):247–50.
27. McArdle CS, Hole DJ. Emergency presentation of colorectal cancer is associated with poor 5-year survival. Br J Surg. 2004;91(5):605–9.
28. Biondo S, Martí-Raguè J, Kresler E, Parés D, Martín A, Navarro M. A prospective study of outcomes of emergency and elective surgeries for complicated colonic cancer. Am J Surg. 2005;189(4):377–83.
29. Alvarez JA, Baldonedo RF, Bear IG, Truán N, Pire G, Alvarez P. Presentation, treatment, and multivariate analysis of risk factors for obstructive and perforative colorectal carcinoma. Am J Surg. 2005;190(3):376–82.
30. Chiarugi M, Galatioto C, Panicucci S, Scasa F, Zocco G, Seccia M. Oncologic colon cancer resection in emergency: are we doing enough? Surg Oncol. 2007;16 Suppl 1:S73–7.
31. MacArdle CS, Hole DJ. Influence of volume and specialization on survival following surgery for colorectal cancer. Br J Surg. 2004;91:610–7.

Pediatric Traumatic Brain Injury: a 5-year descriptive study from the National Trauma Center in Qatar

Ayman El-Menyar[1,2*], Rafael Consunji[3], Hassan Al-Thani[4], Ahammed Mekkodathil[2], Gaby Jabbour[4] and Khalid A. Alyafei[5]

Abstract

Background: The epidemiologic characteristics and outcomes of pediatric traumatic brain injury (pTBI) have not been adequately documented from the rapidly developing countries in the Arab Middle East. We aimed to describe the hospital-based epidemiologic characteristics, injury mechanisms, clinical presentation, and outcomes of pTBI and analyze key characteristics and determinant of pTBI that could help to make recommendations for policies to improve their care.

Methods: We conducted a retrospective observational study in a level 1 trauma center (2010–2014) for all pTBI patients. Data were analyzed and compared according to different patient age groups.

Results: Out of 945 traumatic brain injury patients, 167 (17.7%) were ≤ 18 years old with a mean age of 10.6 ± 5.9 and 81% were males. The rate of pTBI varied from 5 to 14 cases per 100,000 children per year. The most affected group was teenagers (15–18 years; 40%) followed by infants/toddlers (≤ 4 years; 23%). Motor vehicle crash (MVC; 47.3%) was the most frequent mechanism of injury followed by falls (21.6%). MVC accounted for a high proportion of pTBI among teenagers (77.3%) and adolescents (10–14 years; 48.3%). Fall was a common cause of pTBI for infants/toddlers (51.3%) and 5–9 years old group (30.3%). The proportion of brain contusion was significantly higher in adolescents (61.5%) and teenagers (58.6%). Teenagers had higher mean Injury Severity Scoring of 24.2 ± 9.8 and lower median (range) Glasgow Coma Scale of 3 (3–15) ($P = 0.001$ for all). The median ventilatory days and intensive care unit and hospital length of stay were significantly prolonged in the teenage group. Also, pTBI in teenage group showed higher association with pneumonia (46.4%) and sepsis (17.3%) than other age groups ($P = 0.01$). The overall mortality rate was 13% ($n = 22$); 11 died within the first 24 h, 7 died between the second and seventh day and 4 died one week post-admission. Among MVC victims, a decreasing trend of case fatality rate (CFR) was observed with age; teenagers had the highest CFR (85.7) followed by adolescents (75.0), young children (33.3), and infants/toddlers (12.5).

Conclusions: This local experience to describe the burden of pTBI could be a basis to adopt and form an efficient, tailored strategy for safety in the pediatric population.

Keywords: Trauma, Head injury, Pediatric, Brain injury, Road traffic, Falls

* Correspondence: aymanco65@yahoo.com
This study was presented in part at the 45th Critical Care Congress (SCCM) on February 20–24, 2016, Orlando, Florida, USA.
[1]Clinical Research, Trauma Surgery Section, Hamad General Hospital, Doha, Qatar
[2]Clinical Medicine, Weill Cornell Medical School, Doha, Qatar
Full list of author information is available at the end of the article

Background

Traumatic brain injury (TBI) is a main cause of functional disability and death in children worldwide [1, 2]. A report from Europe showed that, among children with blunt head trauma, the rate of fatal and nonfatal TBI was 0.5 and 5.2 per 1000 children, respectively [3]. Younger children are most likely to incur a TBI from falls, whereas adolescents with TBIs are most commonly injured in MVCs and sports-related trauma [4]. An earlier study from Qatar reported MVCs and falls as the most frequent mechanisms of injury among children sustaining severe blunt trauma in 2011 [5].

Some studies have suggested that even children with mild injuries are at increased risk of functional disabilities that might occur in pediatric TBI (pTBI) up to 1 year from the initial injury [6, 7]. Despite the fact that clinical advancements in the care of critically injured children have reduced fatalities in pTBI, the worse functional outcomes are still relying on the severity and type of head injury [8]. To date, the epidemiologic characteristics and outcomes of pTBI have not been adequately documented from the rapidly developing countries in the Arab Middle East. The objectives of this study are to describe the hospital-based epidemiologic characteristics, injury mechanisms, clinical presentation, and outcomes of pTBI in Qatar. We also analyze key characteristics and determinants of pTBI that could, whenever possible, make recommendations for policies to improve their care, reduce their adverse health outcomes, and promote their prevention.

Methods

This is a retrospective review of all pTBI cases, aged ≤ 18 years old, from the prospectively collected trauma registry of the Hamad Trauma Center (HTC), the national trauma center of Qatar, that treats all TBI cases in the country from 1 January 2010 to 31 December 2014. The HTC trauma registry is a mature database that participates in both the National Trauma Data Bank (NTDB) and the Trauma Quality Improvement Program (TQIP) of the American College of Surgeons-Committee on Trauma (ACS-COT).

All pTBIs in the trauma registry were identified by using the ICD-9 codes ranging from 800 to 959.9 (except ICD-9 codes 905-909.9; 910-924.9 and 930-939.9) and included in the study. Collected data included patient demographics, mechanism of injury, use of safety equipment, seating position in and status of ejection from the motor vehicle, Glasgow Coma Scale (GCS) at the scene and emergency department (ED), Injury Severity Score (ISS), head Abbreviated Injury Score (AIS), types of head injury, endotracheal intubation, intracranial pressure monitoring, neurosurgical procedures, hospital and ICU length of stay (LOS), ventilator days, in-hospital complications, and mortality.

Data were classified according to age groups as infants/toddlers (age 0–4 years), school age (5–9 years), adolescents (10–14 years), and teenagers (15–18 years) before analysis. This study was conducted in line with the STROBE checklist (Additional file 1).

The sample size was not prespecified as we intended to enroll all the patients ≤ 18 years who sustained TBI and required admission. Selection bias was minimized as HTC at Hamad General Hospital (HGH), the only tertiary hospital, that deals with significant TBI, however, excluding patients who were not admitted might carry this bias. Data were presented as proportions, mean ± standard deviation (SD) or median as appropriate. Differences in categorical and continuous variables were analyzed using χ^2 test and one-way analysis of variance (ANOVA), as appropriate. Yates' corrected chi-square was used for categorical variables, if the expected cell frequencies were below 5. A significant difference was considered when the two-tailed *P* value was less than 0.05. Data analysis was carried out using the Statistical Package for Social Sciences version 18 (SPSS Inc., Chicago, Illinois, USA).

Results

Out of the 945 TBI patients admitted to HTC during the study period, 167 (17.7%) were children (≤ 18 years) with a mean age of 10.6 ± 5.9 years, 81% were males. Table 1 shows the demographics, injury mechanisms, severity of injury, and outcomes among pTBI patients. MVC (47.3%) was the most frequent mechanism of TBI followed by falls (21.6%) and pedestrian injuries (10.8%). Among MVCs, most frequently injured vehicle occupants were drivers and front seat passengers (23% each). Only 5% were using a seatbelt/restraint system, and 53% were ejected from the vehicle during car crashes.

The median values of injury severity in the study population were indicative that at least half of all the patients had a severe injury and specifically a moderate to severe TBI, i.e., ISS was 19 (1–50), head AIS was 3 (1–5), and scene GCS was 9 (3–15). The majority of cases sustained severe TBI with lower scene GCS (70%) as well as high head AIS (61%), and 82.3% of them had polytrauma (ISS ≥ 16). Based on the GCS at ED, the severity of injury was mild (12.2%), moderate (22.6%), and severe pTBI (65.2%). Skull fracture (61.7%) and brain contusion (49.7%) were the most frequent CT scan findings followed by brain edema (30.7%), subarachnoid hemorrhage (24.2%), subdural hemorrhage (24%), and epidural hemorrhage (13.8%) (Fig. 1).

Table 2 presents the frequency and rate of pTBI per 100,000 populations during the study period, classified by gender. The rate of pTBI was low in 2010 (5.1 cases per 100,000 children per year), and it peaked in 2013

Table 1 Demographics, injury mechanisms, and injury severity among pTBI patients (n = 167)

Variable	Value
Age (years) (mean ± SD)	10.6 ± 5.9
Male gender	136 (81.4%)
Nationality	
Qatari-nationals	78 (46.7%)
Non-nationals	89 (53.3%)
Mechanisms of injury	
Motor vehicle crash	79 (47.3%)
Fall from height	36 (21.6%)
Pedestrians	18 (10.8%)
Motor cycle/bike	7 (4.2%)
All-terrain vehicle crashes	11 (6.6%)
Fall of heavy object	6 (3.6%)
Gunshot wound	2 (1.2%)
Others	5 (3%)
Position in vehicle in MVC	
Driver	18/79 (22.8%)
Front passenger	18/79 (22.8%)
Back passenger	10/79 (12.6%)
Unspecified position	33/79 (41.8%)
Seatbelt use in MVC	4/79 (5.1%)
Ejection from motor vehicle in MVC	42/70 (53.2%)
Head Abbreviated Injury Scale (mean ± SD)/(median, range)	3.5 ± 0.9 / 3 (1–5)
Injury severity score (mean ± SD)/(median, range)	20.7 ± 9.8 / 19 (1–50)
Glasgow Coma Score at Scene (mean ± SD)/(median, range)	8.7 ± 4.3 / 9 (3–15)
Scene time (mean ± SD)	21.4 ± 16.2
Emergency Medical Services time (mean ± SD)	55.3 ± 28
Intubation	129 (77.2%)
On-scene	53 (41%)
Emergency department/Trauma Resuscitation Unit	76 (59%)
Hospital stay	10 (1–131)
ICU stay	5 (1–39)
Ventilator days	1.5 (1–37)
Mortality	22 (13.3%)

(13.8 cases per 100,000 children per year) with a slight drop in the last year of the study period. The rate of pTBI was disproportionately higher among males in comparison to females, but the male to female incidence rate ratio decreased by more than fourfold during the study period, from 13.3 to 3.1 male per female pTBI patient.

Table 3 demonstrates the demographics, mechanism of injury, and characteristics of pTBI patients classified by age group. The predominance of male patients was consistent between all of the age groups. The majority of the local population with TBI was between 15 and 18 years [52.6%]; expatriates, however, had most pTBI patients between 0–4 [32.6%] and 15–18 years [28.1%].

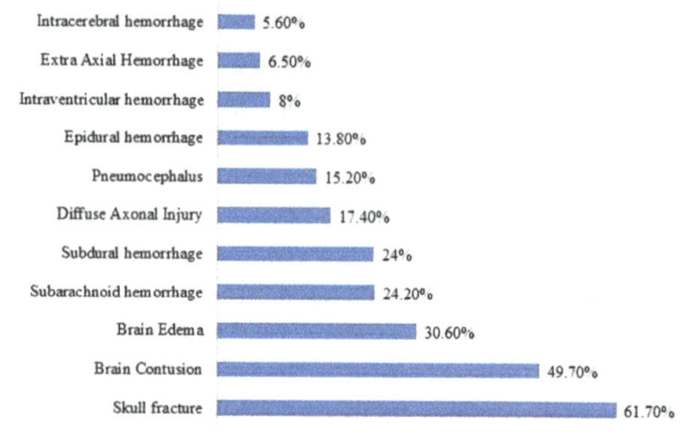

Fig. 1 Type and frequency of head injuries

Table 4 shows the Emergency medical services (EMS) characteristics and interventions, type of head injury, neurosurgical interventions, injury severity, complications, and mortality among pTBI cases. Intubation at the scene was most common in the oldest age group, 15–18 years, whereas the youngest age groups, 0–4 and 5–9 years, were most commonly intubated in the ED. Among the different types of head injuries, brain contusions showed a significantly higher incidence, with the two older age groups of pTBI patients. There were no statistically significant differences between the age groups for the other types of head injuries. Neurosurgical interventions, head AIS, and GCS (at scene) were comparable among different age groups. Although the head AIS showed no significant difference by age groups, it showed a trend towards higher scores in infants/toddlers and teenagers. Teenagers (15–18 years) had significantly higher mean ISS (24.2 ± 9.8) and lower median GCS ED [3 (3–15)] than the younger groups (P = 0.001).

Complications such as pneumonia and sepsis, ICU LOS, and ventilator days were significantly higher in the oldest age group. The overall mortality was 13.3% (n = 22) which was comparable among the different age groups (P = 0.43). Eleven (50%) patients died within the first 24 h, seven (31.8%) died between 2–7 days, and 4 (18.2%) died after 1 week.

The case fatality rate (CFR) by the mechanism of injury in different age groups was presented in Table 5. The highest CFR was traffic-related in the ages between 10 and 18, whereas it was fall-related in younger age (5–9 years).

Discussion

Pediatric TBI remains an important public health concern worldwide, which necessitates the adoption and implementation of strict prevention strategies based on the

Table 2 pTBI rates per 100,000 population across the study duration

Year	Male ≤ 18 years	Female ≤ 18 years	Male to female ratio	Total ≤ 18 years	Male pTBI admissions	Female pTBI admissions	pTBI rates per 100,000 males	pTBI rates per 100,000 females	Male to female ratio (rate per 100,000)	Overall pTBI rates per 100,000 population
2010	150,841	142,632	1.06	293,473	14	1	9.3	0.7	13.3	5.1
2011	160,425	152,427	1.05	312,852	25	3	15.6	2.0	7.8	8.8
2012	169,029	159,408	1.06	328,437	23	6	13.6	3.8	3.6	8.7
2013	183,214	174,098	1.05	357,312	39	11	21.3	6.3	3.4	13.8
2014	204,174	183,461	1.11	387,635	35	10	17.1	5.5	3.1	11.3
Average							15.4	3.6	4.3	9.5

available local epidemiologic characteristics [9]. This is a unique study from the Arab Middle East to describe the epidemiologic characteristics and outcomes of a nationally representative population of pTBI classified by age group. There are several key findings in this study. First, one out of every six victims of TBI in Qatar is a child. Second, the leading mechanism of injury and outcomes of pTBI are age-dependent. Third, the most affected group is teenagers (40%) followed by infants/toddlers (23%). Fourth, two thirds of the cohort has severe pTBI. Fifth, males predominate among the victims but the gender difference is narrowing.

Eighteen percent of all TBI in Qatar, during the study period, were children, and according to the Qatar Statistics Authority, 18% of the population of Qatar are children, aged 18 years or younger [10]. This denotes that children in Qatar do not bear a disproportionate risk for TBI, but at the same time, they are not more protected than adults from TBIs. An analysis of the leading age group-dependent mechanisms of injury, that cause pTBI in Qatar, will inform the creation of focused efforts to prevent these pTBIs.

There are few published studies on pTBI from the Gulf Cooperation Council (GCC) countries including Qatar. In 2012, Hefny et al. [11] reviewed the pediatric trauma research in the GCC and demonstrated a pediatric trauma publication rate of 0.16 publications per 100,000 populations. We have observed a high age-specific incidence and mortality in pTBI cases mainly

Table 3 Demographics and mechanism of injury and severity of pTBI based on different age groups

Variable	0–4 years	5–9 years	10–14 years	15–18 years	*P*
Number	39 (23.4%)	33 (19.8%)	29 (17.4%)	66 (39.5%)	
Age (mean ± SD)	2.6 ± 1.2	6.4 ± 1.2	12.7 ± 1.4	16.6 ± 1.1	0.001
Males	28 (71.8%)	26 (78.8%)	24 (82.8%)	58 (87.9%)	0.22
Nationality					
Qatari-nationals *n* = 78	10 (12.8%)	14 (17.9%)	13 (16.7%)	41 (52.6%)	0.004 for all
Non-nationals *n* = 89	29 (32.6%)	19 (21.3%)	16 (18.0%)	25 (28.1)	
Mechanism of injury					
Motor vehicle crash	8 (20.5%)	6 (18.2%)	14 (48.3%)	51 (77.3%)	0.001 for all
Pedestrian injury	5 (12.8%)	8 (24.2%)	5 (17.2%)	0 (0.0%)	
Falls from height	20 (51.3%)	10 (30.3%)	2 (6.9%)	4 (6.1%)	
Motor cycle crash/bike	0 (0.0%)	3 (9.1%)	2 (6.9%)	2 (3.0%)	
All-terrain vehicle	0(0.0%)	3 (9.1%)	4 (13.8%)	4 (6.1%)	
Fall of heavy object	3 (7.7%)	1 (3.0%)	0 (0.0%)	2 (3.0%)	
Ejection from vehicle	3 (37.5%)	3(50.0%)	4 (28.6%)	29 (56.9%)	0.001
Scene time	12.2 ± 7.3	16.6 ± 11	25.4 ± 14	26.9 ± 19.9	0.002
EMS time	42 ± 20	44 ± 18.7	57.6 ± 22.8	67.6 ± 32.8	0.001
Severe TBI (GCS < 9)	59%	40.6%	67.9%	80%	0.01
Glasgow Coma Score Scene; median(range)	7 (3–15)	10 (3–15)	10 (3–15)	8.5 (3–15)	0.36
Glasgow Coma Score ED; median (range)	7 (3–15)	10 (3–15)	5 (3–15)	3 (3–15)	0.001
Head AIS, mean ± SD	3.6 ± 1.1	3.1 ± 0.8	3.4 ± 0.8	3.6 ± 0.9	0.15
Injury severity score, mean ± SD	19.8 ± 10.1	15.6 ± 8	19.7 ± 8	24.2 ± 9.8	0.001

Table 4 Type of head injury, interventions, and complications among pTBI patients

Variable	0–4 years (*n* = 39)	5–9 years (*n* = 33)	10–14 years (*n* = 29)	15–18 years (*n* = 66)	*P*
Type of head injury (%)					
Skull fracture	69	70	64	53	0.31
Brain contusion	36.4	35.7	61.5	58.6	0.04
Subdural hemorrhage	19.4	17.4	36.4	24.5	0.42
Epidural hemorrhage	12.9	8.7	22.7	13.0	0.56
Extra axial hemorrhage	3.4	12.5	5.3	5.9	0.58
Subarachnoid hemorrhage	22.6	25.0	25.0	24.5	0.99
Intraventricular hemorrhage	10.0	4.3	0.0	11.8	0.36
Intracerebral hemorrhage	3.4	16.7	0.0	3.8	0.06
Pneumocephalus	10.3	21.7	23.8	11.5	0.38
Brain edema	34.4	23.1	27.3	33.3	0.75
Diffuse axonal injury	9.7	15.4	14.3	24.1	0.36
ICP monitor insertion (%)	20.5	6.1	10.3	18.2	0.25
Craniotomy/craniectomy (%)	17.9	3.0	10.3	9.0	0.22
Intubation	26 (66.7%)	20 (60.6%)	22 (75.9%)	61 (92.4%)	0.001
Intubation at scene	15.4	15	41	61	0.001
Intubation at TRU/ED	84.6	85	59	39	0.001
Hospital stay; median(range)	7 (1–98)	7 (1–38)	10.5 (2–76)	19 (1–131)	0.001
ICU stay, median,(range)	2.5 (1–39)	2 (1–11)	3 (1–27)	11 (1–37)	0.001
Ventilator days, median(range)	1 (1–37)	1 (1–6)	1 (1–21)	5 (1–27)	0.001
Pneumonia (%)	6.7	0.0	23.8	46.4	0.001
Sepsis (%)	3.4	0.0	0.0	17.3	0.01

involving teenagers and infants/toddlers. The mean age of pTBI cases in our study was 10 years which is similar to a recent study from a neighboring larger country (Saudi Arabia) with an average age of 8.6 years for pTBI admissions [12]. The present study estimates the hospitalization rate of pTBI to be 9.5 cases per 100,000 children per year, which ranges between 5 and 14 cases per 100,000 children per year. A recent study from Qatar reported the incidence of severe pediatric trauma to be 163 per 280,000 children (≤ 18 years) who visited ED per year [5]. A previous report from our center identified that 28% of the TBI patients were under the age of 20 years old [13].

MVCs were the leading cause of pTBI in our study, accounting for 77.3% of the pTBIs in the 15–18 years old group. A similar figure was reported in the Saudi Arabia (74.4%) for high school students [12]. In our series, the 57% ejection (from the vehicles) rate are inversely proportional to the 5% rate of seatbelt use. A recent publication from our center demonstrated that the underutilization of seatbelt among young vehicle occupants is associated with ejection and higher morbidities and mortality [14]. It has been estimated that seatbelt compliance could possibly result in twofold reduction in severe injury and fourfold reduction of mortality among MVC victims. Grivna et al. [15] reported 24% fatality among unrestrained adolescent (10–14 years) drivers in the UAE. A cross-sectional survey conducted in Kuwait revealed the limited knowledge about child car safety among the parents. Nearly two out of five participants have either seated a child in the front seat or on their

Table 5 pTBI incidence and case fatality rate (CRF) by age groups and mechanism of injury (MOI)

MOI	0–4 years (*n* = 39)	5–9 years (*n* = 33)	10–14 years (*n* = 29)	15–18 years (*n* = 66)	CFR by MOI
MVC	*n* = 8	*n* = 6	*n* = 14	*n* = 51	12.7
Pedestrian injury	*n* = 5	*n* = 8	*n* = 5	*n* = 0	22.2
Fall	*n* = 20	*n* = 10	*n* = 2	*n* = 4	8.3
Other MOI	*n* = 6	*n* = 9	*n* = 8	*n* = 11	14.7
CFR by age group	20.5	9.1	13.8	10.6	

lap while driving [16]. A roadside survey, conducted outside nurseries in Qatar, observed a 38% appropriate utilization with an almost equal 41% incorrect utilization of car seats for children under 5 years. Additionally, 11% of the more than 2000 children observed were improperly seated, unrestrained, and in the front seat [17]. In this study, a higher proportion of injured infants/toddlers, 37.5%, were occupying the front seat of the vehicle, a clear violation of Qatar traffic regulations [17]. This finding highlights the need for more consistent enforcement of the existing laws on child passenger safety and the expansion of these laws that require the use of restraints for all vehicle passengers, children, and adults in all seating locations.

All Terrain Vehicle (ATV)-related pTBIs were most common among adolescents, 10–14 years, in our study, which is in line with a previous study on recreational-related injuries from Qatar [18]. In this study, bicycle-related pTBI was most common in young children, 5–9 years, and the use of helmet was not reported or documented in any. These recreational or sports-related pTBIs among younger children 14 years and under are a call for the widespread education in bicycle and ATV safety in schools and the creation and enforcement of laws requiring the use of helmets and safety gear for all bicycle and ATV users.

During the study period, we noted that the rate of pTBI increased more than the double, from 5.1 to 13.8 cases per 100,000 children per year with a slight decrease in the year 2014. Whether this decrease is sustained will be the subject of future research.

Eighty percent of our pTBI patients were males, and the incidence rate of male pTBI was fourfold higher than females. Similarly, an over-representation of males was also observed in studies from KSA and UAE [12, 19]. The initial gender discrepancy could be partly explained by differential risk exposure which in our study was underage driving by young males. This risk factor has been previously identified and has been the focus of concerted efforts by multi-disciplinary stakeholder groups, but it still remains as a priority area for road safety in Qatar.

The present study shows a frequent association of fall-related pTBI among infants/toddlers which is consistent with an earlier study from Qatar [13]. Studies from Saudi Arabia reported fall to be the most common mechanism for pTBI among children of age less than 6 years (45.6%) and in the age up to 3 years (34%) [12, 20]. Also, our findings showed that pedestrians constituted 11% of total pTBI victims, and the highest association was observed in the young age group (5–9 years). Similarly, Grivna et al. [19] showed that 15% of pTBI involved pedestrian-motor vehicle collisions mainly expatriates of age less than 10 years. Another study from KSA reported a higher frequency of pedestrian (30.3%) sustained pTBI from major trauma [12].

In our study, the CFR was higher in infants/toddlers (20.5%) and adolescents (13.8%). An earlier study from KSA reported a similar mortality rate (20%) in late adolescents [12]. The most fatal mechanism of injury in our study was pedestrian hit by motor vehicle. Further investigation is required in this area using larger sample size.

Creating injury prevention programs to specifically prevent pTBIs must begin with specific evidence on the leading mechanism of disease for each age group. This allows for the application of interventions that are not only proven to work but also appropriate for the developmental stage of the child at risk. A description of the age-specific patterns of road traffic injuries in children in Qatar has been previously presented, and this study further adds to the evidence for child injury programs.

Based on this study, families with infants and young toddlers, 0–4 years of age, should be the beneficiary of education and information campaigns to increase knowledge on ways to improve home safety, to prevent pTBIs from falls and falling objects, and road safety to increase child restraint use and pedestrian safety. For families with older children, 5–9 years, the highest risks for pTBI come from falls, pedestrian injuries, and from the precocious use of the road as pedestrians, cyclists, and ATV riders. Adolescents could be the beneficiary of school-based education in almost all aspects of safe road use, especially as ATV drivers, and the tighter enforcement of the minimum age for driving in Qatar, 18 years and above. Lastly, teenagers must pass through graduated driver licensing programs, the only proven means of reducing their risk from pTBI as drivers. Untested driver education programs must not be implemented as they have actually been proven to increase the odds of young driver involvement in MVCs.

The educational and awareness campaigns must not be limited only to parents but to also include all the caregivers, especially for the younger age groups who are under the supervision of nannies and/or day care center staff. The creation and consistent enforcement of restraint laws for passengers of all ages will be instrumental in reducing the unnecessary toll from pTBIs in Qatar. Lastly, we urge that multi-disciplinary injury prevention programs be implemented and evaluated to reduce pTBI [21]. To highlight the importance of pTBI in our region, we summarized the findings of the present study and other published studies on pediatric head trauma in the Middle Eastern population in Table 6 [12, 20, 22–29].

A potential limitation of this study is the retrospective design. Our registry does not capture comprehensive information on the crash details, height of fall, site of injury and detailed restraint use. Also, we may underestimate the

Table 6 Pediatric head injury studies from the Middle East Region (2007–2016)

Author (year)	Country and Study duration	Study sample size and Inclusion/exclusion criteria	Mechanism of Injury	Injury severity	Incidence/mortality
Iranmanesh (2009) [23]	Iran, 2003–2005	380 head trauma Inclusion: patients admitted with brain injury; age < 18 years Exclusion: not reported	MVC 72%; falls 11%	No GCS reported; abnormal skull radiographs 12%; abnormal brain-CT scans 17%	Head trauma was 32%. Most affected age groups: 7–12 years (43%) and 12–18 years (35%). TBI mortality 7%
Assiry et al. (2014) [20]	KSA, 2012-	71 head trauma Inclusion: pediatric head trauma (age ≤ 16 years). Exclusion: not reported	MVC 63%; falls 32%	Not reported	Most affected age group: > 7–16 years (55%)
Alhabdan et al. (2013) [12]	KSA, 2001–2009	1219 head trauma Inclusion: any head injury in pediatric patients (age ≤ 18 years); patients admitted or died at ED Exclusion: not reported	MVC (34%); pedestrian (30%); falls (28%).	Median (range) GCS 11 (3–15); mean ISS 16.6 (range 1–75)	Most affected age group: < 12 years (66%); Mortality 15%; 50% died on arrival
Fakharian et al. (2014) [24]	Iran, 2004–2010	604 infant head trauma Inclusion: infants (< 24 months) with head trauma; hospitalized for > 24 h. Exclusion: birth trauma	Falls (63%)	GCS: (14–15) 99%; (≤ 13) 1%; mean GCS 14.93 ± 0.8	Head trauma in infants (≤ 24 m) was 21% of all children (< 15 years); mortality 0.8%; in-hospital mortality 6.6 per 100,000 infants.
Lotfi-Sadigh et al. (2015) [25]	Iran, 2011–2014	218 children with blunt head trauma Inclusion: minor blunt head trauma (GCS 14 or 15); presented to ED within 24 h of trauma; age < 2 years. Exclusion: no signs or symptoms of head trauma other than scalp abrasions or lacerations; penetrating trauma; comorbidities (ventricular shunt or bleeding disorders); previous neuroimaging; patients left ED against medical advice	Falls 74%; MVC 14%	Head trauma was defined as GCS 14 or 15; abnormal CT findings in 8%	No mortality was reported due to mild head trauma
Alharthy et al. (2015) [26]	KSA, 2011	289 children with blunt head trauma. Inclusion: blunt head injury; age 1–14 years; GCS 13–15; presentation within 24 h post-injury; CT scan done. Exclusion: penetrating head trauma, local facial signs post trauma, signs of basal skull Fracture; comorbidities that predispose to bleeding tendency; multiple major traumas; prolonged amnesia and LOC (prolonged amnesia and loss of consciousness	Falls 53%; MVC 23%	All cases were with minor head trauma; GCS 15 (94%); 14 (4%); 13 (2%); abnormal brain CT findings in 5% (of these, 53% in falls, 23% in MVC)	TBI in minor head trauma among children (1–14 years) was 5%; no mortality was reported due to mild head trauma

Table 6 Pediatric head injury studies from the Middle East Region (2007–2016) *(Continued)*

Author (year)	Country and Study duration	Study sample size and Inclusion/exclusion criteria	Mechanism of Injury	Injury severity	Incidence/mortality
		for more than 5 min); active seizure on arrival to ED; GCS < 13.			
Yagmur et al. (2016) [27]	Turkey, 2008–2012	203 pre-school children deaths due to head trauma. Inclusion: fatal head trauma in pre-school children (age ≤ 5 years); head trauma with general body trauma if cause of death was head trauma. Exclusion: cause of death other than head trauma	Falls 48%; MVC 33%	All cases were fatal	18% of deaths among children (age ≤ 5 years) were due to head trauma
Klimo et al. (2015) [28]	Iraq, 2004–2012	268 children with severe isolated head trauma in Iraq during Operation Iraqi Freedom (OIF). Inclusion: pediatric head injury; age < 18 years; isolated serious head injury (defined as AIS > 3); during OEF (Operation Enduring Freedom) or OIF (Operation Iraqi Freedom). Exclusion: not reported	Penetrating injuries 61%; caused by IED (38%) or blast (25%).	Median (range) GCS 7 (3–15)	Of the total severe isolated head trauma among children during US military operation in Iraq and Afghanistan, 41% were Iraqi children. Mortality among the severe isolated head trauma in children was 26%
Gofin and Avitzour (2007) [29]	Israel, 2001	472 head trauma in children; Inclusion: pediatric head trauma; age 0–17 years; Israeli citizens; information about mechanism and type of injury were available. Exclusion: not reported TBI definition by ICD-9-CM codes	Falls 46%	GCS was not reported; ISS was >16 in 60%	42% of the head trauma in children (0–17 years) was TBI or possible TBI. Most affected age group: 0–4 years (51% in Jews and 57% in Arabs)
Present study	Qatar, 2010–2014	167 pediatric TBI cases (≤ 18 years); Inclusion: all pTBI cases required admission, ICD-9 codes from 800 to 959.9 Exclusion: codes 905–909.9; 910–924.9 and 930–939.9	MVC 47%; falls 22%	Median (range) GCS at scene: 9 (3–15); Median (range) ISS: 19 (1–50)	18% of the total TBIs were in children; overall rate of TBIs among children in Qatar 9.5 per 100,000; most affected age group was 15–18 years (40%) followed by 0–4 years (23%). Mortality 13%

health burden from pTBI as it does not include patients who died at the scene, child abuse, long-term outcomes, and quality of life. The sample size was not prespecified as we intended to enroll all the patients ≤ 18 years old who sustained TBI and required admissions. Selection bias was minimized as HGH is the tertiary hospital that deal with significant TBI; however, excluding patients who were not admitted might carry this bias.

Conclusions

The present study addresses the local burden of pTBI which could be the basis to develop efficient, tailored strategies and interventions for the community safety in our region. Targeted prevention programs are needed to reduce morbidity and mortality of pTBI.

Acknowledgements

The authors thank the entire registry database team in the Trauma Surgery Section, Hamad General Hospital, Doha, Qatar.

Funding

This research did not receive any specific grant from any funding agency in the public, commercial, or not-for-profit sector.

Author's contributions

AE contributed to the study design, data analysis and interpretation, and drafting and critical review of manuscript. RC was involved in the study design, data acquisition, writing of the manuscript, and review. AM and GJ contributed to the data acquisition, interpretation, and drafting of the manuscript. KA and HA contributed to the study design, data interpretation, and critical review. All authors read and approved the final manuscript.

Competing interests

The authors declare that they have no competing interests.

Author details

[1]Clinical Research, Trauma Surgery Section, Hamad General Hospital, Doha, Qatar. [2]Clinical Medicine, Weill Cornell Medical School, Doha, Qatar. [3]Hamad Injury Prevention Program, Trauma Surgery Section, Hamad General Hospital, Doha, Qatar. [4]Trauma Surgery Section, Hamad General Hospital, Doha, Qatar. [5]Department of Pediatrics, Division of Pediatric Emergency Medicine, Hamad Medical Corporation, Doha, Qatar.

References

1. Zaloshnja E, Miller T, Langlois JA, Selassie AW. Prevalence of long-term disability from traumatic brain injury in the civilian population of the United States, 2005. J Head Trauma Rehabil. 2008;23:394–400.
2. Shao J, Zhu H, Yao H, Stallones L, Yeates K, Wheeler K, et al. Characteristics and trends of pediatric traumatic brain injuries treated at a large pediatric medical centre in China, 2002–2011. PLoS One. 2012;7:e51634. https://doi.org/10.1371/journal.pone.0051634.
3. Da Dalt L, Marchi AG, Laudizi L, et al. Predictors of intracranial injuries in children after blunt head trauma. Eur J Pediatr. 2006;165:142–8.
4. Faul M, Xu L, Wald MM, Coronado VG. Traumatic brain injury in the United States: emergency department visits, hospitalizations and deaths 2002–2006. Atlanta (GA): Centers for Disease Control and Prevention, National Center for Injury Prevention and Control; 2010.
5. Alyafei KA, Toaimah F, El Menyar A, Al Thani H, Youssef B, Mollazehi M, Consunji R. Analysis of pediatric trauma data from a hospital based trauma registry in Qatar. Int J Crit Illn Inj Sci. 2015;5:21–6.
6. Cassidy LD, Potoka DA, Adelson PD, et al. Development of a novel method to predict disability after head trauma in children. J Pediatr Surg. 2003;38:482–5.
7. Rivara FP, Koepsell TD, Wang J, et al. Incidence of disability among children 12 months after traumatic brain injury. Am J Public Health. 2012;102(11):2074–9.
8. deGuise E, LeBlanc J, Feyz M, Meyer K, Duplantie J, Thomas H, Abouassaly M, Champoux MC, Couturier C, Lin H, et al. Long-term outcome after severe traumatic brain injury: the McGill interdisciplinary prospective study. J Head Trauma Rehabil. 2008;23:294–303.
9. Keenan HT, Bratton SL. Epidemiology and outcomes of pediatric traumatic brain injury. Dev Neurosci. 2006;28:256–63.
10. Ministry of Development Planning and Statistics, Population Topics, Retrieved Oct 29 2017 from http://www.mdps.gov.qa.
11. Hefny AF, Grivna M, Abbas AK, Branicki FJ, Abu-Zidan FM. Pediatric trauma research in the Gulf Cooperation Council countries. Asian J Surg. 2012;35:74–80.
12. Alhabdan S, Zamakhshary M, AlNaimi M, et al. Epidemiology of traumatic head injury in children and adolescents in a major trauma center in Saudi Arabia: implications for injury prevention. Ann Saudi Med. 2013;33:52–6.
13. El-Matbouly M, El-Menyar A, Al-Thani H, Tuma M, El-Hennawy H, Abdulrahman H, Parchani A, Peralta R, Asim M, El-Faramawy A, Zarour A, Latifi R. Traumatic brain injury in qatar: age matters- insights from a 4-year observational study. Sci World J. 2013;22:354920.
14. El-Menyar A, Consunji R, Asim M, Abdelrahman H, Zarour A, Parchani A, Peralra R, Al-Thani H. Underutilization of occupant restraint systems in motor vehicle injury crashes: a quantitative analysis from Qatar. Traffic Inj Prev. 2015;17(3):284–91. https://doi.org/10.1080/15389588.2015.1069820.
15. Grivna, M., Barss, P, El-Sadig, M. Epidemiology and prevention of child injuries in the United Arab Emirates: a report for Safe Kids Worldwide, 2008. University Faculty of Medicine & Health Sciences and Roadway Transportation & Traffic Safety Research Center, Al Ain, UAE; 2008.
16. Raman, S.R., Landry, M.D., Ottensmeyer, C.A., Jacob, S., Hamdan, E., & Bouhaimed, M. (in press). Keeping our children safe in motor vehicles: knowledge, attitudes and practice among parents in Kuwait regarding child car safety. Int J Inj Control Saf Promot doi:https://doi.org/10.1080/17457300.2012.745578.
17. Malik S; Saad R; Peralta R; Allen K; Hyder A; Al Thani H; Consunji R. Roadside observational surveys of restraint use by young children in Qatar: initial results and recommendations, Journal of Local and Global Health Science 2015:40 https://doi.org/10.5339/jlghs.2015.itma.40 17
18. Parchani A, El-Menyar A, Al-Thani H, Tuma M, Zarour A, Abdulrahman H, et al. Recreational-related head injuries in Qatar. Brain Inj. 2013;27:1450–3.
19. Grivna M, Eid HO, Abu-Zidan FM. Pediatric and youth traffic-collision injuries in Al Ain, United Arab Emirates: a prospective study. PLoS One. 2013;8(7): e68636. https://doi.org/10.1371/journal.pone.0068636
20. Assiry K, Abdulmutali H, Alqahtani A, Alyahya A, Elawad M. Traumatic head injuries in children: experience from Asir, KSA. Online J Med Med Sci Res. 2014;3(5):44–47. 20.
21. Consunji RJ, Peralta RR, Al-Thani H, Latifi R. The implications of the relative risk for road mortality on road safety programmes in Qatar. Inj Prev. 2015; 21(e1):e105–8. https://doi.org/10.1136/ injuryprev-2013-040939.
22. Dewan MC, Mummareddy N, Wellons JC 3rd, Bonfield CM. Epidemiology of Global Pediatric Traumatic Brain Injury: Qualitative Review. World Neurosurg. 2016;91:497-509.e1.
23. Iranmanesh F. Outcome of head trauma in children. Indian J Pediatr. 2009; 76:929–31.
24. Fakharian E, Mohammadzadeh M, Behdad S, Babamohammadi A, Mirzadeh AS, Mohammadzadeh J. A seven-year study on head injuries in infants, Iran—the changing pattern. Chin J Traumatol. 2014;17(3):153–6.
25. Lotfi Sadigh S, Gholipour C, Vahdati SS, Ghafouri RR, Haghighi AG. Clinical predictors of abnormal computed tomography scan in minor head trauma in children under 2 years old. Anal Res Clin Med. 2015;3:57–63.
26. Alharthy N, Al Queflie S, Alyousef K, Yunus F. Clinical manifestations that predict abnormal brain computed tomography (CT) in children with minor head injury. J Emerg Trauma Shock. 2015;8:88–93.
27. Yagmur F, Celik S, Yener Z, Koral F, Yaman T, Sezer Y, et al. Head trauma-related deaths among preschool children in Istanbul, Turkey. Am J Forensic Med Pathol. 2016;37:35–9.
28. Klimo P Jr, Ragel BT, Jones GM, McCafferty R. Severe pediatric head injury during the Iraq and Afghanistan conflicts. Neurosurgery. 2015;77:1–7. discussion: 7
29. Gofin R, Avitzour M. Outcome of head and other injuries among Israeli children: physical limitations and stress symptoms. Isr Med Assoc J. 2007;9:531–6.

19

Transcatheter thrombolysis combined with damage control surgery for treatment of acute mesenteric venous thrombosis associated with bowel necrosis

Kai Liu[1], Jiaxiang Meng[1], Shuofei Yang[1], Baochen Liu[1], Weiwei Ding[2], Xingjiang Wu[2*] and Jieshou Li[2]

Abstract

Objective: This study aims to evaluate the clinical outcomes of transcatheter thrombolysis in acute superior mesenteric venous thrombosis (ASMVT) associated with bowel necrosis.

Methods: A retrospective study of six patients with ASMVT treated with catheter-directed thrombectomy/thrombolysis and damage control surgery at Jinling Hospital (Nanjing, China) between 2010 and 2013 was conducted. Demographics, past medical history, risk factors, therapeutic methods and effects, mortality, and follow-up of the study population were assessed.

Results: Five of six patients underwent arteriovenous combined thrombolysis, while one patient underwent arterial thrombolysis. All patients required damage control surgery, and four of these patients underwent temporary abdominal closure. All patients survived and were free of recurrence.

Conclusions: Transcatheter thrombectomy/thrombolysis and damage control surgery could help avoid extensive bowel resection, prevent short bowel syndrome and reduce mortality for critically ill patients with acute mesenteric venous thrombosis associated with bowel necrosis.

Keywords: Acute superior mesenteric venous thrombosis, Interventional thrombolysis, Damage control surgery, Bowel necrosis

Introduction

Acute superior mesenteric venous thrombosis (ASMVT) is an uncommon disease that presents no obvious specific symptoms in the early stage [1]. The diagnosis of ASMVT remains elusive until intestinal gangrene and peritonitis occurs [2]. The optimal time for treatment is lost, and eventually massive bowel resection is required, leading to short bowel syndrome [3–5]. Therefore, early diagnosis and prompt therapy is very important to improve the survival rate of patients with ASMVT, with the goal of conserving as much bowel as possible [6–8].

For patients with ASMVT associated with bowel ischemia, the recommended treatment is emergency surgery. However, in venous thrombosis, unlike arterial thrombosis, the line of demarcation is indistinct; leading to massive bowel resection. This is associated with the development of short bowel syndrome and high mortality rates [1, 9]. In order to improve the viability of the ischemic and congested bowel secondary to mesenteric venous thrombosis, a strategy of initial transcatheter thrombolysis followed by surgery has been adopted with success [10, 11].

In this study, we evaluated the outcome of this novel approach in critically ill patients combined with damage control surgery.

* Correspondence: wu_xingjiang@yeah.net
[2]Research Institute of General Surgery, Jinling Hospital, 305 East Zhongshan Road, 210002 Nanjing, Jiangsu, China
Full list of author information is available at the end of the article

Materials and methods

All procedures performed in studies involving human participants were in accordance with the ethical standards of the Ethics Committee of Jinling Hospital and with the 1964 Helsinki declaration and its later amendments or comparable ethical standards. Informed consent was obtained from all individual participants included in the study. Additional informed consent was obtained from all individual participants for whom identifying information is included in this article.

Patient group

This is a retrospective study of patients with ASMVT treated between October 2010 and November 2013. Patients with ASMVT associated with bowel ischemia treated with transcatheter thrombolysis followed by damage control surgery were included in this study. Patient data were retrieved from medical records.

Diagnosis and evaluation

All patients underwent routine blood examination, including: white blood cell, red blood cell, platelet and neutrophilic granulocyte count; hemoglobin, C-reactive protein, serum lactate and procalcitonin levels; and hepatic and renal function including amylase, lipase, aminotransferase, urea, creatinine and phosphocreatine kinase levels. Coagulation was monitored via thrombin time, activated partial thromboplastin time, international normalized ratio, fibrinogen, antithrombin III level, D-dimer and thromboelastogram every 24 h throughout the hospitalization. All patients underwent laboratory testing for thrombophilic states.

All patients underwent Doppler ultrasound scans and multislice spiral computed tomography (MSCT) to confirm ASMVT.

Initial management

Each patient was treated with emergent treatment in the ICU to maintain hemodynamic stability. Vesical pressure was regularly monitored to observe intra-abdominal pressure changes. The use of vasopressors and somatostatin were avoided, because these could exacerbate intestinal ischemia. Systemic anticoagulation for superior mesenteric venous (SMV) thrombosis was carried out by immediate subcutaneous low molecular weight heparin injection. Dextran and alprostadil were used to improve microcirculation.

Thrombolytic technique

Before catheter-directed thrombolytic therapy, the risk of bleeding complications and benefits of catheter-directed thrombectomy and thrombolysis for acute SMV thrombosis were explained to each patient, and informed written consent was obtained. Thrombolytic therapy was used for patients with persistent or worsening abdominal pain despite systemic anticoagulation.

Contraindications to percutaneous thrombolysis included previous stroke, central nervous system malignancies, active bleeding diathesis, and recent gastrointestinal bleeding. Direct portal vein (PV)-SMV thrombolysis was not performed in patients with unfavorable anatomy of the PV, marked atrophy of the liver, or portal venous cavernous transformation.

The route, thrombolytic agent, catheter type, length of treatment, other interventional techniques, and complications are shown in Table 1.

Direct PV-SMV catheterization

The choice between direct-catheter thrombolysis by percutaneous transhepatic or transjugular intrahepatic routes was determined by radiologists and the gastrointestinal surgeon based on the patient's CT findings, vessel status and general condition.

The portal vein was punctured under ultrasonography and fluoroscopic guidance. After the injection of local anesthesia, catheterization of the right hepatic vein was performed using a 10-Fr, 41-cm long sheath (Rösch-Uchida TIPS Puncture Set; Cook, Bloomington, IN, USA) via the right transjugular approach. The catheter was advanced further to puncture the right portal vein. Once the portal puncture was successfully performed, an ultra-smooth guide wire (Terumo Europe, Leuven, Belgium) was introduced into the PV-SMV system. The SMV thrombus was traversed using a 5-Fr Cobra catheter (Cordis, Miami, USA). The thrombus in the PV-SMV system was aspirated as much as possible using an angled 8-Fr guiding catheter (Cordis, Miami, USA) with a 60-ml syringe through the 10-Fr sheath. After most of the thrombi in the PV-SMV were removed, a 5-Fr multiple side-hole catheter (Cordis, Miami, USA) was securely placed within the SMV thrombus.

Alternatively, the right portal vein was punctured directly with a 14-gauge trocar needle (Cook, USA) via the right midaxillary line under ultrasonography guidance. Then, a 6-Fr sheath (Cordis, Miami, USA) was introduced into the PV-SMV system. The rest of the procedure was the same as the prior TIPS method. After thrombolytic treatment, the punctured tract was sealed using a steel ring (Cook, USA) in order to prevent subcapsular hemorrhage.

SMA Catheterization

The right femoral artery was cannulated using the Seldinger technique and a 5-Fr sheath (Cordis, Miami, USA) was placed. A 5-Fr Cobra catheter (Cordis, Miami, USA) was introduced; then, superior mesenteric arteriography and indirect portal and mesenteric vein venography were performed. Subsequently, selective catheterization of the superior mesenteric artery (SMA) was performed with

Table 1 Details of transcatheter thrombolysis therapy

No. of patients	location of thrombosis	Route of thrombolysis	Days of SMA thrombolysis	Agent and dose of SMA thrombolysis	Days of SMV thrombolysis	Agent and dose of SMV thrombolysis	Total dose of thrombolytics	Days of thrombolytic infusion
1	PV + SPV + SMV	SMA (first) + PT (next)	6	Urokinase (3,200,000 IU)	5	Urokinase (2,800,000 IU)	Urokinase (6,000,000 IU)	11
2	PV + SMV + IVC	SMA + PT	3	Urokinase (600,000 IU)	7	Urokinase (2,600,000 IU)	Urokinase (3,200,000 IU)	7
3	SMV	PT + SMA	6	urokinase (1,700,000 IU)	6	Urokinase (1,200,000 IU)	Urokinase (2,900,000 IU)	6
4	PV + SPV + SMV + IVC	SMA	5	Alteplase (60 mg) + urokinase (1,200,000 IU)	-	-	Alteplase (60 mg) + urokinase (1,200,000 IU)	5
5	PV + SMV + IVC	TI + SMA	3	Alteplase (10 mg) + urokinase (600,000 IU)	6	Alteplase (110 mg) + urokinase (400,000 IU)	Alteplase (120 mg) + urokinase (1,000,000 IU)	6
6	PV + SPV + SMV	PT + SMA	5	Alteplase (30 mg)	5	Alteplase (50 mg)	Alteplase (80 mg)	5

SMV superior mesenteric vein, *PV* portal vein, *SPV* splenic vein, *IVC* inferior vena cave, *PT* percutaneous transhepatic route, *TI* transjugular intrahepatic route, *SMA* superior mesenteric arterial route

a 5-Fr multiple side-hole catheter (Cordis, Miami, USA) in order to perform the indirect PV-SMV thrombolytic treatment.

Transcatheter anticoagulant and thrombolytic therapy

Following the mechanical aspiration procedure, a bolus of 5 mg of rt-PA (alteplase; Boehringer Ingelheim GmbH, Germany) was injected via the catheter followed by continuous infusion of 0.625–0.833 mg/h for 24–48 h at the ICU (laboratory analysis and thromboelastogram were performed at 24-h intervals throughout the rt-PA infusion period). Then, rt-PA was replaced with urokinase (Nanjing Nanda Pharmaceutical Co. Ltd. Nanjing, China) at 400,000–600,000 IU/day for 4–6 days.

After completion of the thrombolytic therapy, the indwelling catheter was used to give low molecular heparin infusions at a rate of 417 IU/h; in order to maintain the activated partial thromboplastin time (APTT) at values two times the control value throughout the hospitalization.

Termination of thrombolysis and timing of laparotomy

During transcatheter thrombolytic therapy, PV and SMV patency of patients were assessed every 24 h by ultrasonography. The angiogram was repeated via the infusion catheter at 24, 48 and 72 h and one week following the procedure. Contrast-enhanced CT scan was performed upon completion of thrombolytic therapy or in patients with signs of peritonism or bloody ascites.

Termination of thrombolysis was based on clinical and radiographic findings. Particularly, when CT demonstrated intestinal perforation, transmural bowel necrosis, and abdominal paracentesis revealed bloody ascites. Patients with these findings were treated by laparotomy as soon as possible. Some abnormal serum markers and intra-abdominal pressure are shown in Table 2. During surgery, resection of the gangrenous bowel with double barrel enterostomy was performed. In the presence of intra-abdominal hypertension, the abdomen was left open. Abdominal closure was performed once intra-abdominal pressure returned to normal range. Definite intestinal anastomosis was performed after patients completely recovered from the acute phase and were on a full oral diet (Table 3).

Follow-up

After recovery from transcatheter thrombolysis and damage control surgery, patients were discharged on oral anticoagulation, which was adjusted to maintain prothrombin time at 4–6 s higher than normal values for six months.

Contrast enhanced CT and ultrasonography of the portal vein and SMV was conducted at discharge, followed by repeat imaging every three months for the first year, and every 6–12 months thereafter. Records of hospitalization and clinic visits were reviewed from the time of discharge until October 31, 2014.

Results

Patient demographics

Among these six patients, three were male and three were female; and mean age of patients was 41 ± 14.38 years (range, 20–59 years). Initial symptom of all patients was abdominal pain, which was accompanied by the following symptoms: abdominal distension ($n = 5$), nausea and vomiting ($n = 3$), and hematemesis ($n = 1$). All six patients experienced abdominal pain for less than two weeks (range, 5–14 days; mean, 9 ± 3.82 days). Related past medical history and risk factors in our study are presented in Table 4.

ASMVT was diagnosed and evaluated by MSCT. All patients underwent MSCT to detect SMV thrombosis and bowel affected by ischemia (Figs. 1 and 2). Based on clinical symptoms and CT findings, all patients underwent thrombolytic therapy.

Thrombolytic therapy

Six patients were successfully treated with direct PV-SMV thrombolysis and SMA thrombolysis (Figs. 1 and 2). Patient No. 1 first received trans-SMA thrombolysis for six days, and was treated with trans-SMV thrombolysis for 5 days. Patient No. 4 only received SMA thrombolysis therapy for 5 days due to failure of direct PV-SMV catheterization. Catheter-directed mechanical thrombectomy was performed in three patients. Continuous thrombolysis via the

Table 2 Biochemical and hematological parameters of patients 24 h before exploratory laparotomy

No. of patients	WBC (10^9/L)	CRP (mg/L)	D-dimer (mg/L)	PCT (μg/L)	Albumin (g/L)	Lactate (mmol/L)	LDH (U/L)	LAP (U/L)	IAP (cmH_2O)
1	19	144	2.55	21.16	34.3	19.6	230	61	8
2	19.4	140.6	2.25	23.94	29.4	17.6	171	65	10
3	39.1	190	1.45	12.26	30.5	21.3	339	76	13
4	19.9	189	18.79	55.27	27.9	16.4	437	78	5
5	32.9	150	8.55	5.13	30.0	25.8	980	65	9
6	22.8	151.3	3.54	14.45	24.5	15	959	103.9	6

Reference range: white blood cell (WBC): 3.5–9.5 × 10^9/L, Creactive protein (CRP): 0–8 mg/L, D-dimer: 0–0.55 mg/L, procalcitonin (PCT): 0–0.5 μg/L, Albumin: 40.0–55.0 g/L, Lactate: 0.5–1.6 mmol/L, lactate dehydrogenase (LDH): 109–245 U/L, leukocyte alkaline phosphatase (LAP): 30–120 U/L, intra-abdominal pressure (IAP): 0 kPa. 1 kPa = 10.2 cmH_2O

Table 3 Perioperative and follow up data of patients

No. of patients	Days from thrombolysis to surgery	Initial findings and treatment	Range of small bowel resection	Days of open abdomen (temporary abdominal closure)	Days of hospital stay	Timing of definitive surgery (months)	Findings and definitive surgery	Months of follow-up	Clinical outcome
1	7	Bowel resection, double barrel enterostomy and open abdomen[a]	200 cm	3	27	12	No further intestinal necrosis. double-cavity stoma reversion	37	No recurrence
2	7	Bowel resection, double barrel enterostomy and open abdomen[a]	200 cm	3	47	12	No further intestinal necrosis. double-cavity stoma reversion	32	No recurrence
3	7	Bowel resection, double barrel enterostomy and open abdomen[a]	150 cm	7	29	12	No further intestinal necrosis. double-cavity stoma reversion	25	No recurrence
4	18	Bowel resection and double barrel enterostomy	150 cm	-	70	12	No further intestinal necrosis. double-cavity stoma reversion	20	No recurrence
5	8	Bowel resection, double barrel enterostomy and open abdomen[a]	250 cm	3	38	12	No further intestinal necrosis. double-cavity stoma reversion	16	No recurrence
6	6	Bowel resection and double barrel enterostomy	80 cm	-	40	13	No further intestinal necrosis. double-cavity stoma reversion	11	No recurrence

[a]Open abdomen was treated with temporary abdominal closure using Prolene Mesh

Table 4 Summary of clinical data

No. of patients	Age (years)/ gender	Initial symptoms and signs	Etiologies	Past medical history and risk factors	Indication for intervention	Days from symptoms to admission	Days from symptoms to intervention
1	46/M	Abdominal pain, distention	Portal hypertension	Portal hypertension	Continued pain, despite anticoagulation	5	7
2	51/M	Abdominal pain, distention	Pancreatitis and hypercoagulable state	Pancreatitis, deep venous thrombosis	Progressive pain, despite anticoagulation	14	17
3	29/F	Abdominal pain, distention	Post partum, IgA nephropathyand hypercoagulable state	Post partum, IgA nephropathy, deep venous thrombosis	Worsening pain, despite anticoagulation	7	7
4	41/F	Abdominal pain, nausea, anorexy	Hypercoagulable state with oral contraceptive agent	Oral contraceptive agent	Worsening pain, despite anticoagulation	8	9
5	20/M	Abdominal pain, distention, vomiting, diarrhea, hematemesis	Hypercoagulable state with activated protein C deficiency	Deep venous thrombosis, inferior vena cava thrombosis, pulmonary embolism	Persistent pain, distension, bloody ascites, despite anticoagulation	7	8
6	59/F	Abdominal pain, distention, vomiting, nausea,	Myeloproliferative disorders	None	Worsening pain, distension, despite anticoagulation	7	11

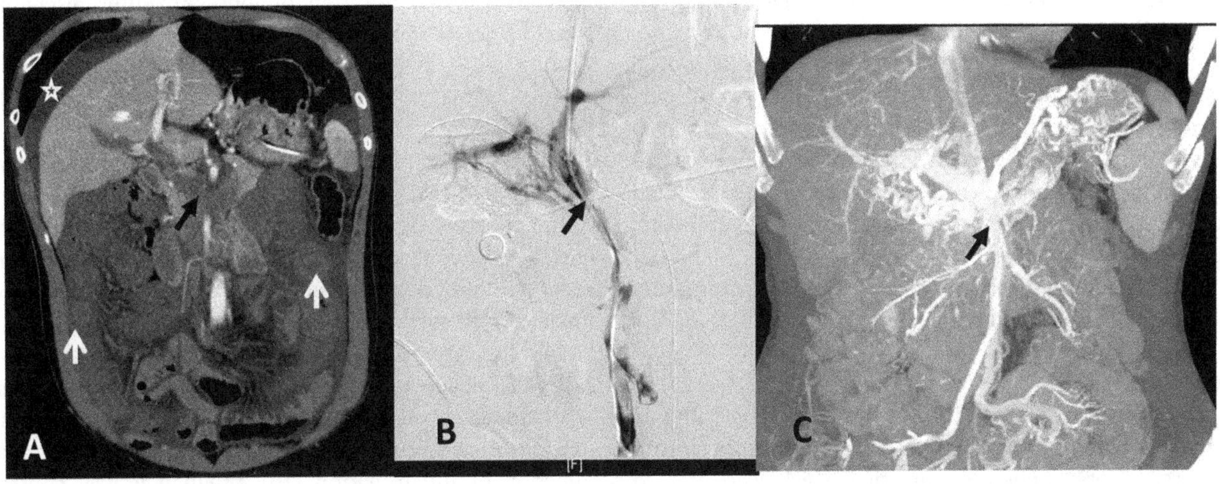

Fig. 1 Patient No. 5: **a** MSCT demonstrates the massive thrombosis of the portal vein (PV) and superior mesenteric vein (SMV) (black arrow), diffuse circumferential bowel wall thickening with "halo sign" (white arrows), and the small amount of ascites (star). **b** Venography of the superior mesenteric and portal veins demonstrates filling defects in the lumen of PV and SMV via the percutaneous transhepatic route (black arrow). **c** MSCT demonstrates partial recanalization of PV and SMV (black arrow) and collateral vessels 12 months after surgery

infusion catheter in the SMV was provided for 5–7 days (average, 5.8 ± 0.84 days). The mean doses of thrombolytics via SMV access were: alteplase, 80 ± 42.43 mg; urokinase, 1.75 ± 1.15,000 000 IU. SMA trans-catheter thrombolysis lasted for 3–6 days (average, 4.67 ± 1.37 days). The mean doses of thrombolytics via SMA access were: alteplase, 33.3 ± 25.12 mg; urokinase, 1.46 ± 1.08,000 000 IU. The total doses of thrombolytics were: alteplase, 86.67 ± 30.55 mg; urokinase, 2.86 ± 2.01,000 000 IU. After completion of the infusion of thrombolytic drugs, venography via the infusion catheter was performed to observe the thrombolytic effect on SMV thrombosis. MSCT images were obtained again before surgery, which revealed the recanalization of SMV and the necrotic intestine.

Damage control surgery

All six patients underwent exploratory laparotomy due to worsening of symptoms with the development of hemodynamic instability. During the procedure, hemorrhagic ascites were found along with intestinal

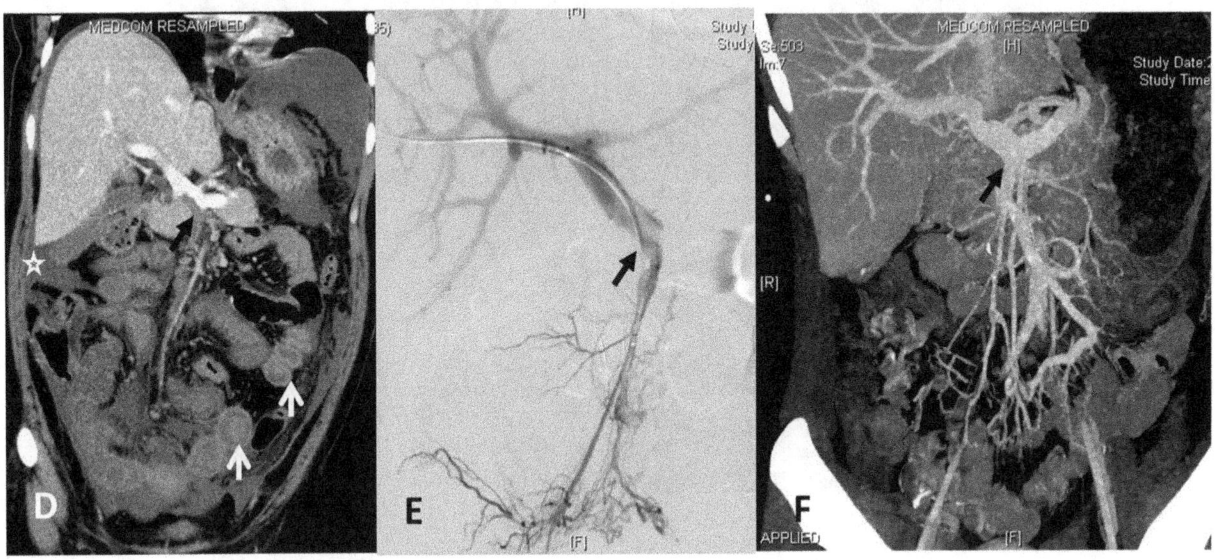

Fig. 2 Patient No. 3: **d** MSCT demonstrates the massive thrombosis of the portal vein (PV) and superior mesenteric vein (SMV) (black arrow), diffuse circumferential bowel wall thickening with "halo sign" (white arrows), and the small amount of ascites (star). **e** Venography of the superior mesenteric and portal veins demonstrates filling defects in the lumen of PV and SMV via the transjugular intrahepatic route (black arrow). **f** MSCT demonstrates partial recanalization of PV and SMV (black arrow) at discharge

gangrene and mesenteric edema. SMA pulsations were palpable, but mesenteric veins of the bowel were dilated and filled with red thrombi. Necrotic bowel resection and double barrel enterostomy were performed in all patients, in which four patients also underwent open abdomen due to sustained intra-abdominal hypertension. Mean length of the resected bowel was 171.67 ± 58.45 cm (range, 80–250 cm; Fig. 3)

Definitive surgery for restoring intestinal continuity was performed 6–12 months later.

Complications

During thrombolytic infusion via the indwelling catheter, a small hematoma was observed in three patients at both the arterial or venous puncture site; which were treated conservatively without stopping thrombolytic therapy. Sepsis occurred in one patient, while intestinal perforation occurred in another patient before open exploration.

Follow-up

None of the patients required long-term parenteral nutrition. In addition, there was no mortality or thrombosis recurrence until the last follow up. Mean duration of hospitalization was 41.83 ± 15.63 days (range, 27–70 days), and mean duration of follow-up after discharge was 23.5 ± 9.81 months (range, 11–37 months).

Discussions

ASMVT is a rare but potentially catastrophic clinical complication that may lead to ischemia and/or infarction of the intestine [1, 4, 5]. The mortality rate of acute mesenteric venous thrombosis is usually up to 50 % [9]. The exact pathophysiology of acute SMV thrombosis remains unclear. However, it has been associated with some risk factors for thrombophilia such as myeloproliferative disease [12], coagulation factor deficiency, factor V Leiden [13] and prothrombin gene mutation [14], portal hypertension, post-splenectomy, malignancy, intra-abdominal infection or inflammation [15], pregnancy, oral contraceptive use, and so on.

Transcatheter thrombolysis is used to treat patients with ASMVT and bowel ischemia to achieve early recognition and mesenteric recanalization, and subsequently salvage the adjacent bowel with reversible ischemia. Operative intervention is reserved for patients with severe and diffuse peritonitis, and transmural bowel infarction [16]. Damage control surgery is performed to remove the gangrenous bowel with minimum surgical stress, in order to

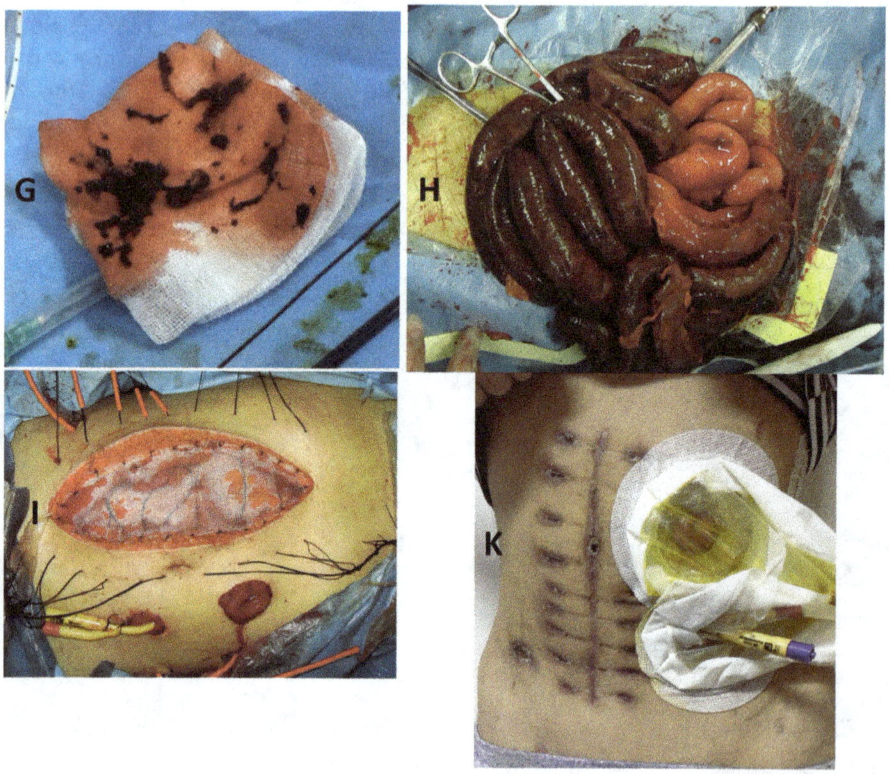

Fig. 3 Patient No. 5: Venous thromboembolus (**g**) aspirated from the superior mesenteric vein via the catheter. Damage control surgery after thrombolysis: obvious transmural necrosis of the small intestine (**h**) temporary abdominal closure, and double stoma (**i**). Abdominal wound (**k**) at discharge after damage control surgery is shown

accelerate recovery from acute illness before performing definitive surgery [17, 18].

In the absence of clear indications for surgery, systemic anticoagulation therapy should be started as soon as possible [6, 8]. Interventional catheter thrombolysis may be more effective than systemic anticoagulation. For acute thrombosis, local thrombolytic therapy via a catheter introduced into the superior mesenteric vein or artery has all been shown to have gratifying results [19–23]. The indirect and continuous infusion of fibrinolytic therapy through the SMA is effective, because it enables the thrombolytic agent to disperse from the capillaries and small venules, tertiary and secondary arcades before reaching the larger veins [22, 23]. Transarterial infusion can reduce the side effects of drugs such as bleeding, and avoid intraperitoneal and hepatic subcapsular bleedings that may result from the association of liver puncture and the use of fibrinolytic agents and heparin [24]. Direct access to the portal system targets SMV thrombosis by a transjugular or transhepatic route, leading to rapid thrombus removal and venous flow re-establishment, and an improvement in symptoms [20–22]. Compared to the indirect method, direct thrombolysis is more efficient, less time-consuming, and provides the opportunity to perform mechanical aspiration and balloon angioplasty with possible stent placement for elastic recoil or persistent stenosis.

We conducted arteriovenous combined thrombolysis for these patients to reduce the need for greater lytic agent doses and longer durations of infusion therapy [22, 23]. There is no consensus on the best fibrinolytic agent to be used and its correct dosage [25]. In our study, alteplase was first used with a significantly smaller initial bolus (5 mg), and was maintained for 24–48 h at the recommended safe 0.625–0.833 mg/h infusion rate. It has been reported that t-PA has demonstrated a higher thrombolytic rate, less plasminogen activation, less α2-antiplasmin consumption and less fibrinogen breakdown when compared to urokinase [25]. Consequently, when the effect of urokinase was not obvious, we switched and used alteplase (tissue-type plasminogen activator), which can selectively dissolve blood clots. However, we cautiously reduced the dose of t-PA when the risk of bleeding was taken into account.

Contrary to previous thinking, surgical exploration is not necessary in all patients with mesenteric venous thrombosis. Premature laparotomy would lead to extensive resection of the small intestine, increase postoperative mortality, and affect the clinical outcome of patients [10, 16].

From our own perspective (Fig. 4), the first step is to evaluate the extent and severity of intestinal ischemia. Unfortunately, there are no precise markers that can identify patients who are at risk for bowel infarction [2]. CT and laparoscopy may play a role in the diagnosis of transmural bowel infarction [7, 26]. Prolonged stasis of venous flow can cause arterial spasm, aggravating intestinal ischemia. Therefore, in patients with suspected acute mesenteric ischemia, revascularization is preferentially started prior to bowel surgery [16]; and anticoagulation treatment should be started immediately [6]. Compared to arterial thrombosis, intestinal ischemia caused by venous thrombosis has a slow development. It

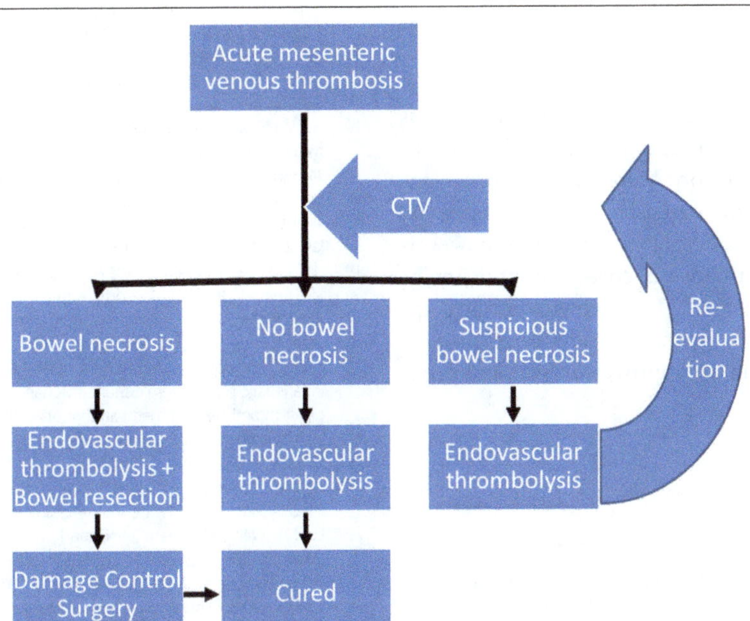

Fig. 4 Proposed treatment strategy for acute mesenteric venous thrombosis is shown

is noteworthy to mention that ischemic lesions occur first in the mucosa, which may be extensive. Thrombolytic therapy should be performed angiographically in an attempt to avoid further infarction. Previous studies have emphasized that longer durations of ischemia prior to treatment are associated with poorer prognosis [27]. Early catheter thrombolysis can restore blood flow to ischemic bowel and achieve maximum retention of the remaining intestine.

If bowel ischemia fails to reverse, intestinal gangrene occurs; leading to sepsis. In such cases, damage control surgery like bowel resection with double barrel enterostomy is preferred over complex definitive procedures in order to reduce second hit phenomenon in such critically ill patients [11, 17].

Double barrel enterostomy allows the observation of the color and vitality of the stoma, which provides an indirect assessment of the intestinal blood supply and avoids a second-look operation. Sometimes, temporary abdominal closure with prolene Mesh (Ethicon, LLC, USA) may be applied when there is severe bowel edema with risk of intra-abdominal hypertension or abdominal compartment syndrome [18].

This study has some limitations. Firstly, this is a retrospective study with a small sample size; hence, further comparative prospective trials are required to validate the findings of this study. Secondly, transcatheter thrombolysis can cause delay in damage control surgery, which can lead to bowel perforation, sepsis and deterioration of the patient's clinical condition; as seen in one of our patients. Hence, continuous close monitoring is required during thrombolytic therapy in order to prevent undue delay in surgery.

Conclusions

For critically ill patients with acute mesenteric venous thrombosis, transcatheter thrombectomy and thrombolysis may be useful to restore blood flow, improve intestinal ischemia, and avoid extensive bowel necrosis. By using the damage control strategy, necrotic bowel is resected, metabolic disturbance is corrected, and finally, definitive surgery is completed. The stepwise surgical approach for ASMVT needs further researches to provide more evidence-based data, to improve survival and prognosis of patients [11].

Competing interests

The authors declare that they have no competing interests.

Authors' contributions

LK, MJX, DWW and WXJ carried out the surgery, and drafted the manuscript. LK, MJX, YSF, participated in the design of the study and performed the statistical analysis. LBC, DWW and LJS conceived of the study, and participated in its design and coordination and helped to draft the manuscript. All authors read and approved the final manuscript.

Author details

[1]Medical School of Nanjing University, Nanjing 210002, Jiangsu Province, P. R. China. [2]Research Institute of General Surgery, Jinling Hospital, 305 East Zhongshan Road, 210002 Nanjing, Jiangsu, China.

References

1. Acosta S, Ögren M, Sternby N-H, Bergqvist D, Björck M. Mesenteric venous thrombosis with transmural intestinal infarction: a population-based study. J Vasc Surg. 2005;41:59–63.
2. Glenister KM, Corke CF. Infarcted intestine: a diagnostic void. ANZ J Surg. 2004;74:260–5.
3. Harnik IG, Brandt LJ. Mesenteric venous thrombosis. Vasc Med. 2010;15:407–18.
4. Kumar S, Sarr MG, Kamath PS. Mesenteric venous thrombosis. N Engl J Med. 2001;345:1683–8.
5. Singal AK, Kamath PS, Tefferi A. Mesenteric venous thrombosis. In: Mayo Clinic Proceedings. Elsevier; 2013. p. 285–94.
6. Amitrano L, Guardascione MA, Scaglione M, Pezzullo L, Sangiuliano N, Armellino MF, et al. Prognostic factors in noncirrhotic patients with splanchnic vein thromboses. Am J Gastroenterol. 2007;102:2464–70.
7. Duran R, Denys AL, Letovanec I, Meuli RA, Schmidt S. Multidetector CT features of mesenteric vein thrombosis. Radiographics. 2012;32:1503–22.
8. Joh J-H, Kim D-I. Mesenteric and portal vein thrombosis: treated with early initiation of anticoagulation. Eur J Vasc Endovasc Surg. 2005;29:204–8.
9. Abdu RA, Zakhour B, Dallis D. Mesenteric venous thrombosis–1911 to 1984. Surgery. 1987;101:383–8.
10. Kim H-K, Chun JM, Huh S. Anticoagulation and delayed bowel resection in the management of mesenteric venous thrombosis. World J Gastroenterol. 2013;19:5025.
11. Yang S, Wu X, Li J. Transcatheter thrombolysis centered stepwise management strategy for acute superior mesenteric venous thrombosis. Int J Surg. 2014;12:442–51.
12. Michiels J, Commandeur S, Hoogenboom G, Wegman J, Scholten L, Van Rijssel R, et al. JAK2V617F positive early stage myeloproliferative disease (essential thrombocythemia) as the cause of portal vein thrombosis in two middle-aged women: therapeutic implications in view of the literature. Ann Hematol. 2007;86:793–800.
13. Famularo G, Minisola G, Nicotra GC, Simone C. Mesenteric and portal vein thrombosis associated with hyperhomocysteinemia and heterozygosity for factor V Leiden mutation. World J Gastroenterol. 2005;11:7700.
14. Vayá A, Plumé G, Bonet E, Carrasco P, Morales-Suárez-Varela MM. Hyperhomocysteinemia and the methylene tetrahydrofolate reductase C677T mutation in splanchnic vein thrombosis. Eur J Haematol. 2011;86:167–72.
15. Hatoum OA, Spinelli KS, Abu-Hajir M, Attila T, Franco J, Otterson MF, et al. Mesenteric venous thrombosis in inflammatory bowel disease. J Clin Gastroenterol. 2005;39:27–31.
16. Acosta S. Surgical management of peritonitis secondary to acute superior mesenteric artery occlusion. World J Gastroenterol. 2014;20:9936.
17. Jansen J, Loudon M. Damage control surgery in a non-trauma setting. Br J Surg. 2007;94:789–90.
18. Waibel BH, Rotondo MM. Damage control surgery: it's evolution over the last 20 years. Rev Col Bras Cir. 2012;39:314–21.
19. da Motta Leal Filho JM, Santos ACB, Carnevale FC, de Oliveira Sousa W, Grillo LSP, Cerri GG. Infusion of recombinant human tissue plasminogen activator through the superior mesenteric artery in the treatment of acute mesenteric venous thrombosis. Ann Vasc Surg. 2011;25:e1-840. e4.
20. Ferro C, Rossi UG, Bovio G, Dahamane MH, Centanaro M. Transjugular intrahepatic portosystemic shunt, mechanical aspiration thrombectomy, and direct thrombolysis in the treatment of acute portal and superior mesenteric vein thrombosis. Cardiovasc Intervent Radiol. 2007;30:1070–4.
21. Kim HS, Patra A, Khan J, Arepally A, Streiff MB. Transhepatic catheter-directed thrombectomy and thrombolysis of acute superior mesenteric venous thrombosis. J Vasc Interv Radiol. 2005;16:1685–91.
22. Liu F-Y, Wang M-Q, Fan Q-S, Duan F, Wang Z-J, Song P. Interventional treatment for symptomatic acute-subacute portal and superior mesenteric vein thrombosis. World J Gastroenterol. 2009;15:5028.
23. Yang S, Liu B, Ding W, He C, Wu X, Li J. Acute Superior Mesenteric Venous Thrombosis: Transcatheter Thrombolysis and Aspiration Thrombectomy Therapy by Combined Route of Superior Mesenteric Vein and Artery in Eight Patients. Cardiovasc Intervent Radiol. 2015;38:88–99.

24. Henao E, Bohannon WT, Silva M. Treatment of portal venous thrombosis with selective superior mesenteric artery infusion of recombinant tissue plasminogen activator. J Vasc Surg. 2003;38:1411–5.
25. Kozuch P, Brandt L. Review article: diagnosis and management of mesenteric ischaemia with an emphasis on pharmacotherapy. Aliment Pharmacol Ther. 2005;21:201–15.
26. Cho YP, Jung SM, Han MS, Jang HJ, Kim JS, Kim YH, et al. Role of diagnostic laparoscopy in managing acute mesenteric venous thrombosis. Surg Laparosc Endosc Percutan Tech. 2003;13:215–7.
27. Park WM, Gloviczki P, Cherry KJ, Hallett JW, Bower TC, Panneton JM, et al. Contemporary management of acute mesenteric ischemia: factors associated with survival. J Vasc Surg. 2002;35:445–52.

Retrospective one-million-subject fixed-cohort survey of utilization of emergency departments due to traumatic causes in Taiwan, 2001–2010

Nan-Ping Yang[1,2,3†], Dinh-Van Phan[4,5†], Yi-Hui Lee[6], Jin-Chyr Hsu[7], Ren-Hao Pan[4,5], Chien-Lung Chan[4,5], Nien-Tzu Chang[6,8†] and Dachen Chu[2,3,9,10*]

Abstract

Background: Epidemiological study was needed to evaluate trends in emergency department (ED) utilization that could be taken into account when making policy decisions regarding the delivery and distribution of medical resources.

Methods: A retrospective fixed-cohort study of emergency medical utilization from 2001 to 2010 was performed based on one-million people sampled in 2010 in Taiwan. Focusing on traumatic cases, the annual incidences in various groups split according to sex and age were calculated, and further information regarding location of trauma and type of trauma was obtained.

Results: In 2010, significantly greater proportions of male and younger subjects were visitors to EDs with a traumatic injury. During 2001–2010, the number of both traumatic cases and non-traumatic cases presenting at EDs significantly increased (average annual percentage change, AAPC 4.7 and 3.6, respectively) and a significantly greater direct medical cost associated with traumatic cases than non-traumatic cases was noted. Focusing on traumatic cases, most of these cases were directed to highest-level hospitals, accounting for 73.5–78.8 % of all traumatic cases, with a significant AAPC of 5.6. The traumatic ED visit annual incidence in males was 58.63 in 2001, which significantly increased to 69.35 per 1000 persons in 2010 (AAPC 1.5); and in females was 38.96 in 2001, which significantly increased to 50.73 per 1000 persons in 2010 (AAPC 2.5). Most of the traumatic cases treated in EDs were minor injuries, such as contusion with the skin intact, open wound of the upper limbs, open wound of the head, neck, or trunk, and other superficial injury (accounting for about 60 % of all cases). The traumatic categories of sprains/strains of joints and adjacent muscles, fractures of upper limbs, fractures of lower limbs, and fractures of the spine/trunk required greater medical resources and significantly positive AAPC values (4.3, 4.0, 4.5 and 6.8, respectively).

Conclusions: Increased ED utilization due to traumatic causes, as assessed by the annual number of cases and incidence, average direct medical cost and highest-level hospital utilization, was observed from 2001 to 2010. Orthopedic-related injuries, including soft tissue trauma of extremities and various fractures, were the categories with the greatest increase in incidence.

Keywords: Emergency department, Trauma, Utilization

* Correspondence: dad57@tpech.gov.tw
†Equal contributors
[2]Faculty of Medicine, School of Medicine, National Yang-Ming University, Taipei, Taiwan
[3]Institute of Public Health and Community Medicine Research Center, National Yang-Ming University, Taipei, Taiwan
Full list of author information is available at the end of the article

Background

Globally, injury is a major cause of death and disability. The burden of injury is greatest in developing countries, and trauma registries are known to be integral in the monitoring and improvement of trauma care [1]. There remains great international variability in terms of patient mix, process of care, and performance of different pre-hospital trauma care systems [2]. To date, the classification, measurement and improvement of data quality in trauma registries have been inconsistent [3]. There is no doubt that injury is a large issue for the health care system, and in particular for emergency management units.

Usually, patients suffering a traumatic injury and other acute diseases constitute the majority of ambulance transports, and adult patients aged 15–60 years are the principal users of Emergency Medical Services (EMSs) [4]. Furthermore, triage, inter-hospital transfer processes and protocols for inter-hospital transfer are also central to trauma systems [5, 6]. From the viewpoints of public health and health policy, epidemiological study is needed in order to evaluate trends in health care utilization, which could inform policy decision-making for the redistribution of medical resources, especially in developing countries.

Methods

Data source, security, and quality control

Taiwan launched a single-payer National Health Insurance (NHI) program on March 1, 1995. As of 2014, 99.9 % of Taiwan's population was enrolled [7]. Foreigners in Taiwan are also eligible for this program. The database of this program contains registration files and original claim data for reimbursement. Large computerized databases derived from this system by the National Health Insurance Administration (the former Bureau of National Health Insurance, BNHI), Ministry of Health and Welfare (the former Department of Health, DOH), Taiwan and maintained by the National Health Research Institutes (NHRI), Taiwan, are provided to scientists in Taiwan for research purposes. Only citizens of the Republic of China who fulfill the requirements of conducting research projects are eligible to apply for the National Health Insurance Research Database (NHIRD). The NHIRD includes nationwide population-based data with good quality control and representation and is provided to scientists in Taiwan for research purposes [8–12].

Ethics approval, and consent for participation or publication

The study design was a retrospective health data analytic study. The protocol was evaluated and approved by the Institutional Review Board (IRB) of Taipei Hospital, Ministry of Health & Welfare, Taiwan, which has been certificated by the Ministry of Health and Welfare, Taiwan (IRB Approval Number: TH-IRB-0015-0003).

The information related to all subjects is encrypted using a double scrambling protocol for research purposes to protect the privacy of patients. Theoretically, it is impossible to query the data alone to identify individuals at any level using this database. No any individual informed consent of all the insured is requested. All researchers who wish to use the NHIRD are required to sign a written agreement declaring that they have no intention of attempting to obtain information that could potentially violate the privacy of patients or care providers. The use of NHIRD is limited to research purposes only. Applicants must follow the Computer-Processed Personal Data Protection Law and related regulations of National Health Insurance Administration and NHRI, and an agreement must be signed by the applicant and his/her supervisor upon application submission.

The application of the present study was reviewed by the NHI Administration, who gave their agreement to the planned analysis of the NHIRD and released the data. (Data approval Number: NHIRD-104-183).

Source and definition of study population

In this retrospective fixed-cohort study, the records of 1 million people in the NHIRD sampled in 2010 were used to perform an epidemiological and descriptive study of emergency medical utilization in Taiwan from 2001 to 2010. This specific longitudinal health insurance dataset (LHID) is the latest cohort data in Taiwan that was named LHID2010 (see Fig. 1) [13]. LHID2010, used as the study population in the present study, contains the entire original claim data of 1,000,000 beneficiaries enrolled in year 2010 randomly sampled from the year 2010 Registry for Beneficiaries (ID) of the NHIRD, where registration data of everyone who was a beneficiary of the National Health Insurance program during the period of Jan. 1st 2010 to Dec. 31 2010 were drawn for random sampling. There are approximately 27.38 million individuals in this registry. All the registration and claim data of these 1,000,000 individuals collected by the National Health Insurance program constitute the LHID2010. There was no significant difference in the gender distribution (p-value = 0.796) between the patients in the LHID2010 and the original NHIRD [13].

The entire medical claim data of the patients enrolled in LHID2010 was collected in the year 2010 and during the period of 2001–2009 retrospectively. All incident ED visits of the 1,000,000 studied subjects in each calendar year were evaluated. The causes of ED visits were divided into 2 groups: traumatic (ICD-9-CM diagnostic codes ranging from 800.X to 959.X) and non-traumatic. Traumatic cases were defined as subjects who visited an ED due to a trauma event once or more in 1 year, while

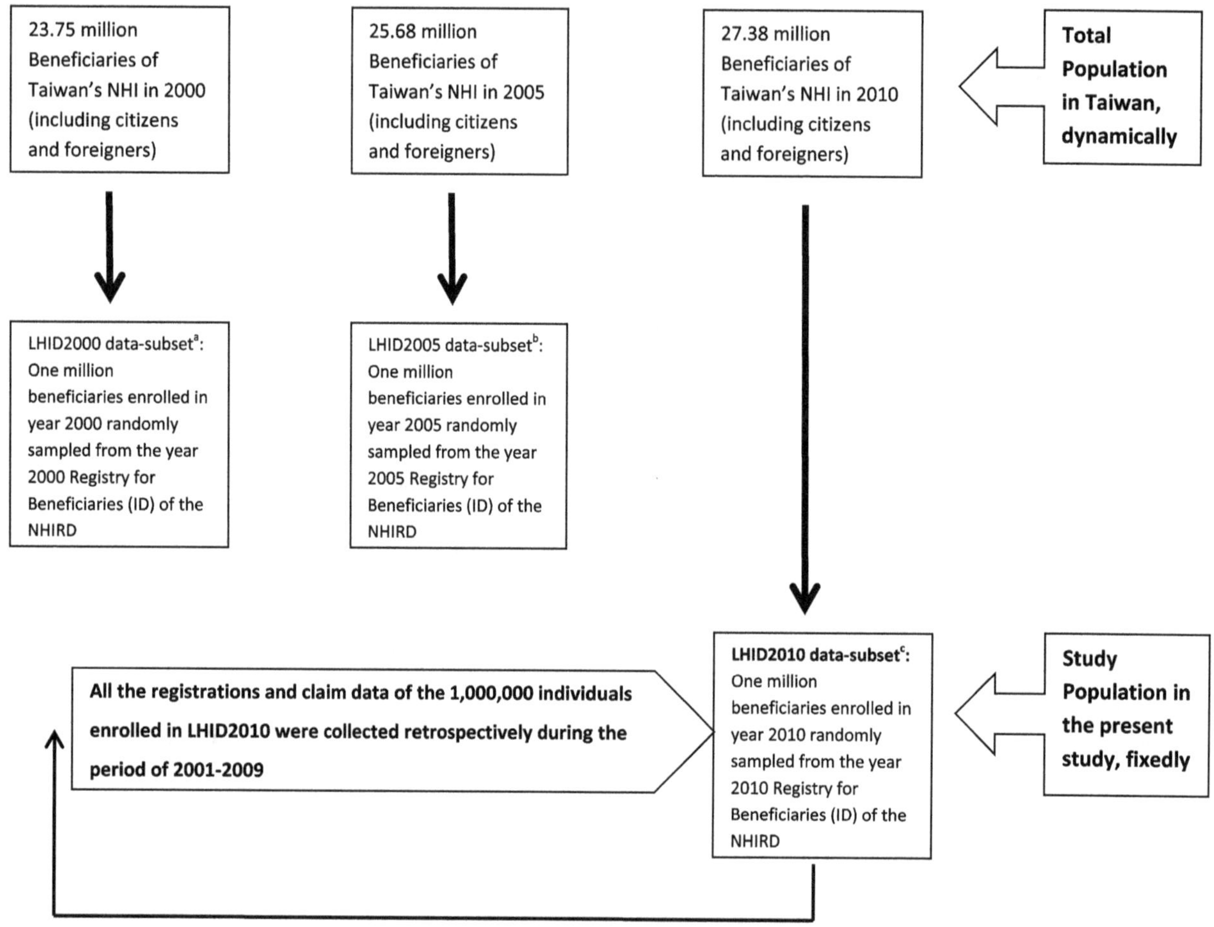

Note:

[a] There was no significant difference in the gender distribution (p=0.187) between the patients in the LHID2000 and the original NHIRD.

[b] There was no significant difference in the gender distribution (p=0.931) between the patients in the LHID2005 and the original NHIRD.

[c] There was no significant difference in the gender distribution (p=0.796) between the patients in the LHID2010 and the original NHIRD.

These three datasets (LHID2000, LHID2005 and LHID2010) are isolated and not traced back to their original NHIRD.

Fig. 1 The relationship of study population and total population in the present study

the non-traumatic cases were defined as subjects who visited an ED for reasons entirely due to a non-traumatic event. Furthermore, each ED visit of the subjects was analyzed to assess the number of annual ED visits and the direct medical cost per ED case. Focusing on traumatic ED cases, the distribution of hospital level, annual incidence by gender, annual incidence by age strata, and detailed information regarding traumatic location/type (classified into 20 categories) [11] were studied.

Statistical analysis

Descriptive statistics are represented by numbers of cases, percentages, and means with standard deviation (SD). The chi-square test or independent *t*-test was used to analyze significant differences between groups for categorical or continuous variables, respectively. The average annual percentage change (AAPC) and its 95 % confidence interval (CI) was calculated using the Join-point Regression Program Ver.4.2.0.2 in order to test for time trends. 95 % CI of cumulative incidence (ci) cab be calculated as the followed formula: ci +/− 1.96√ci(1-ci)/N. All analyses of data were conducted using the Hadoop big data distributed computing environment and the Impala massive parallel processing (MPP) SQL query engine (Cloudera Corporation), and statistical calculations were performed using the Statistical Package for Social Sciences for Windows (SPSS Ver.22.0).

Results

Of the enrolled 1 million people sampled in 2010, 176,126 subjects visited an ED, who were classified into 59,900 traumatic subjects (34 %) and 116,226 non-traumatic subjects (66 %). Significantly greater proportions of male subjects (57 %) and younger patients (64 %) presented as traumatic ED cases (see Table 1).

All ED visits of the subjects were analyzed as individual cases, and the annual number of ED visits, average direct ED medical cost per case, and time trends were evaluated, as shown in Table 2. During 2001–2010 in Taiwan, the numbers of both traumatic cases and non-traumatic cases sent to EDs significantly increased (average annual increase ratio 4.7 % (95 % CI: 3.2–6.2 %) and 3.6 % (95 % CI: 1.0–6.4 %), respectively). Although fewer traumatic cases were seen in EDs than non-traumatic cases, the direct medical cost of traumatic cases was significantly greater than that of non-traumatic cases, and a significant increasing trend of the direct medical cost was observed for both types of case. Focusing on traumatic cases, most (i.e., 73.5–78.8 % of all traumatic cases) were taken to highest-level hospitals, this incidence exhibiting a significant increasing annual trend of 5.6 % during 2001–2010 in Taiwan.

Furthermore, still focusing on traumatic cases, the annual ED visit incidence and the annual trend were analyzed by gender and age. The point estimation of incidence was calculated by the number of subjects visiting ED due to traumatic causes divided by the numbers of various gender and age stratums among the one million study population in each calendar year. Because the study population of 1,000,000 subjects was randomly sampled in 2010 whose information could not be traced back to their original NHIRD, point estimates of cumulative incidences were calculated and their 95 % CIs could be predicted only in 2010. Even though the same fixed one-million subjects were studied during 2001–2009, all the 95 % CIs of point estimates of incidence were not projected accounting for actually dynamic total population rather than an assumedly fixed total population in Taiwan for the past 10 years. As shown in Table 3, the annual incidence of traumatic ED visitors in male subjects was 58.63 per 1000 persons, significantly increasing to 69.35 (95 % CI: 68.85–69.85) per 1000 persons from 2001 to 2010, with an average annual change of 1.5 % (95 % CI: 0.1–2.8 %); that in the female subjects was 38.96 per 1000 persons, significantly increasing to 50.73 (95 % CI: 50.30–51.16) per 1000 persons from 2001 to 2010, with an average annual change of 2.5 % (95 % CI: 1.3–3.7 %). Analyzing the subjects by age, significant increasing trends in the annual incidence of traumatic ED visitors were noted in subjects aged 29 years or under and ones aged 60 years or order. However, as illustrated in Fig. 2, a dramatically increasing linear trend of 43.61/1000 to 70.16/1000 during 2001–2010 was noted in the subject population aged 60 years or older, with an AAPC of 5.7 (95 % CI: 4.7–6.8), which was greater than that in other age strata groups.

Based on the ICD-9-CM diagnostic codes, the trauma locations of the traumatic cases in the present study were classified into 20 categories. Table 4 shows that most of the traumatic patients in EDs were treated for minor injuries, such as contusion with the skin intact, open wound of upper limb, open wound of the head, neck, or trunk, and other superficial injury (accounting for about 60 % of all cases, ranging from 58.5 to 63.3 %). Besides the above-listed and some unspecified injuries, the traumatic categories of sprains/strains of joints and adjacent muscles, fractures of upper limbs, fractures of lower limbs, and fractures of the spine/trunk required greater medical resources and significantly positive AAPC values (4.3, 4.0, 4.5 and 6.8, respectively).

Table 1 Retrospective one-million-subject fixed-cohort survey of utilization of emergency departments (EDs) due to traumatic or non-traumatic causes in Taiwan, 2010

Age (years)/Gender	Traumatic subjects		Non-traumatic subjects			ED-utilized subjects in 2010		One million study subjects based on LHID2010[a]	
	N	(%)	N	(%)	p value of χ^2 test	N	(%)	N (%)	
Total subjects who visited the ED	59,900	34.01	116,226	65.99		176,126	100.00	1,000,000	100
Age (years)									
0–29	25,801	43.07	46,062	39.63	.000	71,863	40.80	372,341	37.23
30–44	12,286	20.51	22,493	19.35		34,779	19.75	251,103	25.11
45–59	11,047	18.44	21,024	18.09		32,071	18.21	223,100	22.31
60+	10,766	17.97	26,647	22.93		37,413	21.24	153,456	15.35
Gender									
Female	25,750	42.99	60,968	52.46	.000	86,718	49.24	507,577	50.76
Male	34,150	57.01	55,258	47.54		89,408	50.76	492,423	49.24

[a]LHID2010: longitudinal health insurance dataset randomly selected in 2010

Table 2 Trends and comparisons of medical utilization in traumatic and non-traumatic ED cases in Taiwan, 2001–2010

	2001–2002	2003–2004	2005–2006	2007–2008	2009–2010	AAPC[a]	95 % CI[b] of AAPC
Annual ED visits, case numbers							
Traumatic cases	63,477	71,221	76,904	80,703	94,176	4.7	3.2, 6.2
Non-traumatic cases	127,988	133,837	141,391	145,217	175,571	3.6	1.0, 6.4
Direct medical cost (US$), per visit							
Traumatic cases, mean (SD)	53.51 (97.20)	60.98 (72.12)	67.86 (86.65)	72.08 (84.97)	78.61 (100.81)	4.8	3.6, 6.0
Non-traumatic cases, mean (SD)	40.53 (94.04)	46.37 (113.32)	56.11 (104.56)	65.24 (110.76)	75.49 (116.98)	8.2	7.5, 9.0
p value for *t* test	0.000	0.000	0.000	0.000	0.000		
Level of hospital visited by traumatic cases, per year							
Medical center, No. (%)	46,647 (73.49)	52,296 (73.43)	57,909 (73.91)	61,737 (76.50)	74,179 (78.77)	5.6	4.0, 7.3
Regional hospital, No. (%)	15,770 (24.84)	17,557 (24.65)	18,590 (23.73)	17,385 (21.54)	18,513 (19.66)	1.6	−1.0, 4.2
Local hospital or other, No. (%)	1061 (01.67)	1369 (01.92)	1852 (02.36)	1581 (01.96)	1484 (01.58)	4.2	−5.1, 14.3

Currency: USD: NTD = 1: 32

[a]*AAPC* average annual percentage change; the AAPC was significantly different from zero at alpha = 0.05

[b]*95 % CI* 95 % confidence interval

Discussion

In the US, publicly-available ED visit data from the National Hospital Ambulatory Medical Care Survey (NHAMCS) from 1997 through 2007 were assessed using codes from the International Classification of Diseases, Ninth Revision (ICD-9). ED visit rates increased from 352.8 to 390.5 per 1000 persons during that time ($P = .001$ for trend), and adults with Medicaid cover accounted for most of the increase in ED visits; in addition, the visit rate increased from 693.9 to 947.2 visits per 1000 enrollees ($p = 0.001$ for trend) between 1999 and 2007 [14]. According to NHAMCS data from 1997 to 2009, the overall adjusted probability of an ED visit being treatable in a primary care setting increased by 0.19 % (95 % CI = 0.10 to 0.28) per year. This probability increased at a rate of 0.52 % per year for Medicare patient visits (95 % CI = 0.38 % to 0.65 %), more than double that for Medicaid patient visits (0.25 % per year, 95 % CI = 0.13 % to 0.37 %). In contrast, there was no significant change from 1997 to 2009 in the average probability of an ED visit being treatable in a primary care setting in privately-insured patients (0.05 % per year, 95 % CI = −0.07 to 0.16) or uninsured individuals (0.00 % per year, 95 % CI = −0.12 to 0.13) [15]. In Taiwan, the ED visit rate, including traumatic and non-traumatic cases, was approximately 190 visits per 1000 persons in 2001, which increased significantly to 270 visits per 1000 persons in 2010 based on one-million sampled patients who were insured under the official Taiwan health insurance system. Therefore, a greater increase in the ED visit rate as measured by the AAPC, and in particular in the ED visit rate for cases due to traumatic causes, was observed in Taiwan, an Asian developing country.

In the US, older adults (aged 75 and over), non-Hispanic black persons, less wealthy people, and those with Medicaid coverage were more likely to have made at least one ED visit within a 12-month period than other subjects. Persons with Medicaid coverage were more likely to have made multiple visits to an ED within a 12-month period than those with private insurance

Table 3 Characteristics of traumatic ED visitors in terms of annual incidence* of the fixed one-million subjects in Taiwan, 2001–2010 retrospectively

	2001 Inc.	2002 Inc.	2003 Inc.	2004 Inc.	2005 Inc.	2006 Inc.	2007 Inc.	2008 Inc.	2009 Inc.	2010 Inc.	95 % CI of Inc. in 2010	AAPC	95 % CI of AAPC
Gender													
Male	58.63	57.09	61.80	68.42	68.59	64.68	64.63	62.44	66.52	69.35	68.85–69.85	1.5	0.1,2.8
Female	38.96	39.62	41.25	45.98	47.00	45.09	46.17	43.87	48.40	50.73	50.30–51.16	2.5	1.3,3.7
Age (years)													
0–29	55.99	56.45	60.65	67.59	67.25	63.54	63.58	61.61	66.20	69.29	68.80–69.79	2.8	0.3,5.3
30–44	42.52	41.65	43.99	48.75	49.84	46.32	45.96	43.29	46.88	48.93	48.51–49.35	2.0	−3.1,7.4
45–59	40.76	39.94	42.15	47.23	47.86	46.69	46.66	44.52	47.69	49.52	49.09–49.94	2.0	0.7,3.2
60 +	43.61	42.56	45.97	51.55	55.80	55.71	61.31	59.52	66.52	70.16	69.66–70.66	5.7	4.7, 6.8

*Incidence (Inc.): cumulative incidence, 1/1000

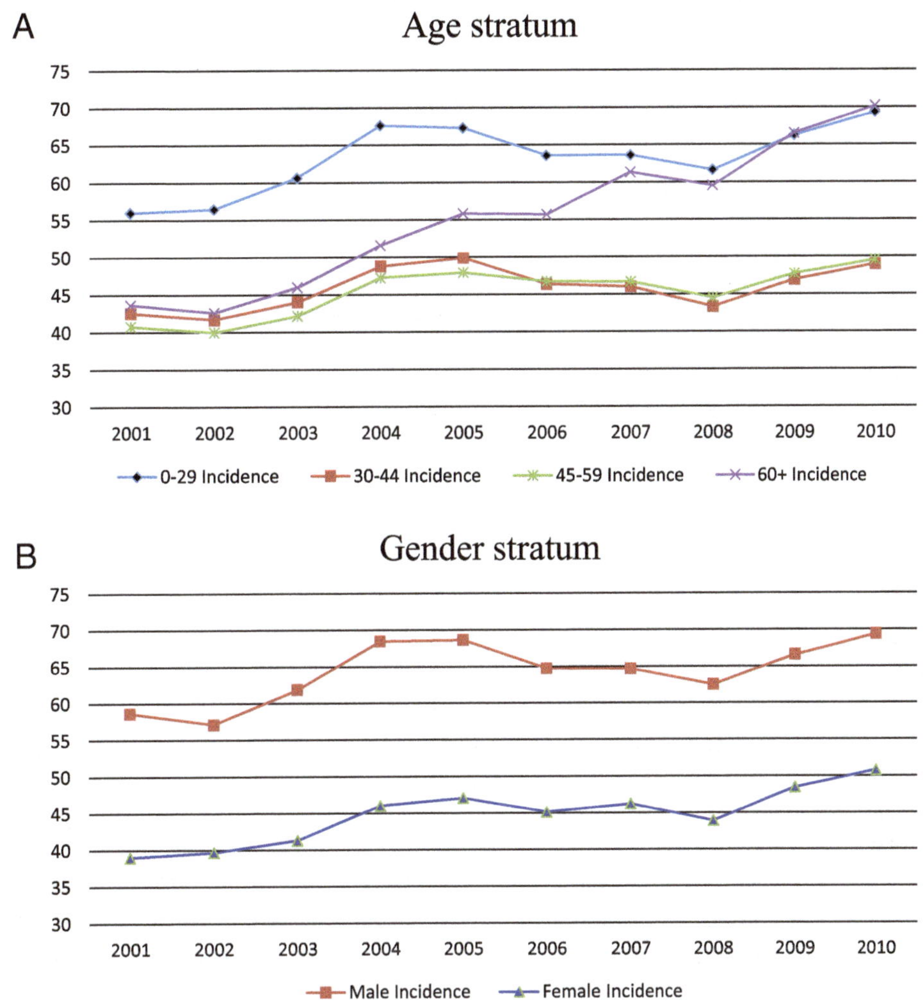

Fig. 2 a, **b** Linear trends of the annual incidence of traumatic ED visiting subjects in various subgroups

and the uninsured [16]. Based on data from the USA National Health Interview Survey in 2012, 18 % of children aged 0–17 years visited the ED, and children with Medicaid coverage were more likely than uninsured children and those with private coverage to have visited the ED at least once in the past year [17]. A recent systematic review concluded that in most healthcare systems, frequent ED users were more likely to be older, female, and have a mental health diagnosis, and previous hospitalizations and high primary care use were associated with future frequent ED use [18]. The main finding of the present study was that female subjects and the elderly (aged 65 years or more) exhibited a greater increase in the incidence of ED visits for traumatic reasons in Taiwan.

Overcrowding of EDs is an important issue, and in order to design strategies aimed at avoiding overcrowding, mathematical models used to predict ED patient volume are considered essential. Most of the models used to predict patient volume are linear regression models, including Poisson regression models or time series models that can include calendar- or climate-related variables. These models explain 31–75 % of the patient-volume variability [19–22]. A significantly increased rate of ED utilization was found in the present study, especially with regards to traumatic cases, of which cases of soft tissue trauma of extremities and various fractures were the categories that exhibited the greatest increasing tendencies. This information is useful to inform Taiwan's health authorities with regards to the delivery and distribution of medical resources.

In Singapore, a statistical report showed that 40.7 % of ambulance arrivals were attributable to trauma, versus 27.3 % of walk-in arrivals. The majority of trauma cases brought in by ambulance was because of road traffic accidents, followed by accidents in the home [23]. In India, traffic crashes and consequent injuries represent a growing public health concern. Open wounds and superficial

Table 4 Distributions of traumatic categories in traumatic ED cases in Taiwan, 2001–2010

Traumatic category*	ICD-9-CM code	2001–2002 No. (%)	2003–2004 No. (%)	2005–2006 No. (%)	2007–2008 No. (%)	2009–2010 No. (%)	AAPC	95 % CI of AAPC
1. Fracture of skull, intracranial injury	800–804 & 850–854	11,060 (11.66)	10,229 (9.77)	8650 (7.60)	7429 (6.47)	7688 (6.09)	−5.5	−8.0, −2.1
2. Fracture of spine and trunk	805–809	870 (0.92)	835 (0.80)	989 (0.87)	1133 (0.99)	1439 (1.14)	6.8	2.2, 11.6
3. Fracture of upper limb	810–819	3058 (3.22)	3305 (3.16)	3539 (3.11)	3819 (3.33)	4193 (3.32)	4.0	3.5, 4.4
4. Fracture of lower limb	820–829	2376 (2.51)	2511 (2.40)	2597 (2.28)	2875 (2.51)	3432 (2.72)	4.5	1.8, 7.2
5. Dislocation	830–839	963 (1.02)	821 (0.78)	846 (0.74)	938 (0.82)	1037 (0.82)	1.4	−3.5, 6.5
6. Sprains and strains of joints and adjacent muscles	840–848	3472 (3.66)	3998 (3.82)	4441 (3.90)	4482 (3.91)	4975 (3.94)	4.3	2.2, 6.3
7. Internal injury of chest	860–862	151 (0.16)	139 (0.13)	128 (0.11)	090 (0.08)	132 (0.10)	−3.5	−12.3, 6.2
8. Internal injury of abdomen and pelvis	863–869	158 (0.17)	144 (0.14)	137 (0.12)	133 (0.12)	153 (0.12)	−0.7	−4.6, 3.3
9. Open wound of head, neck and trunk	870–879	15,579 (16.43)	15,939 (15.22)	15,739 (13.83)	15,062 (13.12)	14,221 (11.26)	−1.2	−2.7, 0.3
10. Open wound of upper limb	880–887	14,278 (15.06)	15,498 (14.80)	16,147 (14.19)	15,072 (13.13)	15,768 (12.48)	0.9	−1.4, 3.2
11. Open wound of lower limb	890–897	7437 (7.84)	7506 (7.17)	7932 (6.97)	7853 (6.84)	8149 (6.45)	1.1	0.4, 1.9
12. Injury to blood vessels	900–904	660 (0.70)	944 (0.90)	671 (0.59)	232 (0.20)	194 (0.15)	−17.5	−33.1, 1.7
13. Late effects of injuries and other external causes	905–909	101 (0.11)	84 (0.08)	75 (0.07)	70 (0.06)	96 (0.08)	−1.4	−9.6, 7.6
14. Superficial injury	910–919	7429 (7.83)	8580 (8.19)	10,376 (9.12)	11,497 (10.02)	13,376 (10.59)	7.6	6.4, 8.8
15. Contusion with intact skin surface	920–924	18,229 (19.22)	23,468 (22.41)	28,704 (25.23)	30,963 (26.98)	36,358 (28.78)	8.6	5.6, 11.8
16. Crush injuries	925–929	1958 (2.06)	2190 (2.09)	2237 (1.97)	2070 (1.80)	2089 (1.65)	0.4	−2.6, 3.4
17. Effects of foreign body entering through orifice	930–939	2359 (2.49)	2661 (2.54)	2844 (2.50)	2794 (2.43)	3023 (2.39)	2.8	0.7, 4.9
18. Burns	940–949	3411 (3.60)	3369 (3.22)	3320 (2.92)	3226 (2.81)	3579 (2.83)	0.3	−1.9, 2.5
19. Injury to nerves and spinal cord	950–957	107 (0.11)	155 (0.15)	163 (0.14)	179 (0.16)	227 (0.18)	8.6	3.6, 13.8
20. Certain traumatic complications and unspecified injuries	958–959	1181 (1.25)	2343 (2.24)	4246 (3.73)	4850 (4.23)	6203 (4.91)	22.4	9.6, 36.7

*Accounting for the 1st main diagnostic code only

injuries to the head (69.3 %), upper extremities (27 %) and lower extremities (24 %) were found to be the most common injuries [24]. Based on data from the statewide trauma registry in Queensland, Australia, from 2006 to 2010, moped/scooter riders sustained a greater percentage of head/neck (+8.6 %), facial (+3.0 %) and abdominal injuries (+2.3 %), whereas motorcycle riders sustained a greater percentage of upper extremity (+4.0 %), thoracic (+3.9 %), spinal (+3.6 %) and lower extremity injuries (+2.6 %) [25]. In Taiwan, the incidence of traffic accident-related hospitalization was between 9.17 and 11.54 %, and in all inpatients admitted due to road traffic accidents, the orthopedic fractures of (1) fracture of upper limb, (2) fracture of lower limb, and (3) fracture of spine/trunk were the most common injuries, accounting for 29.36 % of all injuries [26]. Road traffic accidents involving motorized two-wheeled vehicle (MTV) riders often result in severe morbidity and mortality. Many studies have focused on this specific issue [27, 28]. In the present study, which focused on traumatic injuries, most traumatic cases presenting at EDs had sustained superficial or open-wound injuries; however, the traumatic categories of sprains/strains of joints and adjacent muscles, fractures of upper limbs, fractures of lower limbs, and fractures of the spine/trunk exhibited significant annual increases in incidence. Most traumatic ED cases in the present study were sent to highest-level hospitals, which is contrary to another study performed in Taiwan showing the use of the ED service in the nearest community hospital to be more acceptable in an emergency situation than medical center treatment for dying cancer patients [29]. More detailed evaluation is needed in future studies to examine the causes of accidents and the subsequent morbidity or mortality.

Some limitations were still persisted in the present study. In Taiwan, no researchers can approach all the NHI beneficiaries' inpatient and ambulatory medical records. A longitudinal health dataset of one million fixed cohort populations, including their inpatient and ambulatory medical records, was the most popular research databank. However, more detailed personal information such as occupation, education level, living area, or healthy habitus were absent. Up to now, there were three isolated longitudinal datasets containing LHID2000, LHID2005 and LHID2010 that can provide only point estimates for epidemiological studies due to lack of available data of whole Taiwan's population in each calendar year. In another way, during the study period of 2001–2010, 10 separated cross-sectional surveys in each calendar year might be performed based on the truly dynamic total population but only 0.2 % of the ambulatory care records extracted by systematic sampling method have been allowed to be released to Taiwanese researchers [13]. Finally, the latest longitudinal health dataset (LHID2010) in Taiwan was chosen to perform a descriptive epidemiological analysis that was designed as a retrospective fixed-cohort study.

Conclusions

Focusing on traumatic visits of patients to EDs, increased ED utilization was observed between 2001 and 2010 in Taiwan, as evidenced by the increases in the annual number of cases, annual incidence assessed by gender and age, average direct medical cost, and highest-level hospital utilization. Of the 20 categories into which all traumatic causes were divided, orthopedic-related injuries, including soft tissue trauma of extremities and various fractures, were the categories in which the greatest increases in incidence were observed. Greater numbers of surgical and orthopedic physicians may be needed in EDs, especially in the highest-level hospitals in Taiwan,

Acknowledgments

This study was partially supported by MOST-102-2221-E-155-027-MY3 & MOST-104-2218-E-155-004. The authors would still like to thank Keelung Hospital and the Ministry of Health& Welfare for supporting the study.

Authors' contributions

The study was designed by NPY, CLC and DC; data were gathered and analyzed by NPY, DVP, NTC and RHP; the initial draft of the manuscript was written by NPY, DVP and NTC; the accuracy of the data and analyses was assured by YHL, JCH and DC. All authors participated in the preparation of the manuscript and approved the final version. All authors have read and approved the final manuscript. NPY, DVP and NTC contributed equally to this work.

Competing interests

The authors declare that they have no competing interests.

Author details

[1]Department of Surgery & Orthopedics, Keelung Hospital, Ministry of Health & Welfare, Keelung, Taiwan. [2]Faculty of Medicine, School of Medicine, National Yang-Ming University, Taipei, Taiwan. [3]Institute of Public Health and Community Medicine Research Center, National Yang-Ming University, Taipei, Taiwan. [4]Department of Information Management, Yuan Ze University, Taoyuan, Taiwan. [5]Innovation Center for Big Data and Digital Convergence, Yuan Ze University, Taoyuan, Taiwan. [6]Department of Nursing, School of Nursing, College of Medicine, Chang-Gang University, Taoyuan, Taiwan. [7]Department of Medicine, Taipei Hospital, Ministry of Health & Welfare, Taipei, Taiwan. [8]School of Nursing, College of Medicine, National Taiwan University, Taipei, Taiwan. [9]Department of Neurosurgery, Taipei City Hospital, Taipei, Taiwan. [10]Department of Health Care Management, National Taipei University of Nursing and Health Sciences, Taipei, Taiwan.

References

1. O'Reilly GM, Joshipura M, Cameron PA, Gruen R. Trauma registries in developing countries: a review of the published experience. Injury. 2013;44: 713–21.
2. Roudsari BS, Nathens AB, Arreola-Risa C, Cameron P, Civil I, Grigoriou G, et al. Emergency Medical Service (EMS) systems in developed and developing countries. Injury. 2007;38:1001–13.
3. O'Reilly GM, Gabbe B, Moore L, Cameron PA. Classifying, measuring and improving the quality of data in trauma registries: a review of the literature. Injury. 2016;47:559–67.
4. Man Lo S, Min Yu Y, Larry Lee LY, Eliza Wong ML, Ying Chair S, J Kalinowski E, et al. Overview of the shenzhen emergency medical service call pattern. World J Emerg Med. 2012;3:251–6.
5. Kristiansen T, Lossius HM, Søreide K, Steen PA, Gaarder C, Næss PA. Patients Referred to a Norwegian Trauma Centre: effect of transfer distance on injury patterns, use of resources and outcomes. J Trauma Manag Outcomes. 2011; 5:9.
6. Kristiansen T, Ringdal KG, Skotheimsvik T, Salthammer HK, Gaarder C, Naess PA, et al. Implementation of recommended trauma system criteria in south-eastern Norway: a cross-sectional hospital survey. Scand J Trauma Resusc Emerg Med. 2012;20:5.
7. National Health Insurance Administration, Ministry of Health and Welfare, Taiwan, R.O.C. Background of National Health Insurance Research Database. [http://nhird.nhri.org.tw/en/index.html]. Accessed 1 Aug 2016.
8. Yang NP, Deng CY, Chou YJ, Chen PQ, Lin CH, Chou P, et al. Estimated prevalence of osteoporosis from a Nationwide Health Insurance database in Taiwan. Health Policy. 2006;75:329–37.
9. Yang NP, Chan CL, Yu IL, Lee CY, Chou P. Estimated prevalence of orthopaedic fractures in Taiwan—a cross-sectional study based on nationwide insurance data. Injury. 2010;41:1266–72.
10. Chan CL, Lin W, Yang NP, Huang HT. The association between the availability of ambulatory care and non-emergency treatment in emergency medicine departments: a comprehensive and nationwide validation. Health Policy. 2013;110:271–9.
11. Yang NP, Chan CL, Chu D, Lin JS, Lin KB, Yu CS, et al. Epidemiology of hospitalized traumatic pelvic fractures and their combined injuries in Taiwan: 2000–2011 nationwide surveillance. BioMed Res Int. 2014. Article ID 878601. doi: 10.1155/2014/878601.
12. Lin KB, Lai KR, Yang NP, Chan CL, Liu YH, Pan RH, et al. Epidemiology and socioeconomic features of appendicitis in Taiwan: a 12-year population-based study. World J Emerg Surg. 2015;10:42.
13. National Health Insurance Administration, Ministry of Health and Welfare, Taiwan, R.O.C. Data subset of National Health Insurance Research Database. [http://nhird.nhri.org.tw/en/Data_Subsets.html]. Accessed 1 Aug 2016.
14. Tang N, Stein J, Hsia RY, Maselli JH, Gonzales R. Trends and characteristics of US emergency department visits, 1997–2007. JAMA. 2010;304:664–70.
15. Pukurdpol P, Wiler JL, Hsia RY, Ginde AA. Association of Medicare and Medicaid insurance with increasing primary care-treatable emergency department visits in the United States. Acad Emerg Med. 2014;21:1135–42.
16. Garcia TC, Bernstein AB, Bush MA. Emergency department visitors and visits: who used the emergency room in 2007? NCHS Data Brief. 2010;38:1–8.
17. Gindi RM, Jones LI. Reasons for emergency room use among U.S. children: National Health Interview Survey, 2012. NCHS Data Brief. 2014;160:1–8.
18. Soril LJ, Leggett LE, Lorenzetti DL, Noseworthy TW, Clement FM. Characteristics of frequent users of the emergency department in the general adult population: a systematic review of international healthcare systems. Health Policy. 2016;120:452–61.
19. Wargon M, Guidet B, Hoang TD, Hejblum G. A systematic review of models for forecasting the number of emergency department visits. Emerg Med J. 2009;26:395–9.
20. Au-Yeung SW, Harder U, McCoy EJ, Knottenbelt WJ. Predicting patient arrivals to an accident and emergency department. Emerg Med J. 2009;26: 241–4.

21. Schweigler LM, Desmond JS, McCarthy ML, Bukowski KJ, Ionides EL, Younger JG. Forecasting models of emergency department crowding. Acad Emerg Med. 2009;16:301–8.
22. McCarthy ML, Zeger SL, Ding R, Aronsky D, Hoot NR, Kelen GD. The challenge of predicting demand for emergency department services. Acad Emerg Med. 2008;15:337–46.
23. Seow E, Wong HP, Phe A. The pattern of ambulance arrivals in the emergency department of an acute care hospital in Singapore. Emerg Med J. 2001;18:297–9.
24. Fitzharris M, Dandona R, Kumar GA, Dandona L. Crash characteristics and patterns of injury among hospitalized motorised two-wheeled vehicle users in urban India. BMC Public Health. 2009;9:11.
25. White D, Lang J, Russell G, Tetsworth K, Harvey K, Bellamy N. A comparison of injuries to moped/scooter and motorcycle riders in Queensland, Australia. Injury. 2013;44:855–62.
26. Pan RH, Chang NT, Chu D, Hsu KF, Hsu YN, Hsu JC, et al. Epidemiology of orthopedic fractures and other injuries among inpatients admitted due to traffic accidents: a 10-year nationwide survey in Taiwan. ScientificWorldJournal. 2014;2014:637872.
27. Leijdesdorff HA, Siegerink B, Sier CF, Reurings MC, Schipper IB. Injury pattern, injury severity, and mortality in 33,495 hospital-admitted victims of motorized two-wheeled vehicle crashes in The Netherlands. J Trauma Acute Care Surg. 2012;72:1363–8.
28. Miggins M, Lottenberg L, Liu H, Moldawer L, Efron P, Ang D. Mopeds and scooters: crash outcomes in a high traffic state. J Trauma. 2011;71:217–22.
29. Lee YH, Chu D, Yang NP, Chan CL, Cheng SP, Pai JT, et al. Emergency visits among end-of-life cancer patients in Taiwan: a nationwide population-based study. BMC Palliat Care. 2015;14:25.

21

2017 update of the WSES guidelines for emergency repair of complicated abdominal wall hernias

Arianna Birindelli[1], Massimo Sartelli[2], Salomone Di Saverio[3*], Federico Coccolini[4], Luca Ansaloni[4], Gabrielle H. van Ramshorst[5], Giampiero Campanelli[6], Vladimir Khokha[7], Ernest E. Moore[8], Andrew Peitzman[9], George Velmahos[10], Frederick Alan Moore[11], Ari Leppaniemi[12], Clay Cothren Burlew[8], Walter L. Biffl[13], Kaoru Koike[14], Yoram Kluger[15], Gustavo P. Fraga[16], Carlos A. Ordonez[17], Matteo Novello[1], Ferdinando Agresta[18], Boris Sakakushev[19], Igor Gerych[20], Imtiaz Wani[21], Michael D. Kelly[22], Carlos Augusto Gomes[23,24], Mario Paulo Faro Jr[25], Antonio Tarasconi[26], Zaza Demetrashvili[27], Jae Gil Lee[28], Nereo Vettoretto[29], Gianluca Guercioni[30], Roberto Persiani[31], Cristian Tranà[2], Yunfeng Cui[32], Kenneth Y. Y. Kok[33], Wagih M. Ghnnam[34], Ashraf El-Sayed Abbas[34], Norio Sato[14], Sanjay Marwah[35], Muthukumaran Rangarajan[36], Offir Ben-Ishay[15], Abdul Rashid K Adesunkanmi[37], Helmut Alfredo Segovia Lohse[38], Jakub Kenig[39], Stefano Mandalà[40], Raul Coimbra[41], Aneel Bhangu[42], Nigel Suggett[43], Antonio Biondi[44], Nazario Portolani[45], Gianluca Baiocchi[45], Andrew W Kirkpatrick[46], Rodolfo Scibé[2], Michael Sugrue[47], Osvaldo Chiara[48] and Fausto Catena[26]

Abstract

Emergency repair of complicated abdominal wall hernias may be associated with worsen outcome and a significant rate of postoperative complications. There is no consensus on management of complicated abdominal hernias. The main matter of debate is about the use of mesh in case of intestinal resection and the type of mesh to be used. Wound infection is the most common complication encountered and represents an immense burden especially in the presence of a mesh. The recurrence rate is an important topic that influences the final outcome. A World Society of Emergency Surgery (WSES) Consensus Conference was held in Bergamo in July 2013 with the aim to define recommendations for emergency repair of abdominal wall hernias in adults. This document represents the executive summary of the consensus conference approved by a WSES expert panel. In 2016, the guidelines have been revised and updated according to the most recent available literature.

Keywords: Hernia repair, Emergency surgery, Incarcerated hernia, Strangulated hernia, Mesh repair, Biologic mesh, Bowel resection, Infected field, Contaminated wound, Abdominal wall hernia

Background

A large number of abdominal hernias require emergency surgery. However, these procedures may be associated with poor prognosis and a significant rate of postoperative complications [1].

Abdominal hernias may be classified as groin hernias (femoral or inguinal) and ventral hernias (umbilical, epigastric, Spigelian, lumbar, and incisional).

* Correspondence: salo75@inwind.it; salomone.disaverio@gmail.com
[3]Department of Surgery, Maggiore Hospital, Bologna, Italy
Full list of author information is available at the end of the article

An incarcerated hernia is a hernia in which the content has become irreducible due to a narrow opening in the abdominal wall or due to adhesions between the content and the hernia sac. Moreover, intestinal obstruction may complicate an incarcerated hernia. A strangulated hernia occurs when the blood supply to the contents of the hernia (e.g. omentum, bowel) is compromised [2]. Strangulated hernias remain a significant challenge, as they are sometimes difficult to diagnose by physical examination and require urgent surgical intervention. Early surgical intervention of a strangulated hernia with obstruction is crucial as delayed diagnosis can result in the need for bowel resection with prolonged recovery and increased complication rate. Strangulated hernias may lead to bacterial translocation and intestinal wall necrosis (potentially resulting in bowel perforation). This condition significantly increases the risks in emergency hernia repair that may lead to an increased incidence of surgical site contamination and recurrence.

An interesting topic is the use of laparoscopy in emergency hernia repair. However, its role in acute settings is not well established yet.

Bacteria inherently colonize all surgical wounds, but not all of these contaminations ultimately lead to infection. In most patients, infection does not occur because innate host defences are able to eliminate microbes at the surgical site. However, there is some evidence that the implantation of foreign materials, such as prosthetic mesh, may lead to a decreased threshold for infection [3].

While many factors can influence surgical wound healing and postoperative infection, bacterial burden is the most significant risk factor. According to the likelihood and degree of wound contamination at the time of operation, the Centers for Disease Control and Prevention (CDC) wound classification stratifies the wound as follows [4]:

Class I = clean wounds
Class II = clean-contaminated wounds
Class III = contaminated wounds
Class IV = dirty or infected wounds (Table 1)

The choice of technique repair is based on the contamination of the surgical field, the size of the hernia, and the experience of the surgeon.

In clean-contaminated, contaminated, and dirty surgical procedures, the polymicrobial aerobic and anaerobic flora closely resemble the normal endogenous microflora of the gastrointestinal (GI) tract and are the most frequently observed pathogens. The contaminating pathogens in GI surgery include gram-negative bacilli (e.g. *Escherichia coli*) and gram-positive microbes, such as enterococci and anaerobic organisms. A classification scheme has been demonstrated in multiple studies to predict the relative probability that a given wound will become infected [5, 6].

Several studies show clear advantages of mesh use in elective cases, where infection is uncommon [7]. Mesh is easy to use, has low complication rates, and significantly reduces the rate of hernia recurrence. However, few studies have investigated the outcome of mesh use in an emergency setting, where there is often surgical field contamination due to bowel involvement [8, 9].

The use of biological mesh has many advantages, including a decreased immune response, as well as decreased incidence of fistulae formation, fibrosis, and erosions.

There is, however, a paucity of high-quality evidence on the superiority of biological mesh, and it is still a very expensive device [10].

The role of local anaesthesia in the treatment of complicated inguinal and femoral hernia needs to be taken into consideration because of its multiple advantages, especially in patients with multiple comorbidities.

A World Society of Emergency Surgery (WSES) Consensus Conference was held in Bergamo in July 2013, during the 2nd Congress of the World Society of Emergency Surgery with the goal of defining recommendations for emergency repair of abdominal wall hernias in adults. This document represents the executive summary of the consensus conference approved by a WSES expert panel. In 2017, the guidelines have been revised and updated according to the most recent available literature (Appendix).

Materials and methods

A computerized search was done by the bibliographer in different databanks (MEDLINE, Scopus, Embase), and

Table 1 Surgical wound classification [4]

Class I/clean	An uninfected operative wound in which no inflammation is encountered and the respiratory, alimentary, genital, or uninfected urinary tract is not entered. In addition, clean wounds are primarily closed and, if necessary, drained with closed drainage. Operative incisional wounds that follow non-penetrating (blunt) trauma should be included in this category if they meet the criteria
Class II/clean-contaminated	An operative wound in which the respiratory, alimentary, genital, or urinary tract is entered under controlled conditions and without unusual contamination. Specifically, operations involving the biliary tract, appendix, vagina, and oropharynx are included in this category, provided no evidence of infection or major break in technique is encountered
Class III/contaminated	Open, fresh, accidental wounds. In addition, operations with major breaks in sterile technique (e.g. open cardiac massage) or gross spillage from the gastrointestinal tract, and incisions in which acute, non-purulent inflammation is encountered are included in this category
Class IV/dirty-infected	Old traumatic wounds with retained devitalized tissue and those that involve existing clinical infection or perforated viscera. This definition suggests that the organisms causing postoperative infection were present in the operative field before the operation

citations were included for the period between January 2000 and December 2016 using the primary search strategy: hernia, groin, inguinal, femoral, crural, umbilical, epigastric, spigelian, ventral, incisional, incarcerated, strangulated, acute, emergency, repair, suture, mesh, direct, synthetic, polypropylene, prosthetic, biologic, SSI, wound infection, bowel resection, intestinal resection, complication, morbidity, recurrence, timing, laparoscopy combined with AND/OR. No search restrictions were imposed. The dates were selected to allow comprehensive published abstracts of clinical trials, consensus conference, comparative studies, congresses, guidelines, government publication, multicenter studies, systematic reviews, meta-analysis, large case series, original articles, and randomized controlled trials. Narrative review articles were also analysed to determine other possible studies. Recommendation guidelines are evaluated according to the Grading of Recommendations, Assessment, Development and Evaluation (GRADE), a hierarchical, evidence-based rubric [11, 12] summarized in Table 2.

The guidelines statements have been issued to each class according to the CDC wound classification (Table 1).

In 2016, the guidelines have been revised and updated by the WSES working group on emergency repair of complicated abdominal wall hernias according to the most recent literature available.

Recommendations

Timing of intervention

Patients should undergo emergency hernia repair immediately when intestinal strangulation is suspected (grade 1C recommendation).

Systemic inflammatory response syndrome (SIRS), contrast-enhanced CT findings, as well as lactate, serum creatinine phosphokinase (CPK), and D-dimer levels are predictive of bowel strangulation (grade 1C recommendation).

Unfortunately, morbidity and mortality rates remain high for patients who undergo emergency repair of abdominal hernias. Early diagnosis of strangulated obstruction may be difficult, and delayed diagnosis can lead to septic complications. However, in the case of suspected bowel strangulation, the benefits outweigh the risks of surgery and patients should undergo immediate surgical intervention.

A recent study performed by Martínez-Serrano et al. prospectively analysed morbidity and mortality rates following emergency hernia repair. The study population included 244 patients with complicated abdominal wall hernias requiring surgical repair. In this study, the patients were treated according to standardized protocols with detailed actions taken during the pre-, intra-, and postoperative periods. Clinical outcomes were compared retrospectively to that of 402 patients who had undergone similar procedures before the development and implementation of the protocols outlined in the study. Results showed higher rates of mortality in patients with acute complication as their first hernia-related symptom and whose treatment was delayed for more than 24 h. Thus, the authors concluded that early detection of complicated abdominal hernias may be the best means of reducing the rate of mortality [13].

Similar results were achieved in the study published in 2014 by Koizumi et al., retrospectively analysing the clinical course and outcomes in 93 patients with strangulated inguinal end femoral hernias. The results demonstrated how the elapsed time from onset to surgery was the most important prognostic factor ($P < 0.005$) [14].

In 2007, Derici et al. published a retrospective study using univariate and multivariate analyses to investigate factors affecting morbidity and mortality rates in cases of incarcerated abdominal wall hernias [15]. Using the univariate analysis, results showed that symptomatic periods lasting longer than 8 h, the presence of comorbid disease, high American Society of Anesthesiologists (ASA) scores, the use of general anaesthesia, the presence of strangulation, and the presence of necrosis significantly affect morbidity rates. In contrast, advanced age, the presence of comorbid diseases, high ASA scores, the presence of strangulation, the presence of necrosis, and hernia repair with graft were found to significantly affect mortality rates by univariate analysis; the presence of necrosis, however, was the only factor that appeared to significantly affect mortality rates based on multivariate analysis [16].

A retrospective study evaluated the risk factors associated with bowel resection and treatment outcome in patients with incarcerated groin hernias. The study analysed 182 adult patients with incarcerated groin hernias who underwent emergency hernia repair in the 10-year period from January 1999 to June 2009. Of these patients, bowel resection was required in 15.4% of cases (28/182). A logistic regression model identified three independent risk factors for bowel resection: lack of health insurance (odds ratio (OR) = 5, $P = 0.005$), obvious peritonitis (OR = 11.52, $P = 0.019$), and femoral hernia (OR = 8.31, $P < 0.001$) [17].

Many authors reported that early detection of progression from an incarcerated hernia to a strangulated hernia is difficult to achieve by either clinical or laboratory means, which presents a large challenge in early diagnosis [18–20]. Signs of SIRS including fever, tachycardia, and leukocytosis, as well as abdominal wall rigidity, are considered common indicators of strangulated obstruction. However, an investigation by Sarr et al. demonstrated that the combination of four classic signs of strangulation—continuous abdominal

Table 2 Grading of Recommendations, Assessment, Development and Evaluation (GRADE) from Guyatt and colleagues and Brozek et al. [11, 12]

Grade of recommendation	Clarity of risk/benefit	Quality of supporting evidence	Implications
1A			
Strong recommendation, high-quality evidence	Benefits clearly outweigh risk and burdens, or vice versa	RCTs without important limitations or overwhelming evidence from observational studies	Strong recommendation, applies to most patients in most circumstances without reservation
1B			
Strong recommendation, moderate-quality evidence	Benefits clearly outweigh risk and burdens, or vice versa	RCTs with important limitations (inconsistent results, methodological flaws, indirect analyses, or imprecise conclusions) or exceptionally strong evidence from observational studies	Strong recommendation, applies to most patients in most circumstances without reservation
1C			
Strong recommendation, low-quality or very low-quality evidence	Benefits clearly outweigh risk and burdens, or vice versa	Observational studies or case series	Strong recommendation but subject to change when higher-quality evidence becomes available
2A			
Weak recommendation, high-quality evidence	Benefits closely balanced with risks and burden	RCTs without important limitations or overwhelming evidence from observational studies	Weak recommendation, the best action may differ depending on the patient, treatment circumstances, or social values
2B			
Weak recommendation, moderate-quality evidence	Benefits closely balanced with risks and burden	RCTs with important limitations (inconsistent results, methodological flaws, indirect or imprecise) or exceptionally strong evidence from observational studies	Weak recommendation, the best action may differ depending on the patient, treatment circumstances, or social values
2C			
Weak recommendation, low-quality or very low-quality evidence	Uncertainty in the estimates of benefits, risks, and burden; benefits, risk, and burden may be closely balanced	Observational studies or case series	Very weak recommendation; alternative treatments may be equally reasonable and merit consideration

RCTs randomized controlled trials

pain, fever, tachycardia, and leukocytosis—could not distinguish strangulated from simple obstructions [18]. Furthermore, Shatlla et al. reported a low incidence of these classical findings and stated that their presence indicated an advanced stage of strangulation, which would be of limited value for early diagnosis [19]. In 2004, Tsumura et al. published a retrospective study investigating SIRS as a predictor of strangulated small bowel obstruction. Multivariate analysis revealed that the presence of SIRS alongside abdominal muscle guarding was independently predictive of strangulated small bowel obstruction [21].

Among possible diagnostic tests, CPK appears to be a relatively reliable indicator of early intestinal strangulation [22, 23]. Icoz et al. published a prospective study investigating the relevance of serum D-dimer measurement as a potential diagnostic indicator of strangulated intestinal hernia. The authors concluded that D-dimer assays should be performed on patients presenting with intestinal emergencies to better evaluate and predict ischemic events. Despite having low specificity, elevated D-dimer levels measured upon admission were found to correlate strongly with intestinal ischaemia [24].

In 2012, an interesting retrospective study examining whether various laboratory parameters could predict the viability of strangulation in patients with bowel obstruction was published. Forty patients diagnosed with bowel strangulation operated within 72 h of the start of symptoms were included in the study. Lactate level was the only laboratory parameter significantly associated with a lack of viability ($P < 0.01$, Mann–Whitney U test). Other laboratory data did not show statistically significant associations. The authors concluded that an arterial blood lactate level of 2.0 mmol/L or greater was a useful predictor of non-viable bowel strangulation [25].

Early diagnostic methods to detect bowel strangulation have advanced substantially following the development and refinement of radiological techniques, such as computed tomography (CT) scanning [26]. Jancelewicz et al. published a retrospective analysis demonstrating that CT findings of reduced wall enhancement were the most significant independent predictor of bowel strangulation, with 56% sensitivity and 94% specificity. By contrast, elevated white blood cell (WBC) count and guarding on physical examination were only moderately predictive. It should be noted, however, that an elevated WBC was the only variable found to be independently predictive of bowel strangulation in patients with small bowel obstruction [27].

In 2014, Kahramanca et al. retrospectively analysed the role of WBC count and fibrinogen as predictive factors of incarcerated abdominal hernia. Comparing 100 patients with incarcerated hernia with 100 patients with uncomplicated hernia, the results showed that high levels of WBC and fibrinogen were significantly predictive of morbidity and cost burden ($P < 0.001$) [28].

Laparoscopic approach

Diagnostic laparoscopy may be a useful tool with the target of assessing bowel viability after spontaneous reduction of strangulated groin hernias (grade 2B recommendation).

Repair of incarcerated hernias—both ventral and groin—may be performed with a laparoscopic approach in the absence of strangulation and suspicion of the need of bowel resection, where an open pre-peritoneal approach is preferable (grade 2C recommendation).

Few studies have focused on the laparoscopic approach to hernia repair in an emergency setting.

In 2004, Landau and Kyzer published a retrospective study investigating the use of laparoscopy in the repair of incarcerated incisional and ventral hernias. The authors argued that laparoscopic repair was feasible and could be safely used to treat patients presenting with incarcerated incisional and ventral hernias [29].

In 2007, a series of patients with large irreducible groin hernias (omentoceles), treated by laparoscopy without conversions, was published. The authors described a technique to facilitate complete removal of the hernia contents. A laparoscopic transperitoneal repair for large irreducible scrotal hernias, removing as much omentum as possible, was performed. Then, a small groin incision was made to excise the adherent omentum from the distal sac [30].

Another retrospective study published in 2008 investigated the role of laparoscopy in the management of incarcerated (non-reducible) ventral hernias. The authors concluded that laparoscopic repair of ventral abdominal wall hernias could be safely performed with low subsequent complication rates, even in the event of an incarcerated hernia. Careful bowel reduction with adhesiolysis and mesh repair in an uncontaminated abdomen (without inadvertent enterotomy) using a 5-cm-mesh overlap was an important factor predictive of successful clinical outcome [31].

In 2009, a retrospective study investigating laparoscopic techniques used to treat incisional hernias in an emergency setting was published. The results of this series also demonstrated the feasibility of laparoscopic surgery to treat incarcerated incisional hernias in an emergency setting [32].

Additionally, a systematic literature review performed in 2009 identified articles reporting on laparoscopic treatment, reduction, and repair of incarcerated or strangulated inguinal hernias from 1989 to 2008. It included seven articles on this topic, reporting on 328 cases treated with total extraperitoneal (TEP) or transabdominal preperitoneal (TAPP) repair. Laparoscopy can also be used to resect bowel, if necessary, or to repair an occult contralateral hernia, present in 11.2–50% of cases. The authors concluded that the laparoscopic repair is a feasible procedure with acceptable results; however, its efficacy needs to be studied further, ideally with larger, multicentre randomized controlled trials [33].

The retrospective 4-year analysis of 188 patients who underwent emergency surgical repair of strangulated groin hernias (57 laparoscopic and 131 open, including one and ten bowel resections, respectively, $P = 0.117$) revealed a significant lower wound infection rate ($P < 0.018$) in the laparoscopic group, without a higher recurrence rate ($P < 0.815$) [34].

Hernioscopy is a mixed laparoscopic–open surgical technique for incarcerated inguinal hernias. Specifically, it is effective in evaluating the viability of the herniated loop, thus avoiding unnecessary laparotomy [35].

A prospective randomized study in 2009 aimed to evaluate the impact of hernia sac laparoscopy on the morbidity and mortality of cases with a spontaneous reduction of the strangulated hernia content before the assessment of its viability. Ninety-five patients were randomly assigned to two groups: group A (21 patients managed using hernia sac laparoscopy) and group B (20 patients managed without laparoscopy). The median hospital stay was 28 h for group A and 34 h for group B. Four patients of group B had major complications, whereas there was none observed in group A. Two unnecessary laparotomies and two deaths occurred in group B. The authors concluded that hernia sac laparoscopy seems to be an accurate and safe method of preventing unnecessary laparotomy, and in high-risk patients, it contributes to decreased morbidity [36]..

Emergency hernia repair in "clean surgical field" (CDC wound class I)

The use of mesh in clean surgical fields (CDC wound class I) is associated with lower recurrence rate, if compared to tissue repair, without an increase in the wound infection rate. Prosthetic repair with a synthetic mesh is recommended for patients with intestinal incarceration and no signs of intestinal strangulation or concurrent bowel resection (clean surgical field) (grade 1A recommendation).

Ventral hernias

For patients with intestinal incarceration and no signs of intestinal strangulation or concurrent bowel resection, the surgical field is presumed clean and the infectious risk for synthetic mesh is low. The absence of intestinal wall ischaemia makes patients less prone to bacterial translocation.

Advantages have demonstrated using a mesh for hernia repair in clean fields; such advantages include low rate of long-term complications and reduction of recurrence [37–42].

A wide variety of small-sized retrospective studies comparing mesh use to suture repair in the treatment of acute irreducible hernias have been published [39, 43, 44]. The prospective randomized trial by Abdel-Baki et al. compared the use of mesh repair (group 1, 21 patients) and tissue repair (group 2, 21 patients) in 42 cases with acute para-umbilical hernia. The wound infection rate between the two groups was not statistically significant. At follow-up (mean 16 ± 5.5 months), there were four recurrences in group 2 (4/21, 19%) and no recurrences in group 1 ($P < 0.05$) [42].

The prospective 6-year study by Abd Ellatif et al. included 115 patients who underwent acutely incarcerated abdominal wall hernia repair. The results showed low rates of wound infection (4.3%) and recurrence (4.3%), with a mean follow-up of 42 months. The authors therefore concluded that mesh hernioplasty is crucial to prevent recurrence and that it is safe for repairing acutely incarcerated hernias [45].

Groin hernias

The retrospective study by Venara et al. compared the 30-day outcome after acute hernia (inguinal, femoral, and umbilical) repair with or without mesh. The study included 166 patients, of which 64 were treated with and 102 without mesh repair. Among the 64 patients who underwent mesh repair, four patients had concomitant bowel resection. Among the 102 patients who underwent primary repair, 21 patients had concomitant bowel resection. The mesh repair was neither related to a significant increase of complications ($P = 0.89$) nor related to surgical site infection (SSI) ($P = 0.95$), overall morbidity (OR = 1.5, confidence interval (CI) = 95%, $P = 0.458$), and major complications (OR = 1.2, CI = 95%, $P = 0.77$) [37].

A recent prospective study included 202 patients with acutely incarcerated groin hernias. The results showed extremely low rates of wound infection, mesh infections, and recurrence. The authors concluded that the use of mesh in incarcerated hernias is safe [46].

Emergency hernia repair in "clean-contaminated surgical field" (CDC wound class II)

For patients having a complicated hernia with intestinal strangulation and/or concomitant need of bowel resection without gross enteric spillage (clean-contaminated surgical field, CDC wound class II), emergent prosthetic repair with a synthetic mesh can be performed (without any increase in 30-day wound-related morbidity) and is associated with a significant lower risk of recurrence, regardless the size of hernia defect (grade 1A recommendation).

The use of prosthetic grafts in clean-contaminated settings is seldom described. Most studies on the subject focus on elective repair.

Ventral hernias

In 2000, Mandalà et al. published a series of patients with incisional hernias treated with non-absorbable prostheses and associated visceral surgery. The low incidence of suppurative complications, with neither removal of the patch nor recurrences in the short term, showed that non-absorbable mesh repair in potentially contaminated fields was safe [47].

Retrospective studies by Vix et al., Birolini et al., and Geisler et al. report wound-related morbidity rates of 10.6, 20, and 7%, respectively, following mesh use in both clean-contaminated and contaminated procedures [48–50].

The retrospective study by Campanelli et al. analysed ten prosthetic hernia repairs in potentially contaminated fields and reported no major or minor complications after a 21-month follow-up period [51].

On the other hand, in 2010, Xourafas et al. retrospectively examined the impact of mesh use on ventral hernia repairs with simultaneous bowel resections attributable to either cancer or bowel occlusion. Researchers found a significantly higher incidence of postoperative infection in patients with a prosthetic mesh compared to those without mesh. According to the multivariate regression analysis, prosthetic mesh use was the only significant risk factor, irrespective of other variables such as drain use, defect size, or type of bowel resection [52].

The large-sized US National Surgical Quality Improvement Program (NSQIP) study by Choi et al., analysed and compared postoperative outcome following ventral hernia repair, in the 5-year period from 1 January 2005 to 4 April 2010, including 6721 clean-contaminated cases, of which 3879 underwent mesh repair and 2842 underwent non-mesh repair. The results did not show a significant statistical difference in the rate of deep incisional SSI and return to OR within 30 days, between the mesh and non-mesh groups [53].

One of the few available studies investigating acute hernia repair is the small-sized retrospective analysis by Nieuwenhuizen et al. including 23 patients who underwent acute hernia repair with intestinal resection, and surprisingly, it revealed a higher incidence of wound infection in the primary suture group (5/14, 35%) than in the mesh group (2/9, 22%) [54].

Another retrospective analysis of emergency prosthetic repair of incarcerated incisional hernias with simultaneous bowel resection in potentially contaminated fields including 60 patients demonstrated that the intestinal resection was associated with high rates of wound infection (38%) [55].

The prospective 6-year study by Abd Ellatif et al. included 163 patients who underwent acutely incarcerated abdominal wall hernia mesh repair, of which 48 required intestinal resection and anastomosis and 155 did not. No significant difference was found in terms of postoperative morbidities, wound infection, and recurrence rate between the two groups. The authors therefore concluded that mesh hernia repair is crucial to prevent recurrence and that it is safe for repairing acutely incarcerated hernias, even in case of intestinal resection [45].

In 2013, a prospective study to present a 7-year experience with the use of prosthetic mesh repair in the management of the acutely incarcerated and/or strangulated ventral hernias was published. Resection–anastomosis of non-viable small intestine was performed in 18 patients (23%) and was not regarded as a contraindication for prosthetic repair [43].

Haskins et al. evaluated the outcomes after emergency ventral hernia repair in 1357 patients with CDC wound class II from the American College of Surgeons (ACS) NSQIP database and did not find any statistical significance in wound-related or additional 30-day patient morbidity or mortality, between mesh and non-mesh emergency ventral hernia repair. The authors concluded that emergency ventral hernia repair with a mesh can be safely performed without an increase in wound-related or additional early patient morbidity or mortality in CDC wound class II [56].

The randomized trial by Kassem and El-Haddad compared the use of onlay polypropylene mesh positioned and supported by omentum and/or peritoneum versus inlay implantation of polypropylene-based composite mesh in 60 patients with complicated wide-defect ventral hernias, including 12 bowel resections. Postoperatively, seven patients developed a wound infection (11.6%) and two patients developed a recurrence (3%), after 3 and 8 months, respectively [57].

Groin hernias

Some studies have asserted that prosthetic repair of abdominal hernias can be safely performed alongside simultaneous colonic operations. Such joint procedures, they argue, exhibit acceptable rates of infectious complications and recurrence, and consequently, they stated that there is insufficient evidence to advocate the avoidance of prosthetic mesh in clean-contaminated fields, assuming that the appropriate technique is used [44, 58].

Also, the results of the retrospective study by Ueda et al. including 27 patients operated for strangulated groin hernia with small bowel resection (ten patients with mesh and 17 without mesh) did not show any statistically significant differences in terms of morbidity between the two groups and led to the conclusion that strangulated inguinal hernia cannot be considered a contraindication to the mesh repair even in case of intestinal resection [59].

A recent prospective study by Bessa et al. enrolled 234 patients with acutely or strangulated groin hernias of which 34 underwent resection and anastomosis of non-viable intestine. The results did not show any significant difference (P = 0.7) in the rate of wound or mesh infection between hernias with viable versus non-viable contents. The authors concluded that the presence of non-viable intestine could not be regarded as a contraindication for prosthetic repair [46].

In the retrospective study by Venara et al. including a subgroup of 25 patients who underwent acute hernia repair with concomitant bowel resection (four with mesh repair and 21 with primary repair), bowel resection appeared to be a risk factor for overall postoperative complications (P > 0.0001) and major complications (P = 0.003), but not for postoperative SSI (P = 0.42). The authors concluded that mesh repair appeared to be safe in the treatment of incarcerated hernia, since after multivariate analysis, mesh placement was not a significant predictor of postoperative complication (P = 0.458) [37].

In 2014, a SR and meta-analysis including nine studies has been published, investigating the optimal technique to treat strangulated inguinal hernia (mesh vs non-mesh repair). The wound infection rate has been found to be lower in the mesh group than in the control group (OR = 0.46, CI = 95%, P = 0.07). The recurrence rate was found to be lower in the mesh repair group (OR = 0.2, CI = 95%, P = 0.02). Nonetheless, the authors concluded that the study did not allow to currently recommend the use of mesh in case of bowel resection, despite the finding of similar SSI rates with either mesh repair or non-mesh techniques, when comparing bowel resection and no bowel resection (OR = 1.50, P = 0.73) [60].

Emergency hernia repair in "contaminated-dirty surgical field" (CDC wound classes III and IV)

For stable patients with strangulated hernia with bowel necrosis and/or gross enteric spillage during intestinal resection (contaminated, CDC wound class III) or peritonitis from bowel perforation (dirty surgical field, CDC wound class IV), primary repair is recommended when the size of the defect is small (< 3 cm); when direct suture is not feasible, a biological mesh may be used for repair (grade 2C recommendation).

The choice between a cross-linked and a non-cross-linked biological mesh should be evaluated depending on the defect size and degree of contamination (grade 2C recommendation).

If a biological mesh is not available, either polyglactin mesh repair or open wound management with delayed repair may be a viable alternative (grade 2C recommendation).

In cases of bacterial peritonitis, patients must undergo contaminated surgical intervention, which means that the surgical field is infected and the risk of surgical site infection is very high.

High infection rates are reported after emergency hernia repairs with a polypropylene mesh of CDC wound class III. A retrospective study by Kelly and Behrman reported a 21% infection rate in a series of emergency and elective incisional hernia repairs [61]. Recently, a retrospective study by Carbonell et al. investigated open ventral hernia repairs performed with a polypropylene mesh in the retro-rectus position in clean-contaminated and contaminated fields: the 30-day surgical site infection rate was 7.1 and 19.0%, respectively [62].

Some authors investigated the use of absorbable prosthetic materials [64]. However, the use of absorbable prosthesis exposes the patient to an inevitable hernia recurrence. These meshes, once implanted, induce an inflammatory reaction that, through a hydrolytic reaction, digests and removes and digests the implanted prosthetic material completely. In this case, the high risk of hernia recurrence is explained by the complete dissolution of the prosthetic support [63].

Biological mesh prosthetics are most commonly used in infected fields involving large, complex abdominal wall hernia repairs. The use of biological mesh, which becomes vascularized and remodelled into autologous tissue after implantation, may offer a low-morbidity alternative to prosthetic mesh products in these complex settings, with good results also in immune-compromised patients [64]. By incorporating a biological mesh, surgeons hope to provide a collagen-based extracellular matrix scaffold by which host fibroblasts can induce angiogenesis and deposit new collagen. The non-synthetic material of biological mesh makes it less susceptible to infection, and several biological grafts are available in the current market. The classification of biological meshes is based on the species of origin (allogenic or xenogenic), the type of collagen matrix utilized (dermis, pericardium, or intestinal submucosa), the decellularization process, the presence or absence of cross-linkage, temperature-related storage requirements, and the use of rehydration [65]. On the basis of either the presence or not of the cross-linking, biological prostheses are divided into two subgroups: the partially remodelling ones (cross-linked) and the completely remodelling ones (not cross-linked). Thanks to the presence of additional links, the partially remodelling ones resist better and for a longer period to mechanical stress [64].

Many retrospective studies have explored the promising role of biological mesh in contaminated fields, but most of these investigations did not focus on emergency repair of incarcerated hernias [66–86]. Although a biological mesh in these situations is safe, long-term durability has still not been demonstrated [87–89].

A recent multicentre large-sized retrospective study compared suture, synthetic mesh, and biologic matrix in contaminated ventral hernia repair. On multivariate analysis, a biologic matrix was associated with a non-significant reduction in both SSI and recurrences, whereas a synthetic mesh was associated with fewer recurrences compares to suture and non-significant increase in SSI [90].

A prospective study by Catena et al. published in 2007 focused on complicated incisional hernia repair using mesh prosthetics made of porcine dermal collagen (PDC). Incisional hernioplasty using PDC grafts was found to be a safe and efficient approach to difficult contaminated cases [81].

Coccolini et al. published the results of the first 193 patients of the Italian Register of Biological Prosthesis (IRBP) [86]. This prospective multicentre study suggests the usefulness, versatility, and ease of using biological prosthesis in many different situations, including contaminated surgical fields.

The literature review by Coccolini et al. covered the use of biological meshes for abdominal reconstruction in emergency and elective setting in transplanted patients and reported a complication rate of 9.4% [84].

In 2014, Han et al. published a retrospective study including 63 patients who underwent emergency surgery for acute incarcerated abdominal wall hernias with human acellular dermal matrix (ADM) repair with a very low rate of infection (1.6%) as well as recurrences (15.9%) in a follow-up of 43 months. Bowel resection, performed in 33 patients, did not significantly affect the bulge and recurrence rate (P = 0.262). Interestingly, multivariate analysis demonstrated three factors to be significantly related to bulge and recurrence: BMI (P = 0.008), defect size (P = 0.016), and numbers of biological meshes used (P = 0.027) [91].

The systematic review by Lee et al. included a total of 32 studies regarding the use of synthetic and biologic materials for abdominal wall reinforcement in contaminated fields. In contaminated and/or dirty fields, wound infection rates were similar, but pooled hernia rates were 27.2% (95% CI = 9.5–44.9) with biological and 3.2% (95% CI = 0.0–11.0) with synthetic non-absorbable meshes. Other outcomes were comparable [92].

The recent multicentre prospective observational study by De Simone et al. included 71 patients who underwent emergency ventral hernia repair with a biological mesh. The surgical field resulted contaminated in 27 patients (38%), potentially contaminated in 19 patients (26.7%), and dirty in 25 patients (35.2%). Early postoperative (3rd–7th postoperative days) wound infection occurred in 21 patients (29.57%). High ASA score (≥ 3) (OR = 2.82, CI = 1.85–6.43, P = 0.03), smoking (OR = 4.1, CI = 1.73–6.35, P = 0.02), diabetes (OR = 3.23, CI = 1.92–4.38, P = 0.04), chronic immunosuppression (OR = 2.41, CI = 0.33–5.25, P = 0.003), previous hernia repair (OR = 1.99, CI = 1.5–2.9, P = 0.002), dirty surgical field (OR = 1.87, CI = 0.35–4.4, P = 0.04), sublay extraperitoneal bio-prosthesis placement (OR = 0.45, CI = 0.27–1.13, P = 0.009), and no anterior fascia closure (OR = 0.33, CI = 0.2–2.3, P = 0.04) were associated with wound complications. After a mean follow-up time of 27.2 months, hernia recurrence occurred in 19 patients (26.76%) [93].

Haskins et al. evaluated the outcomes after emergency ventral hernia repair in 1092 patients from the ACS NSQIP database and did not find any statistical significance in wound-related or additional 30-day patient morbidity or mortality, between mesh and non-mesh emergency ventral hernia repair. The authors concluded that emergency ventral hernia repair with a mesh can be safely performed without an increase in early wound-related or additional 30-day patient morbidity or mortality in CDC wound classes III and IV [56].

The use of biological materials in clinical practice has led to innovative methods of treating abdominal wall defects in contaminated surgical fields, although there is still an insufficient level of high-quality evidence on their value, and there is still a very huge price difference between the synthetic and biological meshes [10]. All literature reviews found in the MEDLINE database supported biologic mesh use in the setting of contaminated fields, but the literature included in these reviews consisted of case series and case reports with low levels of evidence [94]. Despite the lack of a cohesive body of evidence, published studies on biological mesh suggest that cross-linked mesh prosthetics have the lowest failure rate in contaminated and outright infected fields. To better guide surgeons, prospective randomized trials should be undertaken to evaluate the short- and long-term outcomes associated with biological meshes [90, 95].

For unstable patients (experiencing severe sepsis or septic shock), open management is recommended to prevent abdominal compartment syndrome; intra-abdominal pressure may be measured intraoperatively (grade 2C recommendation).

A prospective study published by Beltrán et al. examined 81 consecutively unselected patients presenting with complicated hernias and intestinal obstruction. The researchers used intra-abdominal pressure, measured with the intravesicular pressure method, to assess the clinical severity of strangulated hernias and predict intestinal strangulation [96]. Patients with intestinal strangulation and peritonitis are critically ill cases, commonly shocked and at high risk of septic complications; these patients may experience high intraoperative intra-abdominal pressure. Such hypertension may be the underlying cause of increased pulmonary pressures, reduced cardiac output, splanchnic hypoperfusion, and oliguria, leading to an abdominal compartment syndrome. Increased pressure within the constricting abdominal compartment in conjunction with unchanging or more likely disease-induced reduced abdominal compliance will also greatly reduce visceral perfusion within the abdominal compartment leading to an acute bowel injury [97–99]. This "acute bowel injury" results in release of pro-inflammatory mediators into the peritoneum and systemic circulation, leading to neutrophil priming, increased intestinal wall permeability, extravasation of fluid into the bowel wall and mesentery, translocation of intestinal bacteria, and absorption of bacterial endotoxin [100–103]. Even relatively mild intra-abdominal hypertension (IAH) (e.g. an IAP of 15 mmHg) has been reported to decrease intestinal microcirculatory blood flow, increase bowel wall permeability, and induce irreversible gut histopathological changes, bacterial translocation, and multi-organ dysfunction syndrome [103–105].

Prophylactic treatment to avoid abdominal compartment syndrome involves refraining from abdominal closure when fascial approximation becomes problematic due to excessive tension ("open abdomen") [106, 108]. In this setting, negative pressure peritoneal therapy may play a role in mitigating the bio-mediator effects that cause distant organ failure and is an additional potential benefit of an open abdomen.

Even in cases where the abdominal wall can be closed after a laparotomy involving the discovery of diffuse contamination, fulfilling the World Society of Emergency Surgery criteria for severe complicated intra-abdominal sepsis [107, 108], there is controversy as to whether the abdominal wall should be closed or left open. It is financially cheaper and would be preferable from a patient's standpoint to have a single operation and to not be submitted to longer critical care unit management if it was possible to primarily close the abdomen [109]. However, there is a now developing biologic rationale with early clinical evidence that the open abdomen after severe complicated intra-abdominal sepsis may be preferable due to its ability to allow negative pressure peritoneal therapy which may modulate the course of systemic inflammation with progressive organ dysfunction [110, 111] and to provide a survival signal that needs to be confirmed in larger studies [112, 113].

Following stabilization of the patient, surgeons should attempt early, definitive closure of the abdomen. Primary fascial closure may be possible only when the risk of excessive tension or recurrent IAH is minimal (grade 2C recommendation).

When early definitive fascial closure is not possible, progressive closure can be gradually attempted at every surgical wound revision. Cross-linked biological meshes may be considered as a delayed option for abdominal wall reconstruction (grade 2C recommendation).

After the patient's stabilization, the primary objective is early and definitive closure of the abdomen to minimize complications. For many patients, primary fascial closure may be possible within a few days of the first operation. In other patients, early definitive fascial closure may not be possible. In these cases, surgeons must resort to progressive closure, in which the abdomen is incrementally closed each time the patient undergoes a surgical revision. Many methods of fascial closure have been described in the medical literature [94, 114–117].

In 2012, a retrospective analysis evaluating the use of vacuum-assisted closure and mesh-mediated fascial traction (VACM) as temporary abdominal closure was published. The study compared 50 patients treated with VACM and 54 using non-traction techniques (control group). VACM resulted in a higher fascial closure rate and lower planned hernia rate than methods that did not provide fascial traction [117].

Occasionally, abdominal closure is only partially achieved, resulting in large, debilitating hernias of the abdominal wall that will eventually require complex surgical repair. Bridging meshes will often result in bulging or recurrences [118]. The Italian Biological Prosthesis Working Group (IBPWG) proposed a decisional algorithm in using biological meshes to restore abdominal wall defects [64].

When definitive fascial closure cannot be achieved, a skin-only closure is a viable option and subsequent eventration can be managed at a later stage with delayed abdominal closure and synthetic mesh repair (grade 1C recommendation).

Damage control surgery has been widely used in trauma patients, and its use is rapidly expanding in the setting of acute care surgery. Damage control surgery can be used in patients with strangulated obstruction and peritonitis caused by bowel perforation with enteric spillage due to a complicated abdominal wall hernia. These patients are often considered critically ill due to septic complications. Ordonez et al. described a series of 217 non-trauma patients with severe peritonitis and who were managed with damage control surgery. Definitive fascia closure was achieved in 51% of the patients. Failure of definitive fascia closure occurred in 106 patients; of these, 72 (68%) were managed with skin-only closure. Skin-only closure could be an alternative for patients with failure of definitive fascia closure, reducing the risk of complications of open abdomen and abdominal compartmental syndrome. Patients could be deferred for delayed definitive abdominal closure with synthetic mesh repair [119].

The component separation technique may be a useful and low-cost option for the repair of large midline abdominal wall hernias (grade 1B recommendation).

The component separation technique (CST) for reconstructing abdominal wall defects without the use of prosthetic material was described in 1990 by Ramirez et al. [120]. The technique is based on enlargement of the abdominal wall surface by translation of the muscular layers without damaging the muscle innervation and blood supply [121]. In most series, several modifications to the original technique have been performed, including the use of prosthetic material [122–125]. In a prospective randomized trial comparing CST with bridging the defect with a prosthetic material, CST was found to be superior, although a similar recurrence rate was found after a 24-month follow-up [126]. However, high recurrence rates (up to 38.7%) after component separation have recently been reported [127].

The microvascular tensor fasciae latae (TFL) flap is a feasible option for reconstruction of exceptionally large abdominal wall defects. This technique can also be combined with other methods of reconstruction. Vascularized flaps provide healthy autologous tissue coverage without implantation of foreign material at the closure site. A close collaboration between plastic and abdominal surgeons is important for this reconstruction [128].

Antimicrobial prophylaxis

In patients with intestinal incarceration with no evidence of ischaemia and no bowel resection (CDC wound class I), short-term prophylaxis is recommended (grade 2C recommendation).

In patients with intestinal strangulation and/or concurrent bowel resection (CDC wound classes II and III), 48-h antimicrobial prophylaxis is recommended (grade 2C recommendation).

Antimicrobial therapy is recommended for patients with peritonitis (CDC wound class IV, grade 2C recommendation).

In aseptic hernia repair, *Staphylococcus aureus* from the exogenous environment or the patient's skin flora is typically the source of infection. In patients with intestinal strangulation, the surgical field may be contaminated by bacterial translocation [8, 9] from intestinal villi of incarcerated ischemic bowel loops as well as by concomitant bowel resections. In patients with peritonitis, both antimicrobial therapy and surgery are always recommended.

Anaesthesia

Local anaesthesia (LA) can be used, providing effective anaesthesia with less postoperative complications for emergency inguinal hernia repair in the absence of bowel gangrene (grade 1C recommendation).

LA is one of the most commonly used anaesthetic methods in inguinal hernia repair [129–131]. However, the role of LA in emergency inguinal hernia repair is still controversial [132–134]. The recent retrospective 5-year experience by Chen et al. reported that LA could provide effective anaesthesia and patient safety in emergency inguinal hernia repair, with less cardiac complications ($P = 0.044$) and respiratory complications ($P = 0.027$), shorter ICU stay ($P = 0.035$) and hospital stay ($P = 0.001$), as well as lower cost ($P = 0.000$) and faster recovery time ($P = 0.000$) than general anaesthesia [135].

However, general anaesthesia should be preferred in the case of suspected bowel gangrene and need of intestinal resection and always in the case of peritonitis.

Conclusions

Emergency repair of complicated abdominal hernias remains one of the most common and challenging surgical emergencies and is associated with a significant burden for health care systems worldwide. These comprehensive guidelines on the emergency repair of complicated hernia have been developed by a panel of experts through a Web-based discussion and consensus. This document provides evidence-based recommendations on the timing of intervention, laparoscopic approach, surgical repair according to the CDC wound classification, and antimicrobial prophylaxis on the topic of emergency repair of complicated abdominal wall hernias. One of the novel aspects of the present guidelines is the stratification of the management recommendations according to the CDC wound classification, which is a widely used and standardized classification of the surgical wounds. In addition, this 2017 revision includes a new topic on the role of local anaesthesia.

Appendix

Table 3 Resume of recommendation guidelines

GoR	Recommendation
Timing of intervention	
1C	Patients should undergo emergency hernia repair immediately when intestinal strangulation is suspected
1C	Systemic inflammatory response syndrome (SIRS), contrast-enhanced CT findings, as well as lactate, CPK, and D-dimer levels are predictive of bowel strangulation
Laparoscopic approach	
2B	Diagnostic laparoscopy may be a useful tool with the target of assessing bowel viability after spontaneous reduction of strangulated groin hernias
2C	Repair of incarcerated hernias—both ventral and groin—may be performed with a laparoscopic approach in the absence of strangulation and suspicion of the need of bowel resection, where an open preperitoneal approach is preferable
Emergency hernia repair in "clean surgical field" (CDC wound class I)	
1A	The use of mesh in clean surgical fields (CDC wound class I) is associated with a lower recurrence rate, if compared to tissue repair, without an increase in the wound infection rate. Prosthetic repair with a synthetic mesh is recommended for patients with intestinal incarceration and no signs of intestinal strangulation or concurrent bowel resection (clean surgical field)
Emergency hernia repair in "clean-contaminated surgical field" (CDC wound class II)	
1A	For patients having complicated hernia with intestinal strangulation and/or concomitant need of bowel resection without gross enteric spillage (clean-contaminated surgical field, CDC wound class II), emergent prosthetic repair with synthetic mesh can be performed (without any increase in 30-day wound-related morbidity) and is associated with a significant lower risk of recurrence, regardless of the size of hernia defect
Emergency hernia repair in "contaminated-dirty surgical field" (CDC wound classes III and IV)	
2C	For stable patients with strangulated hernia with bowel necrosis and/or gross enteric spillage during intestinal resection (contaminated, CDC wound class III) or peritonitis from bowel perforation (dirty surgical field, CDC wound class IV), primary repair is recommended when the size of the defect is small (< 3 cm); when direct suture is not feasible, a biological mesh may be used for repair
2C	The choice between a cross-linked and a non-cross-linked biological mesh should be evaluated depending on the defect size and degree of contamination
2C	If biological mesh is not available, either polyglactin mesh repair or open wound management with delayed repair may be a viable alternative
2C	For unstable patients (experiencing severe sepsis or septic shock), open management is recommended to prevent abdominal compartment syndrome; intra-abdominal pressure may be measured intraoperatively
2C	Following stabilization of the patient, surgeons should attempt early, definitive closure of the abdomen. Primary fascial closure may be possible only when the risk of excessive tension or recurrent intra-abdominal hypertension (IAH) is minimal
2C	When early definitive fascial closure is not possible, progressive closure can be gradually attempted at every surgical wound revision. Cross-linked biological meshes may be considered as a delayed option for abdominal wall reconstruction
1C	When definitive fascial closure cannot be achieved, a skin-only closure is a viable option and subsequent eventration can be managed at a later stage with delayed abdominal closure and synthetic mesh repair
1B	The component separation technique may be a useful and low-cost option for the repair of large midline abdominal wall hernias
Antimicrobial prophylaxis	
2C	In patients with intestinal incarceration with no evidence of ischaemia and no bowel resection (CDC wound class I), short-term prophylaxis is recommended
2C	In patients with intestinal strangulation and/or concurrent bowel resection (CDC wound classes II and III), 48-h antimicrobial prophylaxis is recommended
2C	Antimicrobial therapy is recommended for patients with peritonitis (CDC wound class IV)
Anaesthesia	
1C	LA can be used, providing effective anaesthesia with less postoperative complications for emergency inguinal hernia repair in the absence of bowel gangrene

Abbreviations

CDC: Centers for Disease Control and Prevention; OR: odds ratio; RCT: randomized controlled trial; WSES: World Society of Emergency Surgery

Acknowledgements

Not applicable.

Funding

No authors received any funding resource. The paper received a WSES Institutional waiver for this publication.

Authors' contributions

AB, SDS, and MN revised the manuscript. All authors reviewed and approved the final manuscript.

Competing interests

The authors declare that they have no competing interests.

Author details

[1]Department of Surgery, University of Bologna, Bologna, Italy. [2]Department of Surgery, Macerata Hospital, Macerata, Italy. [3]Department of Surgery, Maggiore Hospital, Bologna, Italy. [4]Department of General Surgery, Papa Giovanni XXIII Hospital, Bergamo, Italy. [5]Department of Surgery, Red Cross Hospital Beverwijk, Erasmus University Medical Center, Rotterdam, Netherlands. [6]Department of Surgical Science, Istituto Clinico Sant'Ambrogio, Milan, Italy. [7]Department of General Surgery, Mozyr City Hospital, Mazyr, Belarus. [8]Denver Health, University of Colorado, Denver, CO, USA. [9]Department of Surgery, University of Pittsburgh School of Medicine, Pittsburgh, USA. [10]Division of Trauma, Emergency Surgery and Surgical Critical Care, Massachusetts General Hospital, Harvard Medical School, Boston, MA, USA. [11]Department of Surgery, University of Florida, Gainesville, FL, USA. [12]Department of Abdominal Surgery, University Hospital Meilahti, Helsinki, Finland. [13]Department of Surgery, University of Hawaii, Honolulu, HI, USA. [14]Department of Primary Care and Emergency Medicine, Kyoto University Graduate School of Medicine, Kyoto, Japan. [15]Division of General Surgery, Rambam Health Care Campus, Haifa, Israel. [16]Division of Trauma Surgery, Hospital de Clinicas, School of Medical Sciences, University of Campinas, Campinas, Brazil. [17]Department of Surgery, Universidad del Valle, Fundacion Valle del Lili, Cali, Colombia. [18]General Surgery Clinic, Azienda ULSS 5 "Polesana", Adria, RO, Italy. [19]General Surgery Clinic, University Hospital St. George/Medical University of Plovdiv, Plovdiv, Bulgaria. [20]Department of Surgery 1, Lviv Regional Hospital, Danylo Halytsky Lviv National Medical University, Lviv, Ukraine. [21]Department of Surgery, Sheri-Kashmir Institute of Medical Sciences, Srinagar, India. [22]Griffith Base Hospital, Griffith, NSW, Australia. [23]Federal University of Juiz de Fora (UFJF), Juiz de Fora, MG, Brazil. [24]Faculdade de Ciências Médicas e da Saúde de Juiz de Fora (SUPREMA), Juiz de Fora, MG, Brazil. [25]Department of General Surgery, Trauma and Emergency Surgery Division, ABC Medical School, Santo André, SP, Brazil. [26]Department of Emergency Surgery, Maggiore Parma Hospital, Parma, Italy. [27]Department of Surgery, Tbilisi State Medical University, Tbilisi, Georgia. [28]Department of Surgery, Yonsei University College of Medicine, Seoul, South Korea. [29]Department of Surgery, Montichiari Hospital, ASST Spedali Civili Brescia, Brescia, Italy. [30]Department of Surgery, Mazzoni Hospital, Ascoli Piceno, Italy. [31]Catholic University of the Sacred Heart, Rome, Italy. [32]Department of Surgery, Tianjin Nankai Hospital, Nankai Clinical School of Medicine, Tianjin Medical University, Tianjin, China. [33]Department of Surgery, RIPAS Hospital, Bandar Seri Begawan, Brunei. [34]Department of Surgery Mansoura, Faculty of Medicine, Mansoura University, Mansoura, Egypt. [35]Department of Surgery, Pt. BDS Post Graduate Institute of Medical Sciences, Rohtak, India. [36]Department of Laparoscopic and Bariatric Surgery, Health City Cayman Islands, Grand Cayman, Cayman Islands. [37]Department of Surgery, College of Health Sciences, Obafemi Awolowo University Hospital, Ile-Ife, Nigeria. [38]II Cátedra de Clínica Quirúrgica, Hospital de Clínicas, Facultad de Ciencias Médicas, Universidad Nacional de Asunción, San Lorenzo, Paraguay. [39]3rd Department of General Surgery, Jagiellonian University Collegium Medium, Krakow, Poland. [40]Department of Surgery, G. Giglio Hospital Cefalù, Palermo, Italy. [41]Department of Surgery, Division of Trauma, Surgical Care, Burns and Acute Care Surgery, UC San Diego Medical Center, San Diego, CA, USA. [42]Academic Department of Surgery, University Hospitals Birmingham NHS Foundation Trust, Edgabaston, Birmingham, UK. [43]Department of Colorectal Surgery, New Queen Elizabeth Hospital Birmingham, University Hospitals Birmingham NHS Foundation Trust, Edgbaston, Birmingham, UK. [44]University of Catania, Catania, Italy. [45]Department of Surgery, Brescia Hospital, Brescia, Italy. [46]Departments of Critical Care Medicine and Surgery, Foothills Medical Centre, Calgary, AB, Canada. [47]Letterkenny Hospital, Donegal, Ireland. [48]Niguarda Hospital, Milan, Italy.

References

1. Helgstrand F, Rosenberg J, Kehlet H, Bisgaard T. Outcomes after emergency versus elective ventral hernia repair: a prospective nationwide study. World J Surg. 2013;37(10):2273–9. doi:10.1007/s00268-013-2123-5.
2. Miserez M, Alexandre JH, Campanelli G, et al. The European hernia society groin hernia classication: simple and easy to remember. Hernia. 2007;11(2): 113–6. doi:10.1007/s10029-007-0198-3.
3. Horan TC, Gaynes RP, Martone WJ, Jarvis WR, Grace ET. CDC definitions of nosocomial surgical site infections, 1992: a modification of CDC definitions of surgical wound infections. AJIC Am J Infect Control. 1992;20(5):271–4. doi: 10.1016/S0196-6553(05)80201-9.
4. Garner J. CDC guideline for prevention of surgical wound infections, 1985. Infect Control. 1986;7(3):193–200.
5. Cruse P, Foord R. The epidemiology of wound infection. A ten-year prospective study of 62,939 wounds. Surg Ckin North Am. 1980;60:27–40.
6. Olson M, O'Connor M, Schwartz M. A 5-year prospective study of 20,193 wounds at the Minneapolis VA Medical Center. Ann Surg. 1984;199:253–9.
7. Breuing K, Butler CE, Ferzoco S, et al. Incisional ventral hernias: review of the literature and recommendations regarding the grading and technique of repair. Surgery. 2010;148(3):544–58. doi:10.1016/j.surg.2010.01.008.
8. Samel S, Keese M, Kleczka M, et al. Microscopy of bacterial translocation during small bowel obstruction and ischemia in vivo—a new animal model. BMC Surg. 2002;2:6. http://www.pubmedcentral.nih.gov/articlerender.fcgi?artid=126214&tool=pmcentrez&rendertype=abstract
9. Akcay MN, Capan MY, Gundogdu C, Polat M, Oren D. Bacterial translocation in experimental intestinal obstruction. J Int Med Res. 1996;24(1):17–26.
10. Montgomery A. The battle between biological and synthetic meshes in ventral hernia repair. Hernia. 2013;17(1):3–11. doi:10.1007/s10029-013-1043-5.
11. Guyatt G, Gutterman D, Baumann MH, et al. Grading strength of recommendations and quality of evidence in clinical guidelines: report from an American College of Chest Physicians task force. Chest. 2006; 129(1):174–81. doi:10.1378/chest.129.1.174.
12. Brozek JL, Akl EA, Compalati E, et al. Grading quality of evidence and strength of recommendations in clinical practice guidelines. Part 3 of 3. The GRADE approach to developingrecommendations. Allergy. 2011; 64(8):1109–16. doi:10.1111/j.1398-9995.2010.02530.x.
13. Martínez-Serrano MA, Pereira JA, Sancho J, Argudo N, López-Cano M, Grande L. Specific improvement measures to reduce complications and mortality after urgent surgery in complicated abdominal wall hernia. Hernia. 2012;16(2):171–7. doi:10.1007/s10029-011-0875-0.
14. Koizumi M, Sata N, Kaneda Y, et al. Optimal timeline for emergency surgery in patients with strangulated groin hernias. Hernia. 2014;18(6): 845–8. doi:10.1007/s10029-014-1219-7.
15. Derici H, Unalp HR, Bozdag AD, Nazli O, Tansug T, Kamer E. Factors affecting morbidity and mortality in incarcerated abdominal wall hernias. Hernia. 2007;11(4):341–6. doi:10.1007/s10029-007-0226-3.
16. Wolf LL, Scott JW, Zogg CK, et al. Predictors of emergency ventral hernia repair: targets to improve patient access and guide patient

selection for elective repair. In: Surgery (United States), vol. 160; 2016. p. 1379–91. doi:10.1016/j.surg.2016.06.027.
17. Ge BJ, Huang Q, Liu LM, Bian HP, Fan YZ. Risk factors for bowel resection and outcome in patients with incarcerated groin hernias. Hernia. 2010;14(3): 259–64. doi:10.1007/s10029-009-0602-2.
18. Sarr MG, Bulkley GB, Zuidema GD. Preoperative recognition of intestinal strangulation obstruction. Prospective evaluation of diagnostic capability. Am J Surg. 1983;145(1):176–82. doi:10.1016/0002-9610(83)90186-1.
19. Shatlla A, Chamberlain B, Webb W. Current status of diagnosis and management of strangulation obstruction of the small bowel. Am J Sur. 1978;132:299–303.
20. Bizer LS, Liebling RW, Delany HM, Gliedman ML. Small bowel obstruction. The role of nonoperative treatment in simple intestinal obstruction and predictive criteria for strangulation obstruction. Surgery. 1981;89(4):407–13.
21. Tsumura H, Ichikawa T, Hiyama E, Murakami Y, Sueda T. Systemic inflammatory response syndrome (SIRS) as a predictor of strangulated small bowel obstruction. Hepato-Gastroenterology. 2004;51(59):1393–6.
22. Graeber G, O'Neil J, Wolf R, Wukich D, Caffery P, Harman J. Elevated levels of peritoneal serum creatine phosphokinase with strangulated small bowel obstruction. Arch Surg. 1983;118:837–40.
23. Davies MG, Hagen PO. Systemic inflammatory response syndrome. Br J Surg. 1997;84(7):920–35. doi:10.1080/17415349.2015.1113150.
24. Icoz G, Makay O, Sozbilen M, et al. Is D-dimer a predictor of strangulated intestinal hernia? World J Surg. 2006;30(12):2165–9. doi:10.1007/s00268-006-0138-x.
25. Tanaka K, Hanyu N, Iida T, et al. Lactate levels in the detection of preoperative bowel strangulation. Am Surg. 2012;78(1):86–8.
26. Balthazar EJ. CT of small-bowel obstruction. Am J Roentgenol. 1994;162: 255–61. doi:10.2214/ajr.162.2.8310906.
27. Jancelewicz T, Vu LT, Shawo AE, Yeh B, Gasper WJ, Harris HW. Predicting strangulated small bowel obstruction: an old problem revisited. J Gastrointest Surg. 2009;13(1):93–9. doi:10.1007/s11605-008-0610-z.
28. Kahramanca S, Kaya O, Ozgehan G, et al. Are fibrinogen and complete blood count parameters predictive in incarcerated abdominal hernia repair? Int Surg. 2014;99(6):723–8. doi:10.9738/INTSURG-D-13-00107.1.
29. Landau O, Kyzer S. Emergent laparoscopic repair of incarcerated incisional and ventral hernia. Surg Endosc Other Interv Tech. 2004;18(9): 1374–6. doi:10.1007/s00464-003-9116-7.
30. Palanivelu C, Rangarajan M, John SJ. Modified technique of laparoscopic intraperitoneal hernioplasty for irreducible scrotal hernias (omentoceles): how to remove the hernial contents. World J Surg. 2007;31(9):1889–91. doi: 10.1007/s00268-007-9157-5.
31. Shah RH, Sharma A, Khullar R, Soni V, Baijal M, Chowbey PK. Laparoscopic repair of incarcerated ventral abdominal wall hernias. Hernia. 2008;12(5): 457–63. doi:10.1007/s10029-008-0374-0.
32. Olmi S, Cesana G, Erba L, Croce E. Emergency laparoscopic treatment of acute incarcerated incisional hernia. Hernia. 2009;13(6):605–8. doi:10.1007/ s10029-009-0525-y.
33. Deeba S, Purkayastha S, Paraskevas P, Athanasiou T, Darzi A, Zacharakis E. Laparoscopic approach to incarcerated and strangulated inguinal hernias. JSLS J Soc Laparoendosc Surg. 2009;13(3):327–31. http://www.ncbi.nlm.nih.gov/pubmed/19793471%5Cn. http://www.pubmedcentral.nih.gov/articlerender.fcgi?artid=PMC3015964.
34. Yang GPC, Chan CTY, Lai ECH, Chan OCY, Tang CN, Li MKW. Laparoscopic versus open repair for strangulated groin hernias: 188 cases over 4 years. Asian J Endosc Surg. 2012;5(3):131–7. doi:10.1111/j.1758-5910.2012.00138.x.
35. Sajid MS, Ladwa N, Colucci G, Miles WF, Baig MK, Sains P. Diagnostic laparoscopy through deep inguinal ring: a literature-based review on the forgotten approach to visualize the abdominal cavity during emergency and elective groin hernia repair. Surg Laparosc Endosc Percutan Tech. 2013; 23:251–4. doi:http://dx.doi.org/10.1097/SLE.0b013e31828dacc5
36. Sgourakis G, Radtke A, Sotiropoulos GC, Dedemadi G, Fouzas I, Karaliotas C. Assessment of strangulated content of the spontaneously reduced inguinal hernia via hernia sac laparoscopy: preliminary results of a prospective randomized study. Surg Laparosc Endosc Percutaneous Tech. 2009;19:133–7. doi:http://dx.doi.org/10.1097/SLE.0b013e31819d8b8b
37. Venara A, Hubner M, Le Naoures P, Hamel JF, Hamy A, Demartines N. Surgery for incarcerated hernia: short-term outcome with or without mesh. Langenbeck's Arch Surg. 2014;399(5):571–7. doi:10.1007/s00423-014-1202-x.
38. Burger JWA, Luijendijk RW, Hop WCJ, Halm JA, Verdaasdonk EGG, Jeekel J. Long-term follow-up of a randomized controlled trial of suture versus mesh repair of incisional hernia. Ann Surg. 2004;240(4):575–8. doi:10.1097/01.sla.0000141193.08524.e7.
39. Luijendijk RW, Hop WCJ, van den Tol MP, et al. A comparison of suture repair with mesh repair for incisional hernia. N Engl J Med. 2000;343(6): 392–8. doi:10.1056/NEJM200008103430603.
40. Korenkov M, Sauerland S, Arndt M, Bograd L, Neugebauer EAM, Troidl H. Randomized clinical trial of suture repair, polypropylene mesh or autodermal hernioplasty for incisional hernia. Br J Surg. 2002;89(1):50–6. doi:10.1046/j.0007-1323.2001.01974.x.
41. Sanjay P, Reid TD, Davies EL, Arumugam PJ, Woodward A. Retrospective comparison of mesh and sutured repair for adult umbilical hernias. Hernia. 2005;9(3):248–51. doi:10.1007/s10029-005-0342-x.
42. Abdel-Baki NA, Bessa SS, Abdel-Razek AH. Comparison of prosthetic mesh repair and tissue repair in the emergency management of incarcerated para-umbilical hernia: a prospective randomized study. Hernia. 2007;11(2): 163–7. doi:10.1007/s10029-007-0189-4.
43. Bessa S, Abdel-Razek A. Results of prosthetic mesh repair in the emergency management of the acutely incarcerated and/or strangulated ventral hernias: a seven years study. Hernia. 2013;17(1):59–65.
44. Lohsiriwat V, Sridermma W, Akaraviputh T, et al. Surgical outcomes of Lichtenstein tension-free hernioplasty for acutely incarcerated inguinal hernia. Surg Today. 2007;37(3):212–4. doi:10.1007/s00595-006-3380-9.
45. Abd Ellatif ME, Negm A, Elmorsy G, Al-Katary M, Yousef AEAM, Ellaithy R. Feasibility of mesh repair for strangulated abdominal wall hernias. Int J Surg. 2012;10(3):153–6. doi:10.1016/j.ijsu.2012.02.004.
46. Bessa SS, Abdel-fattah MR, Al-Sayes IA, Korayem IT. Results of prosthetic mesh repair in the emergency management of the acutely incarcerated and/or strangulated groin hernias: a 10-year study. Hernia. 2015;19(6): 909–14. doi:10.1007/s10029-015-1360-y.
47. Mandalà V, Bilardo G, Darca F, et al. Some considerations on the use of heterologous prostheses in incisional hernias at risk of infection. Hernia. 2000;4:268–71.
48. Vix J, Meyer C, Rohr S, Bourtoul C. The treatment of incisional and abdominal hernia with a prosthesis in potentially infected tissues? A series of 47 cases. Hernia. 1997;1(4):157–61. doi:10.1007/BF01234750.
49. Birolini C, Massazo Utiyama E, Junqueira Rodrigues A, Birolini D. Elective colonic operation and prosthetic repair of incisional hernia: does contamination contraindicate abdominal wall prosthesis use? J Am Coll Surg. 2000;191(4):366–72. doi:10.1016/S1072-7515(00)00703-1.
50. Geisler DJ, Reilly JC, Vaughan SG, Glennon EJ, Kondylis PD. Safety and outcome of use of nonabsorbable mesh for repair of fascial defects in the presence of open bowel. Dis Colon rectum. 2003;46(8):1118–23. doi:10.1007/ s10350-004-7290-x.
51. Campanelli G, Nicolosi F, Pettinari D, Avesani E. Prosthetic repair, intestinal resection, and potentially contaminated areas: safe and feasible? Hernia. 2004;8:190–2.
52. Xourafas D, Lipsitz SR, Negro P, Ashley SW, Tavakkolizadeh A. Impact of mesh use on morbidity following ventral hernia repair with a simultaneous bowel resection. Arch Surg. 2010;145(8):739–44. doi:10.1001/archsurg.2010.144.
53. Choi JJ, Palaniappa NC, Dallas KB, Rudich TB, Colon MJ, Divino CM. Use of mesh during ventral hernia repair in clean-contaminated and contaminated cases: outcomes of 33,832 cases. Ann Surg. 2012;255(1):176–80. doi:10.1097/ SLA.0b013e31822518e6.
54. Nieuwenhuizen J, Van Ramshorst GH, Ten Brinke JG, et al. The use of mesh in acute hernia: frequency and outcome in 99 cases. Hernia. 2011;15(3):297–300. doi:10.1007/s10029-010-0779-4.
55. Zafar H, Zaidi M, Qadir I, Memon A. Emergency incisional hernia repair: a difficult problem waiting for a solution. Ann Surg Innov Res. 2012;6:1. doi:10.1186/1750-1164-6-1.
56. Haskins IN, Amdur RL, Lin PP, Vaziri K. The use of mesh in emergent ventral hernia repair: effects on early patient morbidity and mortality. J Gastrointest Surg. 2016;20(11):1899–903. doi:10.1007/s11605-016-3207-y.
57. Kassem MI, El-Haddad HM. Polypropylene-based composite mesh versus standard polypropylene mesh in the reconstruction of complicated large abdominal wall hernias: a prospective randomized study. Hernia. 2016;20(5): 691–700. doi:10.1007/s10029-016-1526-2.
58. Wysocki A, Kulawik J, Poźniczek M, Strzałka M. Is the Lichtenstein operation of strangulated groin hernia a safe procedure? World J Surg. 2006;30(11): 2065–70. doi:10.1007/s00268-005-0416-z.
59. Ueda J, Nomura T, Sasaki J, et al. Prosthetic repair of an incarcerated groin hernia with small intestinal resection. Surg Today. 2012;42(4):359–62. doi:10. 1007/s00595-011-0019-2.

60. Hentati H, Dougaz W, Dziri C. Mesh repair versus non-mesh repair for strangulated inguinal hernia: systematic review with meta-analysis. World J Surg. 2014;
61. Kelly ME, Behrman SW. The safety and efficacy of prosthetic hernia repair in clean-contaminated and contaminated wounds. Am Surg. 2002;68(6):524–8.
62. Carbonell AM, Criss CN, Cobb WS, Novitsky YW, Rosen MJ. Outcomes of synthetic mesh in contaminated ventral hernia repairs. J Am Coll Surg. 2013; 217(6):991–8. doi:10.1016/j.jamcollsurg.2013.07.382.
63. Finan KR, Vick CC, Kiefe CI, Neumayer L, Hawn MT. Predictors of wound infection in ventral hernia repair. Am J Surg. 2005;190(5):676–81. doi:10.1016/j.amjsurg.2005.06.041.
64. Coccolini F, Agresta F, Bassi A, et al. Italian Biological Prosthesis Work-Group (IBPWG): proposal for a decisional model in using biological prosthesis. World J Emerg Surg. 2012;7(1):34. doi:10.1186/1749-7922-7-34.
65. Dunne JR, Malone DL, Tracy JK, Napolitano LM. Abdominal wall hernias: risk factors for infection and resource utilization. J Surg Res. 2003;111(1):78–84. doi:10.1016/S0022.
66. Saettele TM, Bachman SL, Costello CR, et al. Use of porcine dermal collagen as a prosthetic mesh in a contaminated field for ventral hernia repair: a case report. Hernia. 2007;11(3):279–85. doi:10.1007/s10029-006-0186-z.
67. Smart N, Immanuel A, Mercer-Jones M. Laparoscopic repair of a Littre's hernia with porcine dermal collagen implant (Permacol). Hernia. 2007;11(4): 373–6. doi:10.1007/s10029-007-0197-4.
68. Liyanage SH, Purohit GS, Frye JNR, Giordano P. Anterior abdominal wall reconstruction with a Permacol implant. J Plast Reconstr Aesthet Surg. 2006; 59(5):553–5. http://www.ncbi.nlm.nih.gov/pubmed/16749204
69. Gupta A, Zahriya K, Mullens PL, Salmassi S, Keshishian A. Ventral herniorrhaphy: experience with two different biosynthetic mesh materials. Surgisis and Alloderm Hernia. 2006;10(5):419–25. doi:10.1007/s10029-006-0130-2.
70. Albo D, Awad SS, Berger DH, Bellows CF. Decellularized human cadaveric dermis provides a safe alternative for primary inguinal hernia repair in contaminated surgical fields. Am J Surg. 2006;192(5 SPEC. ISS) doi:10.1016/j.amjsurg.2006.08.029.
71. Schuster R, Singh J, Safadi BY, Wren SM. The use of acellular dermal matrix for contaminated abdominal wall defects: wound status predicts success. Am J Surg. 2006;192(5 SPEC. ISS):594–7. doi:10.1016/j.amjsurg.2006.08.017.
72. Alaedeen DI, Lipman J, Medalie D, Rosen MJ. The single-staged approach to the surgical management of abdominal wall hernias in contaminated fields. Hernia. 2007;11(1):41–5. doi:10.1007/s10029-006-0164-5.
73. Kim H, Bruen K, Vargo D. Acellular dermal matrix in the management of high-risk abdominal wall defects. Am J Surg. 2006;192(6):705–9. doi:10.1016/j.amjsurg.2006.09.003.
74. Diaz JJ, Guy J, Berkes MB, Guillamondegui O, Miller RS. Acellular dermal allograft for ventral hernia repair in the compromised surgical field. Am Surg. 2006;72(12):1181–7. doi:10.1680/udap.2010.163.
75. Patton JH, Berry S, Kralovich KA. Use of human acellular dermal matrix in complex and contaminated abdominal wall reconstructions. Am J Surg. 2007;193(3):360–3. doi:10.1016/j.amjsurg.2006.09.021.
76. Bellows CF, Albo D, Berger DH, Awad SS. Abdominal wall repair using human acellular dermis. Am J Surg. 2007;194(2):192–8. doi:10.1016/j.amjsurg.2006.11.012.
77. Jin J, Rosen MJ, Blatnik J, et al. Use of acellular dermal matrix for complicated ventral hernia repair: does technique affect outcomes? J Am Coll Surg. 2007;205(5):654–60. doi:10.1016/j.jamcollsurg.2007.06.012.
78. Franklin ME, Gonzalez JJ, Michaelson RP, Glass JL, Chock DA. Preliminary experience with new bioactive prosthetic material for repair of hernias in infected fields. Hernia. 2002;6(4):171–4. doi:10.1007/s10029-002-0078-9.
79. Jr MEF, Jr ÆJJG, Franklin ME, Gonzalez JJ, Glass JL. Use of porcine small intestinal submucosa as a prosthetic device for laparoscopic repair of hernias in contaminated fields: 2-year follow-up. Hernia. 2004;8(3):186–9. doi:10.1007/s10029-004-0208-7.
80. Helton WS, Fisichella PM, Berger R, Horgan S, Espat NJ, Abcarian H. Short-term outcomes with small intestinal submucosa for ventral abdominal hernia. Arch Surg. 2005;140(6):549-560-562. doi:10.1001/archsurg.140.6.549.
81. Catena F, Ansaloni L, Gazzotti F, et al. Use of porcine dermal collagen graft (Permacol) for hernia repair in contaminated fields. Hernia. 2007;11(1):57–60. doi:10.1007/s10029-006-0171-6.
82. Treviño JM, Franklin ME, Berghoff KR, Glass JL, Jaramillo EJ. Preliminary results of a two-layered prosthetic repair for recurrent inguinal and ventral hernias combining open and laparoscopic techniques. Hernia. 2006;10(3): 253–7. doi:10.1007/s10029-006-0085-3.
83. Shaikh FM, Giri SK, Durrani S, Waldron D, Grace PA. Experience with porcine acellular dermal collagen implant in one-stage tension-free reconstruction of acute and chronic abdominal wall defects. World J Surg. 2007;31(10): 1966–72. doi:10.1007/s00268-007-9174-4.
84. Coccolini F, Catena F, Bertuzzo VR, Ercolani G, Pinna A, Ansaloni L. Abdominal wall defect repair with biological prosthesis in transplanted patients: single center retrospective analysis and review of the literature. Updat Surg. 2013;65(3):191–6. doi:10.1007/s13304-013-0212-5.
85. Cavallaro A, Menzo E Lo, di Vita M, et al. Use of biological meshes for abdominal wall reconstruction in highly contaminated fields. World J Gastroenterol 2010;16(15):1928-1933. doi:10.3748/wjg.v16.i15.1928.
86. Coccolini F, Poiasina E, Bertoli P, et al. The Italian Register of Biological Prostheses. Eur Surg Res. 2013;50(3–4):262–72. doi:10.1159/000351333.
87. Smart NJ, Marshall M, Daniels IR. Biological meshes: a review of their use in abdominal wall hernia repairs. Surgeon. 2012;10(3):159–71. doi:10.1016/j.surge.2012.02.006.
88. Rosen MJ, Krpata DM, Ermlich B, Blatnik J. A 5-year clinical experience with single-staged repairs of infected and contaminated abdominal wall defects utilizing biologic mesh. Ann Surg. 2013;257(6):991–6. doi:10.1097/SLA.0b013e3182849871.
89. Primus FE, Harris HW. A critical review of biologic mesh use in ventral hernia repairs under contaminated conditions. Hernia. 2013;17(1):21–30. doi:10.1007/s10029-012-1037-8.
90. Bondre IL, Holihan JL, Askenasy EP, et al. Suture, synthetic, or biologic in contaminated ventral hernia repair. J Surg Res. 2016;200(2):488–94. doi:10.1016/j.jss.2015.09.007.
91. Han JG, Pang GY, Wang ZJ, Zhao Q, Ma SZ. The combined application of human acellular dermal matrix and vacuum wound drainage on incarcerated abdominal wall hernias. Int J Surg. 2014;12(5):452–6. doi:10.1016/j.ijsu.2014.03.019.
92. Lee L, Mata J, Landry T, et al. A systematic review of synthetic and biologic materials for abdominal wall reinforcement in contaminated fields. Surg Endosc Other Interv Tech. 2014;28(9):2531–46. doi:10.1007/s00464-014-3499-5.
93. De Simone B, Catena F, Biondi A, et al. Incisional Hernia Repair in Contaminated Surgical fields (I.H.R.C.S.) study using biological prostheses in emergency surgery setting with contaminated hernias: a multicenter prospective observational study. J Peritoneum (and other serosal surfaces). 2016;1(2) doi:10.4081/joper.2016.26.
94. Leppäniemi A, Tukiainen E. Planned hernia repair and late abdominal wall reconstruction. World J Surg. 2012;36:511–5. doi:10.1007/s00268-011-1177-5.
95. Harth KC, Krpata DM, Chawla A, Blatnik JA, Halaweish I, Rosen MJ. Biologic mesh use practice patterns in abdominal wall reconstruction: a lack of consensus among surgeons. Hernia. 2013;17(1):13–20. doi:10.1007/s10029-012-1029-8.
96. Beltrán M, Villar R, Cruces KS. Abdominal compartment syndrome in patients with strangulated hernia. Hernia. 2008;12(6):613–20. doi:10.1007/s10029-008-0394-9.
97. Shah SK, Jimenez F, Letourneau PA, et al. Strategies for modulating the inflammatory response after decompression from abdominal compartment syndrome. Scand J Trauma Resusc Emerg Med. 2012;20(1):25. doi:10.1186/1757-7241-20-25.
98. Roberts DJ, Ball CG, Kirkpatrick AW. Increased pressure within the abdominal compartment: intra-abdominal hypertension and the abdominal compartment syndrome. Curr Opin Crit Care. 2016;22(2):174–85. doi:10.1097/MCC.0000000000000289.
99. Blaser AR, Björck M, De Keulenaer B, Regli A. Abdominal compliance: a bench-to-bedside review. J Trauma Acute Care Surg. 2015;78(5):1044–53. doi:10.1097/TA.0000000000000616.
100. FACS JACMDF. Abdominal compartment syndrome: a decade of progress. J Am Coll Surg. 2013;216(1):135–46. doi:10.1016/j.jamcollsurg.2012.09.004.
101. Diebel LN, Dulchavsky SA, Brown WJ. Splanchnic ischemia and bacterial translocation in the abdominal compartment syndrome. J Trauma. 1997; 43(5):852–5. http://www.ncbi.nlm.nih.gov/pubmed/9390500.
102. Victoni T, Coelho FR, Soares AL, et al. Local and remote tissue injury upon intestinal ischemia and reperfusion depends on the TLR/MyD88 signaling pathway. Med Microbiol Immunol. 2010;199(1):35–42. doi:10.1007/s00430-009-0134-5.

103. Leng Y, Zhang K, Fan J, et al. Effect of acute, slightly increased intra-abdominal pressure on intestinal permeability and oxidative stress in a rat model. PLoS One. 2014;9(10) doi:10.1371/journal.pone.0109350.
104. Cheng J, Wei Z, Liu X, et al. The role of intestinal mucosa injury induced by intra-abdominal hypertension in the development of abdominal compartment syndrome and multiple organ dysfunction syndrome. Crit Care. 2013;17(6):R283. doi:10.1186/cc13146.
105. Kirkpatrick AW, Roberts DJ, De Waele J, Laupland K. Is intra-abdominal hypertension a missing factor that drives multiple organ dysfunction syndrome? Crit Care. 2014;18(2):124. doi:10.1186/cc13785.
106. Jernigan TW, Fabian TC, Croce M, et al. Staged management of giant abdominal wall defects: acute and long-term results. Ann Surg. 2003;238(3): 349-55-7. doi:10.1097/01.sla.0000086544.42647.84.
107. Sartelli M, Abu-Zidan FM, Catena F, et al. Global validation of the WSES Sepsis Severity Score for patients with complicated intra-abdominal infections: a prospective multicentre study (WISS Study). World J Emerg Surg. 2015;10:61. doi:10.1186/s13017-015-0055-0.
108. Sartelli M, Catena F, Ansaloni L, et al. Complicated intra-abdominal infections in a worldwide context: an observational prospective study (CIAOW Study). World J Emerg Surg. 2013;8:1. doi:10.1186/1749-7922-8-1.
109. van Ruler O, Mahler CW, Boer KR, et al. Comparison of on-demand vs planned relaparotomy strategy in patients with severe peritonitis: a randomized trial. JAMA. 2007;298(8):865–72. doi:10.1001/jama.298.8.865.
110. Kubiak BD, Albert SP, Gatto L, et al. Peritoneal negative pressure therapy prevents multiple organ injury in a chronic porcine sepsis and ischemia/reperfusion model. Shock. 2010;34(5):525–34. doi:10.1097/SHK.0b013e3181e14cd2.
111. Emr B, Sadowsky D, Azhar N, et al. Removal of inflammatory ascites is associated with dynamic modification of local and systemic inflammation along with prevention of acute lung injury: in vivo and in silico studies. Shock. 2014;41(4):317–23. doi:10.1097/SHK.0000000000000121.
112. Kirkpatrick AW, Roberts DJ, Faris PD, et al. Active negative pressure peritoneal therapy after abbreviated laparotomy: the intraperitoneal vacuum randomized controlled trial. Ann Surg. 2015;262(1):38–46. doi:10.1097/sla.0000000000001095.
113. Cheatham ML, Demetriades D, Fabian TC, et al. Prospective study examining clinical outcomes associated with a negative pressure wound therapy system and Barker's vacuum packing technique. World J Surg. 2013; 37(9):2018–30. doi:10.1007/s00268-013-2080-z.
114. Tsuei BJ, Skinner JC, Bernard AC, Kearney PA, Boulanger BR. The open peritoneal cavity: etiology correlates with the likelihood of fascial closure. Am Surg. 2004;70:652–6.
115. Reimer MW, Yelle JD, Reitsma B, Doumit G, Allen MA, Bell MS. Management of open abdominal wounds with a dynamic fascial closure system. Can J Surg. 2008;51(3):209–14.
116. Urbaniak RM, Khuthaila DK, Khalil AJ, Hammond DC. Closure of massive abdominal wall defects: a case report using the abdominal reapproximation anchor (ABRA) system. Ann Plast Surg. 2006;57(5):573–7. doi:10.1097/01.sap.0000237052.11796.63.
117. Kissane NA, Itani KMF. A decade of ventral incisional hernia repairs with biologic acellular dermal matrix: what have we learned? Plast Reconstr Surg. 2012;130(5 Suppl 2):194S–202S. doi:10.1097/PRS.0b013e318265a5ec.
118. Boele Van Hensbroek P, Wind J, Dijkgraaf MGW, Busch ORC, Carel Goslings J. Temporary closure of the open abdomen: a systematic review on delayed primary fascial closure in patients with an open abdomen. World J Surg. 2009;33(2):199–207. doi:10.1007/s00268-008-9867-3.
119. Ordonez C, Badiel M, Parra M, et al. The open abdomen in acute care surgery: factors associated with success of definitive fascial closure. 2013.
120. Ramirez OM, Ruas E, Dellon AL. "Components separation" method for closure of abdominal-wall defects: an anatomic and clinical study. Plast Reconstr Surg. 1990;86(3):519–26. doi:10.1097/00006534-199009000-00023.
121. DiBello JN, Moore JH. Sliding myofascial flap of the rectus abdominus muscles for the closure of recurrent ventral hernias. Plast Reconstr Surg. 1996;98(3):464–9. doi:10.1097/00006534-199609000-00016.
122. Girotto JA, Ko MJ, Redett R, Muehlberger T, Talamini M, Chang B. Closure of chronic abdominal wall defects: a long-term evaluation of the components separation method. Ann Plast Surg. 2000;44(1):109.
123. Shestak KC, Edington HJ, Johnson RR. The separation of anatomic components technique for the reconstruction of massive midline abdominal wall defects: anatomy, surgical technique, applications, and limitations revisited. Plast Reconstr Surg. 2000;105:731–738; quiz 739. doi:10.1097/00006534-200002000-00041.
124. Lowe JB, Garza JR, Bowman JL, Rohrich RJ, Strodel WE. Endoscopically assisted "components separation" for closure of abdominal wall defects. Plast Reconstr Surg. 2000;105(2):720–729; quiz 730. doi:10.1097/00006534-200002000-00039.
125. Cohen M, Morales R, Fildes J, Barrett J. Staged reconstruction after gunshot wounds to the abdomen. Plast Reconstr Surg. 2001;108(1):83–92. doi:10.1097/00006534-200107000-00014.
126. Reilingh TSDV, Van Goor H, Charbon JA, et al. Repair of giant midline abdominal wall hernias: "components separation technique" versus prosthetic repair: interim analysis of a randomized controlled trial. World J Surg. 2007;31:756–63. doi:10.1007/s00268-006-0502-x.
127. Slater NJ, Van Goor H, Bleichrodt RP. Large and complex ventral hernia repair using "components separation technique" without mesh results in a high recurrence rate. Am J Surg. 2015;209(1):170–9. doi:10.1016/j.amjsurg.2014.02.013.
128. Tukiainen E, Leppäniemi A. Reconstruction of extensive abdominal wall defects with microvascular tensor fasciae latae flap. Br J Surg. 2011;98(6): 880–4. doi:10.1002/bjs.7489.
129. Nordin P, Zetterström H, Carlsson P, et al. Cost-effectiveness analysis of local, regional and general anaesthesia for inguinal hernia repair using data from a randomized clinical trial. Br J Surg. 2007;94(4):500–5. doi:10.1002/bjs.5543.
130. O'Dwyer PJ, Serpell MG, Millar K, et al. Local or general anesthesia for open hernia repair: a randomized trial. Ann Surg. 2003;237(4):574–9. doi:10.1097/01.SLA.0000059992.76731.64.
131. Reece-Smith AM, Maggio AQ, Tang TY, Walsh SR. Local anaesthetic vs. general anaesthetic for inguinal hernia repair: systematic review and meta-analysis. Int J Clin Pract. 2009;63(12):1739–42. doi:10.1111/j.1742-1241.2009.02131.x.
132. Simons MP, Aufenacker T, Bay-Nielsen M, et al. European Hernia Society guidelines on the treatment of inguinal hernia in adult patients. Hernia. 2009;13(4):343–403. doi:10.1007/s10029-009-0529-7.
133. Nordin P, Hernell H, Unosson M, Gunnarsson U, Nilsson E. Type of anaesthesia and patient acceptance in groin hernia repair: a multicentre randomised trial. Hernia. 2004;8(3):220–5. doi:10.1007/s10029-004-0234-5.
134. Teasdale C, McCrum a M, Williams NB, Horton RE. A randomised controlled trial to compare local with general anaesthesia for short-stay inguinal hernia repair. Ann R Coll Surg Engl 1982;64(4):238-242.
135. Chen T, Zhang Y, Wang H, et al. Emergency inguinal hernia repair under local anesthesia: a 5-year experience in a teaching hospital. BMC Anesthesiol. 2016;16:17. doi:10.1186/s12871-016-0185-2.

22

Foregut caustic injuries: results of the world society of emergency surgery consensus conference

Luigi Bonavina[1*], Mircea Chirica[2], Ognjan Skrobic[3], Yoram Kluger[4], Nelson A. Andreollo[5], Sandro Contini[6], Aleksander Simic[3], Luca Ansaloni[7], Fausto Catena[8], Gustavo P. Fraga[5], Carlo Locatelli[9], Osvaldo Chiara[10], Jeffry Kashuk[11], Federico Coccolini[7], Yuri Macchitella[1], Massimiliano Mutignani[12], Cesare Cutrone[13], Marco Dei Poli[14], Tino Valetti[15], Emanuele Asti[1], Michael Kelly[16] and Predrag Pesko[3]

Abstract

Introduction: Lesions of the upper digestive tract due to ingestion of caustic agents still represent a major medical and surgical emergency worldwide. The work-up of these patients is poorly defined and no clear therapeutic guidelines are available.

Purpose of the study: The aim of this study was to provide an evidence-based international consensus on primary and secondary prevention, diagnosis, staging, and treatment of this life-threatening and potentially disabling condition.

Methods: An extensive literature search was performed by an international panel of experts under the auspices of the World Society of Emergency Surgery (WSES). The level of evidence of the screened publications was graded using the Oxford 2011 criteria. The level of evidence of the literature and the main topics regarding foregut caustic injuries were discussed during a dedicated meeting in Milan, Italy (April 2015), and during the 3rd Annual Congress of the World Society of Emergency Surgery in Jerusalem, Israel (July 2015).

Results: One-hundred-forty-seven full papers which addressed the relevant clinical questions of the research were admitted to the consensus conference. There was an unanimous consensus on the fact that the current literature on foregut caustic injuries lacks homogeneous classification systems and prospective methodology. Moreover, the non-standardized definition of technical and clinical success precludes any accurate comparison of therapeutic modalities. Key recommendations and algorithms based on expert opinions, retrospective studies and literature reviews were proposed and approved during the final consensus conference. The clinical practice guidelines resulting from the consensus conference were approved by the WSES council.

Conclusions: The recommendations emerging from this consensus conference, although based on a low level of evidence, have important clinical implications. A world registry of foregut caustic injuries could be useful to collect a homogeneous data-base for prospective clinical studies that may help improving the current clinical practice guidelines.

* Correspondence: luigi.bonavina@unimi.it
[1]Department of Surgery, IRCCS Policlinico San Donato, University of Milan Medical School, Piazza Malan 1, 20097 San Donato Milanese (Milano), Italy
Full list of author information is available at the end of the article

Introduction

A wide variety of chemical agents including mineral and organic acids and alkalis, oxidizing agents, denaturants, hydrocarbons and other chemicals may cause corrosive injuries. Although the mechanism, the severity, and the timing of the injury may vary, all these substances cause damage to living tissue on contact. Accidental or intentional ingestion of corrosive substances cause life-threatening injuries of the upper digestive tract. The degree of injury is related to the concentration, amount, viscosity, and duration of exposure to the caustic agent. The large majority of caustic agents are liquids. Strong acids and alkali are readily available as household cleaners. Lye is a generic term for the alkali used to make soap, either potassium hydroxide or sodium hydroxide. Acids cause coagulation necrosis, whereas alkali combine with tissue proteins and cause liquefaction necrosis which penetrates deep into tissues. Concentrated alkali ingestion may lead to more serious injury and complications by penetrating tissues and leading to full-thickness damage of the esophageal/gastric wall. Liquid household bleach, although often reported, does rarely cause severe injuries. Children under the age of 5 years account for more than 80 % of accidental caustic ingestion, whereas adult injuries are more often intentional and suicidal [1–3].

Foregut caustic ingestion is certainly an under-reported public health issue. Primary prevention of these dramatic injuries was initiated in the United States by Chevalier Jackson who began a campaign that led to the Federal Caustic Act (1927) which mandated proper labeling of these harmful compounds. Subsequent acts have enforced proper labeling, antidote instructions, concentration restrictions, and child-resistant packaging. The effects of these changes have decreased but not eliminated the incidence and severity of caustic ingestions in the United States [4]. Nowadays, most information on foregut caustic injuries comes from countries where legislation is less restrictive or even absent, such as Africa, Turkey, India, Eastern Europe, Southeast Asia, and France [5].

Caustic ingestion can result in a number of injuries ranging in severity from mild oral burns to minimal mucosal erythema or transmural necrosis of the esophagus and stomach with visceral perforation. Emergency surgery is indicated for hemorrhage, free perforation, mediastinitis or peritonitis. Full thickness esophagogastric necrosis is a severe form of injury associated with considerable morbidity and mortality. It may occur due to ingestion of a large amount or highly concentrated corrosive substance. The injury may extend and involve adjacent viscera such as the duodenum, small intestine, colon, pancreas, and gallbladder. Complications such as hemorrhage, perforation, aorto-enteric fistula, or gastrocolic fistula may occur in patients surviving the initial event during the first 2–3 weeks after ingestion. Patients who have survived severe caustic injury of the foregut are at high risk of luminal strictures. After recovery from the initial injury, collagen deposition and fibrosis continue for months and scar retraction results in esophageal shortening and stricture. The incidence of esophageal stricture following grade IIB and grade III esophageal burns is in the range of 50–80 % [6, 7]. Concomitant gastric outlet obstruction occurs in up to 30 % of patients with esophageal stricture [8, 9]. In the long term, development of pharyngeal, esophageal, or gastric strictures may compromise nutritional outcome. Interestingly, the risk of squamous-cell cancer of the damaged esophagus is estimated to be 1000 times higher than that of the general population, and the latent period for the malignant change is 15–40 years [10, 11].

Currently, in most referral centers therapeutic algorithms for the management of patients with caustic injuries rely on the findings of upper digestive endoscopy. Despite the use of different endoscopic classification systems, therapeutic approaches are similar and include conservative management of patients with mild injuries, while patients with severe injuries undergo emergency surgical exploration. Although there are studies describing the short and long-term outcomes of reconstruction for established caustic strictures of the esophagus, there is limited literature on the early and long term outcomes of patients managed in an emergency setting for corrosive induced acute esophagogastric and/or adjacent organ necrosis.

Methods

Two independent MEDLINE and EMBASE searches were performed to identify relevant papers published between 1990 and 2015. The following medical subject headings terms were used in the searches: caustic ingestion, caustic lesions, corrosive injuries, esophagus, stomach, esophageal dilatation, gastric outlet obstruction. The search terms were identified in the title, abstract, or medical subject heading. Initially, 2143 abstracts of the retrieved studies were reviewed and screened for exclusion criteria. At the end of the search, 1113 abstracts that fulfilled the inclusion criteria were selected. Finally, 147 full papers which addressed the relevant clinical questions of the research were admitted to the consensus conference. The level of evidence for each recommendation statement was assigned by using the grading system proposed by the Oxford Centre for Evidence-Based Medicine [12]. A preliminary manuscript was prepared by an international panel of 12 experts including anesthesiologists, endoscopists, surgeons, and toxicologists. The key recommendations and algorithms were discussed at a dedicated meeting held in Milan in April 2015, and at the 3rd Congress of the World Society of

Emergency Surgery held in Jerusalem in July 2015. Finally, evidence based guidelines for the management of foregut caustic injuries were developed to outline clinical recommendations.

Recommendations

Initial therapeutic approach [13–57]

Pre-hospital management

- Establish the diagnosis of caustic agent ingestion. Identify the involved agent. Collect the product on the scene and bring it to the emergency department. If difficult product identification try to evaluate pH (<2; > 10), but be aware that some agents cause a pH-independent corrosive injury. (Level 4–5)
- Evaluate the ingestion scenario by: a) ascertain ingestion; b) determine the accidental or voluntary character; c) detect co-ingestion of alcohol and/or drugs; d) try to evaluate ingested quantity (in adults assess normal sip (30–50 ml) vs. large gulp (60–90 ml); e) assess delay from ingestion. (Level 4–5)
- Identification of additional risk factors such as extreme ages (young children, elderly), pregnancy, underlying disease, and the form of the ingested agent (solid, liquid, gel, vapors-concomitant aspiration). (Level 5)
- Supportive care rather than specific antidotes is the mainstay of treatment. Secure airway patency and hemodynamic stabilization. Prevent vomiting, repeat esophageal passage, and aspiration by: a) use of antiemetics (metoclopramide); b) seated 45° position during transport; c) avoid gastric lavage and induced emesis; d) avoid diluents (milk, water). (Level 5)
- Avoid increasing damage by exothermic reaction: attempts at pH neutralization with either a weak alkali or acid are prohibited. (Level 5)

Emergency department management

- Continue symptomatic treatment including adequate pain relief while waiting to evaluate the severity of caustic injuries. If airway support is required favor fiberoptic laryngoscopy over blind intubation; perform tracheotomy if necessary. (Level 5)
- Laboratory tests should include WBC, hemoglobin, platelet count, CRP, pH, and serum levels of Na, K, Cl, Ca, Mg, urea, creatinin, LDH, CPK, AST, ALT, lactates, alcohol. β-HCG levels should be measured in young women. (Level 5)
- Contact Poison Control Centers to evaluate systemic toxicity of the ingested agents. (Level 4–5)
- Avoid nasogastric tube positioning as their validity to prevent vomiting and stricture formation has never been proven; nasogastric tubes have been reported to increase risks of gastric perforation, gastroesophageal reflux, and pneumonia. (Level 5)
- The efficacy of proton-pump inhibitors and H2 blockers in minimizing esophageal injury by suppressing acid reflux has not been proven. (Level 5)
- The utility of corticosteroid in terms of stricture prevention is controversial and systematic administration is not recommended. Steroids should be reserved for patients with symptoms involving the airway. (Level 3)
- Administration of broad-spectrum antibiotics should not be done on a systematic basis. Antibiotics are advised in grade 3 injuries if corticosteroids are initiated or if lung involvement is identified. (Level 5)

Management algorithm

- Patients with clinical signs of peritonitis and hemodynamic instability require immediate surgical exploration. Although symptoms such as chest pain, dysphagia, odynophagia, drooling, hemorrhage are usually associated with severe injuries after voluntary ingestion, the absence of oropharyngeal damage does not exclude the possibility of severe esophagogastric injuries. (Level 4)
- Results of laboratory tests such as WBC, platelet count, CRP, pH, AST, ALT, creatinin, and lactate can help decision making in difficult situations. (Level 5)
- Endoscopy is the cornerstone of management of caustic injuries. Endoscopy is usually performed 3 to 6 h after ingestion, and injuries are graded according to the Zargar classification. Patients with severe (grade 3b) esophagogastric injuries are considered for surgery while patients with low grade injuries (≤ grade 3a) are offered non-operative treatment. Endoscopy grading can also predict the risk to develop an esophageal stricture during follow-up. Inability of endoscopy to predict accurately the depth of intramural necrosis may result in either futile surgery, with negative effects on survival, digestive function and management costs, or in patient death due to inappropriate non operative treatment. Moreover, emergency endoscopy is futile in up to 30 % of patients who do not have injuries of the upper digestive tract following ingestion of bleach or corrosive agents other than strong acids or alkali. (Level 4)
- Computed tomography helps palliate shortcomings of endoscopy based algorithms. The use of CT is helpful in guiding indications for esophagectomy in patients with grade 3b caustic injury (Fig. 1). In a recent study CT did better than endoscopy in selecting patients for surgery or non-operative

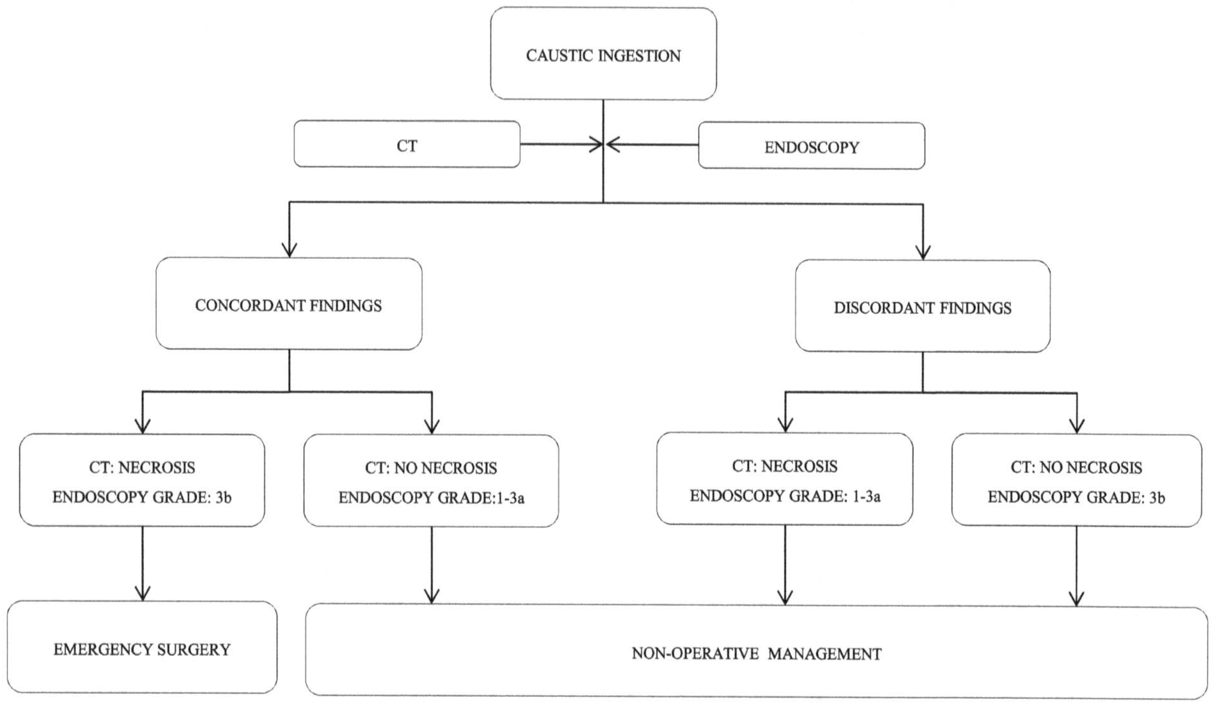

Fig. 1 Management algorithm for caustic ingestion based on computed tomography and endoscopic findings

treatment, suggesting that CT can replace endoscopy in the management of caustic injuries. CT criteria of transmural esophageal necrosis include esophageal-wall blurring and periesophageal-fat blurring on unenhanced images, and absence of post-contrast esophageal-wall enhancement; transmural necrosis of the stomach was defined as the absence of post-contrast gastric-wall enhancement. (Level 3)

Emergency surgery for caustic injuries

- Emergency surgery is eventually required in a small number of patients with transmural necrosis to avoid involvement of adjacent organs and death. Laparotomy is usually performed but laparoscopic exploration has been reported as feasible and safe. (Level 4)
- Transhiatal esophagectomy and total gastrectomy are the most frequently employed surgical procedures in the acute setting. Meanwhile, esophagectomy with gastric preservation and total gastrectomy with esophagojejunostomy can be performed if transmural necrosis is limited to the esophagus or the stomach, respectively. (Level 4)
- Feeding jejunostomy should be systematically constructed at the end of the operation, regardless of the type of surgical procedure performed. (Level 4)
- Extended surgery (beyond esophagogastrectomy) should be attempted in case of existing injuries on other abdominal organs. All injured organs should be resected during the first operation as caustic lesions invariably progress. Mortality rates are high, but surgery may be only choice for these patients. (Level 4)
- If the patient's conditions allow, immediate biliary and pancreatic reconstruction should be attempted after pancreatoduodenectomy for caustic necrosis. (Level 5)
- Transmural esophageal necrosis may lead to subsequent tracheobronchial extension in a small number (<10 %) of patients. Preoperative bronchoscopy should be performed in all patients considered for surgery. In the presence of tracheobronchial necrosis, esophagectomy should be performed by a right thoracic approach. Tracheobronchial necrosis can be successfully treated with pulmonary patch technique. (Level 4)
- Massive intestinal necrosis should be a reason for the surgeon to stop due to inability of later reconstruction and nutrition. (Level 5)
- Mortality rates are high, but surgery may be only choice for these patients. Factors which have a negative impact on outcome include advanced age, tracheobronchial injuries, emergency esophagectomy, need for extended resections and severe modifications of laboratory tests (pH < 7.2, AST > 2 N, renal failure, etc.). (Level 4)
- The need to perform emergency surgery for caustic injuries has a persistent long-term negative

impact both on survival and functional outcome. Moreover, esophageal resection is an independent negative predictor of survival after emergency surgery. (Level 4)

Nutritional approach

- Caustic ingestion can induce SIRS or sepsis with a severe hypermetabolic and catabolic response. Negative nitrogen balance and weight loss are related to injury severity. (Level 3–4)
- Use as soon as possible the gastrointestinal tract for nutrition. Patients with low grade injuries should resume oral alimentation as soon as they are able to swallow. In patients with severe burns, enteral feeding through jejunostomy or nasojejunal tube is recommended rather than a gastrostomy due to the possibility of a hidden gastric outlet obstruction (Level 5)

Endoscopic treatment of esophageal stricture [58–98]

- Esophageal caustic strictures are frequently complex, i.e. long (>2 cm), angulated, irregular, and multiple. In addition, the "remodeling time", i.e. the time to stricture stabilization ranges between 6 months to 3 years. As a consequence, the reported success rate of dilatation is lower than for other benign esophageal strictures. The optimum time for dilatation is after healing of the acute injury, usually in the 3rd week. Late management is usually associated with marked esophageal wall fibrosis and collagen deposition, which requires more endoscopic sessions for adequate dilatation. This is a crucial issue in developing countries, where late presentations are more than 50 %. (Level 3–4)
- Dilatation can be carried out with balloon dilators or Savary bougies. A prospective randomized study has shown no clear advantage of each method in peptic esophageal strictures. Savary dilators are considered more reliable and effective than balloon dilators in consolidated strictures. Moreover, Savary bougies offer the advantage of "feeling" the resistance to dilatation under the operator's hands. (Level 4)
- "Rules of the thumb": 1)To begin with dilators that are one or two French sizes smaller than the estimated diameter of the stricture, 2)Not to dilate more than two to three sizes larger than the size of the first dilator meeting resistance. (Level 4)
- The perforation rate after dilatation for caustic strictures ranges from 0.4 to 32 %, higher than for other benign strictures. Fluoroscopy during dilatation may help in difficult cases. Although comparative trials are not available, selective use of fluoroscopy is supported by extensive clinical experience. (Level 4)
- The interval between dilatations varies from less than 1 week to 2–3 weeks. Although three or four sessions may provide durable results, the number of dilatation required is unpredictable and the endoscopic treatment may continue for years. A cut-off value for stopping dilatations is not clear and is influenced by patient, physician and geographic factors. In adult studies, the maximal esophageal wall thickness at CT scan and the involvement of muscolaris propria at endoscopic ultrasound were found to be significant predictors of stricture development, more difficult dilatations, and recurrent stricture. Gastroesophageal reflux and alterations in esophageal motility due to esophageal wall fibrosis can contribute to persistent dysphagia, in spite of apparently successful dilatations. (Level 4)
- A sustained esophageal lumen patency is not the only therapeutic goal: especially in children, an associated improvement in nutritional status should be considered an important end-point. (Level 3–4)
- Gastrostomy feeding may be life-saving, especially in developing countries. Moreover, gastrostomy allows a retrograde approach for dilatation. In challenging strictures, a nylon thread left between the nose and the gastrostomy maintains luminal access and facilitates further dilatations. (Level 3–4)
- Use of intralesional steroids and Mitomycin C applied endoscopically have been evaluated in several studies. Apparently, intralesional steroids favour a longer symptom-free time interval between dilatations but seem less effective in caustic strictures. Overall, there is no convincing evidence of the efficacy of these procedures. (Level 5)
- There is no convincing evidence that intraluminal stenting as an alternative to repeat dilatations is beneficial. Early stenting has been proposed to prevent stricture in uncontrolled studies. The number of dilatations and the duration of treatment were reduced. Notably, 50 % of children in whom a home-made stent was placed after the first dilatation, did not require further treatment. (Level 5)
- Long-term outcomes of stent placement for refractory benign esophageal strictures are poor. Partially covered SEMS are almost abandoned, in spite of their superior anchoring capacity, because of the associated hyperplastic ingrowth or overgrowth, with consequent difficult removal and recurrent dysphagia. Fully covered Self Expanding Polyflex Stents (SEPS) and Self Expanding Metallic Stents (SEMS) show a reduced reactive hyperplasia at a price of a higher migration rate. Biodegradable (BD) stents

begin to degrade after 4–5 weeks and to dissolve within 2–3 months. Although the migration rate is reduced owing to the uncovered design, BD stents are only temporarily effective and sequential stenting has been suggested to avoid serial dilations. Moreover, hyperplastic tissue reactions have emerged as a significant problem. A recent systematic review of patients with a benign esophageal stricture (25 % caustic) treated by SEPS showed that only 52 % of the patients were dysphagia-free after a median follow-up of 13 months. A recent publication evaluated the results of stenting in benign strictures from twelve prospective studies. The stent was successfully placed in 98.7 %, but the overall clinical success rate was 24.2 %. (Level 4)

Management of gastric outlet obstruction [99–118]

- Grade three injury to the stomach is an independent risk factor for gastric outlet obstruction that can occur from a few days up to 6 years after caustic ingestion. Distal obstructions account for 60–100 % of the lesions and are located in the prepyloric area. Endoscopic balloon dilatation is safe and successful in the management of a subgroup of patients with gastric outlet obstruction. Progressive endoscopic dilatation can safely be initiated even at 2 weeks from ingestion, especially in short strictures (<25 mm). (Level 3–4)
- There is no clear evidence supporting the use of stents in the management of gastric outlet obstruction. (Level 5)
- Early surgery seems to decrease morbidity and mortality, but elective surgery earlier than 3 months is considered risky because of the poor nutritional status, adhesions, edematous gastric wall, difficult assessment of the extent of gastric resection due to ongoing fibrosis. (Level 5)
- Pyloroplasty may be performed in patients with moderate/localized strictures, but the risk of recurrent stricture is high. (Level 5)
- Gastrojejunostomy is indicated in the presence of extensive perigastric adhesions, unhealthy duodenum, and poor general condition; marginal ulcerations are reported. In selected patients the operation can safely be performed through a laparoscopic approach. (Level 5)
- The indication for gastric resection as prophylaxis against malignancy has been probably overstated in the literature. Partial gastric resection seems preferred by most surgeons. The type of surgery should be chosen according to local and general conditions. (Level 5)

Esophageal reconstruction [119-156]

- When esophageal dilatation is not possible or fails to provide an adequate esophageal caliber in the long-term, esophageal replacement by retrosternal stomach or, preferably, colonic interposition should be considered. (Level 3–4)
- A laryngoscopic examination is mandatory prior to all esophageal reconstructions for caustic injuries. (Level 4–5)
- The surgical bypass should be performed at least 6 months after caustic ingestion or emergency surgery since the “remodeling time”, i.e. time to stricture stabilization, is rather long. (Level 3–4)
- Removal of the native esophagus in adult patients is largely debated. It seems advisable in children because of the higher risk of cancer in the long-term. (Level 5)
- No randomized studies address the issue of which type of esophagoplasty is preferable. There are pros and cons for either right or left colon. An expert surgeon should do what he/she is used to do. (Level 5)
- One-stage esophageal resection and replacement with a gastric conduit, instead of a bypass, is feasible and safe in patients with isolated distal esophageal strictures. (Level 5)
- Minimally invasive/hybrid surgical techniques have been used with favourable results in selected patients. (Level 5)
- Angiographic study of the vascular pedicle is not routinely recommended before colon interposition or bypass, with the exception of patients with previously failed surgical attempts. (Level 5)
- Surgical revision is effective in patients who present with redundancy of the interposed colon years after retrosternal or mediastinal reconstruction. (Level 4)
- Pharyngeal strictures are difficult to manage and require special expertise. Endoscopic laser therapy of pharyngo-laryngeal adhesions may prove useful in selected patients before definitive surgical treatment. Colopharyngoplasty for strictures involving the pharynx is a safe and effective procedure. In such circumstances, the restoration of upper digestive tract continuity requires concomitant esophageal and pharyngeal reconstruction with resection of all scar tissue. Treatment of pharyngeal and laryngeal injuries should be done at the same surgical session. Supraglottic laryngectomy and suprahyoid pharyngectomy are required if the epiglottis and/or the base of the tongue are involved (Level 4–5)
- Temporary tracheostomy is mandatory during the rehabilitation training period after colopharyngoplasty. The postoperative re-education

process is long and difficult and requires full cooperation from a psychiatric stable patient. (Level 5)

- Advanced age has a negative impact on esophageal reconstruction. Patients older than 55 years are likely to experience severe complications, worse functional outcomes, and decreased long-term survival. For these reasons colopharyngoplasty should not be offered after this age limit. (Level 4)
- Use of myocutaneous flaps and free jejunal grafts should be considered for salvage cervical esophageal reconstruction and restoration of alimentary transit after previously failed surgical attempts. (Level 4)

Conclusions

The recommendations of these clinical practice guidelines are based on an extensive review of the literature and expert advice. Published data lack homogeneous classification systems and prospective methodology, the majority of papers being retrospective case reports, case series, or literature reviews. Moreover, the non-standardized definition of technical and clinical success precludes any accurate comparison of therapeutic modalities. There has been only one negative controlled trial assessing the effect of steroids to prevent esophageal stricture after caustic ingestion in children [157]. For all the above reasons, the extrapolated recommendations are mainly based on expert opinions, retrospective studies, and literature reviews with a low level of evidence.

Despite all these limitations, the value of this consensus conferences was to gather a panel of recognized experts and over 200 physicians attending the two meetings. Among the debated issues, an unanimous consensus has emerged on the fact that use of CT scan in the initial patient staging may indeed represent a true change of paradigm. The new diagnostic algorithm may allow to avoid endoscopy in selected patients, to increase the rate of esophageal preservation, and it could translate into a better long-term patients outcome and quality of life. Interestingly, a previous WSES survey has found that 80 % of the responders to a questionnaire treat fewer than ten cases of caustic ingestion per year [158], indicating the utility to apply and share clinical practice guidelines to improve patients' care.

Caustic ingestion continues to be a complex clinical problem and a burden for the healthcare systems worldwide. Emergency surgery and subsequent alimentary tract reconstruction are a formidable challenge in these patients. On the light of the consensus that has emerged among experts in Milan and Jerusalem, the World Society of Emergency Surgery will be running a World Registry of foregut caustic injuries (www.clinicalregisters.org). This could be the first step toward a more standardized data collection and the implementation of prospective clinical studies.

Competing interests
The authors declare that they have no competing interests.

Authors' contribution
LB MC and OS designed the guidelines. LB and MC wrote the manuscript. All authors reviewed and approved the final manuscript

Author details
[1]Department of Surgery, IRCCS Policlinico San Donato, University of Milan Medical School, Piazza Malan 1, 20097 San Donato Milanese (Milano), Italy. [2]Department of Digestive Surgery, Saint-Louis Hospital, Paris, France. [3]Department of Surgery, University of Belgrade, Belgrade, Serbia. [4]Department of General Surgery, Rambam Health Care Campus, Haifa, Israel. [5]Department of Surgery, University of Campinas, Campinas, Brasil. [6]University of Parma, Parma, Italy. [7]General Surgery I, Papa Giovanni XXIII Hospital, Bergamo, Italy. [8]Emergency Surgery Department, Maggiore Parma Hospital, Parma, Italy. [9]Institute of Toxicology, University of Pavia, Pavia, Italy. [10]Emergency Department, Niguarda Hospital, Milan, Italy. [11]Department of Surgery, University of Jerusalem, Jerusalem, Rehovot, Israel. [12]Department of Endoscopy, Niguarda Hospital, Milan, Italy. [13]Department of Otolaryngology, Azienda Ospedaliera, Padova, Italy. [14]Intensive Care Unit, IRCCS Policlinico San Donato, San Donato Milanese, Italy. [15]Department of Anesthesiology, Papa Giovanni XXIII Hospital, Bergamo, Italy. [16]Department of Surgery, Wagga Wagga Hospital, Wagga Wagga, Australia.

References

1. Sarfati E, Gossot D, Assens P, Celerier M. Management of caustic ingestion in adults. Br J Surg. 1987;74:146–8.
2. Kikendall JW. Caustic ingestion injuries. Gastroenterol Clin N Am. 1991;20(4):847–57.
3. Hugh TB, Kelly MD. Corrosive ingestion and the surgeon. J Am Coll Surg. 1999;189(5):508–22.
4. Leape LL, Ashcraft KW, Scarpelli DG, Holder TM. Hazard to health-liquid lye. N Engl J Med. 1971;284:578–81.
5. Contini S, Scarpignato C. Caustic injury of the upper gastrointestinal tract: a comprehensive review. World J Gastroenterol. 2013;19(25):3918–30.
6. Mehta SK, Mehta S, Nagi B, Kochlar R, Zargar SA. Ingestion of strong corrosive alkalis: spectrum of injury to upper gastrointestinal tract and natural history. Am J Gastroenterol. 1992;87(3):337–41.
7. Cheng HT, Cheng CL, Lin CH, Tang JH, Chu YY, Liu N, et al. Caustic ingestion in adults: the role of endoscopic classification in predicting outcome. BMC Gastroenterol. 2008;8:1.
8. Peracchia A, Bardini R, Bonavina L, Pavanello M, Asolati M, Buin F. Lesioni da caustici dell'esofago. Esperienza su 143 casi osservati. Chirurgia. 1989;2(1–2):1–6.
9. Knezevic JD, Radovanovic NS, Simic AP, Kotarac MM, Skrobic OM, Konstantinovic VD, et al. Colon interposition in the treatment of esophageal caustic strictures: 40 years of experience. Dis Esophagus. 2007;20(6):530–4.
10. Imre J, Kopp M. Arguments against long-term conservative treatment of oesophageal strictures due to corrosive burns. Thorax. 1972;27(5):594–8.
11. Appelqvist P, Salmo M. Lye corrosion carcinoma of the esophagus: a review of 63 cases. Cancer. 1980;45(10):2655–8.
12. OCEBM Levels of Evidence Working Group. The Oxford 2011 levels of evidence. htpp://www.cebm.net/index.aspx?o=5653.
13. Andreoni B, Farina ML, Biffi R, Crosta C. Esophageal perforation and caustic injury: emergency management of caustic ingestion. Dis Esophagus. 1997;10:95–100.
14. Benjamin B, Agueb R, Vuarnesson H, Trachart H, Munoz Bongard N, Sarfati E, et al. Chirica M. Ann Surg: Tracheobronchial necrosis after caustic injury; 2015. PMID:25775065.
15. Berthet B, Castellani P, Brioche MI, Assadourian R, Gauthier A. Early operation for severe corrosive injury of the upper gastrointestinal tract. Eur J Surg. 1996;162(12):951–5.
16. Boybeyi O, Karnak I, Tanyel FC, Senocak ME. Management of unusually extensive esophagogastric corrosive injuries: emergency measures and gastric reconstruction. J Pediatr Surg. 2009;44(5):1022–6.
17. Braga M, Ljungqvist O, Soeters P, Fearon K, Weinmann A, Bozzetti F. ESPEN guidelines on parenteral nutrition: Surgery. Clin Nutr. 2009;28:378–86.

18. Bonnici KS, Wood DM, Dargan PI. Should computerised tomography replace endoscopy in the evaluation of symptomatic ingestion of corrosive substances? Clin Toxicol (Phila). 2014;52(9):911–25.
19. Cabral C, Chirica M, de Chaisemartin C, Gornet JM, Munoz-Bongrand N, Halimi B, et al. Caustic injuries of the upper digestive tract: a population observational study. Surg Endosc. 2012;26(1):214–21.
20. Cattan P, Munoz Bongrand N, Berney T, Halimi B, Sarfati E, Celerier M. Extensive abdominal surgery after caustic ingestion. Ann Surg. 2000;519:523.
21. Celik B, Nadir A, Sahin E, Kaptanoglu M. Is esophagoscopy necessary for corrosive ingestion in adults? Dis Esophagus. 2009;22:638–41.
22. Ozokutan BH, Gündüz F, Gözen A, Ceylan H. Gastric perforation after corrosive ingestion. Pediatr Surg Int. 2011;27(6):649–53.
23. Chiba S, Brichkov I. Pulmonary Patch Repair of Tracheobronchial Necrosis With Perforation Secondary to caustic ingestion. Ann Thorac Surg. 2014;97:2205–7.
24. Chirica M, Kraemer A, Petrascu E, Vuarnesson H, Pariente B, Halimi B, et al. Esophagojejunostomy after total gastrectomy for caustic injuries. Dis Esophagus. 2014;27(2):122–7.
25. Chirica M, Resche-Rigon M, Munoz Bongrand N, Zohar S, Halimi B, Gornet JM, et al. Surgery for caustic injuries of the upper gastrointestinal tract. Ann Surg. 2012;256:994–1001.
26. Chirica M, Resche-Rigon M, Pariente B, Fieux F, Sabatier F, Loiseaux F, et al. Computed tomography evaluation of high-grade esophageal necrosis after corrosive ingestion to avoid unnecessary esophagectomy. Surg Endosc. 2015;29(6):1452–61.
27. Chirica M, Vuarnesson H, Zohar S, Faron M, Halimi B, Munoz Bongrand N, et al. Similar outcomes after primary and secondary esophagocoloplasty for caustic injuries. Ann Thorac Surg. 2012;93(3):905–12.
28. Chou SH, Chang YT, Li HP, Huang MF, Lee CH, Lee KW. Factors predicting the hospital mortality of patients with corrosive gastrointestinal injuries receiving esophagogastrectomy in the acute stage. World J Surg. 2010;34:2383–88.
29. Dapri G, Himpens J, Mouchart A, Ntounda R, Claus M, Dechamps P, et al. Laparoscopic transhiatal esophago-gastrectomy after corrosive injury. Surg Endosc. 2007;21(12):2322–5.
30. Díaz-Sánchez A, Carrión G, Barreiro A, Ortiz C, De Fuenmayor ML, Gimeno M, et al. Massive gastric necrosis from hydrochloric acid ingestion. Eur J Surg. 2001;167:195–8.
31. Di Saverio S, Biscardi A, Piccinini A, Mandrioli M, Tugnoli G. Different possible surgical managements of caustic ingestion: diagnostic laparoscopy for Zargar's grade 3a lesions and a new technique of "duodenal damage control" with "4-tube ostomy" and duodenal wash-out as an option for extensive 3b lesions in unstable patients. Updates Surg 2015: DOI 10.1007/s13304-015-0313-4
32. Fulton JA, Hofman RS. Steroids in second degree caustic burns of the esophagus: a systematic pooled analysis of fifty years of human data:1956–2006. Clin Toxicol (Phila). 2007;45:402–8.
33. Ganepola GA, Bhuta K. A case of total esophago-gastro-duodeno-jejunectomy and partial pancreatectomy for lye burns, and reconstruction with colon interposition. J Trauma. 1984;24(10):913–6.
34. Gupta SK, Rana AS, Gupta D, Jain G, Kalra P. Unusual presentation of caustic ingestion and its surgical treatment: a case report. J Maxillofac Oral Surg. 2011;10(1):74–6.
35. Horvath OP, Olah T, Zentai G. Emergency esophagogastrectomy for treatment of hydrochloric acid injury. Ann Thorac Surg. 1991;52:98–101.
36. Huscher CG, Mingoli A, Mereu A, Sgarzini G. Laparoscopy can be very effective in reducing mortality rate for caustic ingestion in suicide attempt. World J Surg. 2011;35:2363–64.
37. Jaillard S, Nseir S, Métois D, Marquette C, Darras J, Porte H, et al. Extensive corrosive injuries of the upper airways and gastrointestinal tract. J Thorac Cardiovasc Surg. 2002;123:186–8.
38. Jain RK, Gouda NB, Sharma VK, Dubey TN, Shende A, Malik R, et al. Esophageal complications following aluminium phosphide ingestion: an emerging issue among survivors of poisoning. Dysphagia. 2010;25(4):271–6.
39. Javed A, Pal S, Krishnan E, Sanhi P, Chattopadhyay T. Surgical management and outcomes of severe gastrointestinal injuries due to corrosive ingestion. World J Gastroenterol. 2012;4(5):121–5.
40. Karagiozoglou-Lampoudi T, Agakidis CH, Chryssostomidou S, Arvanitidis K, Tsepis K. Conservative management of caustic substance ingestion in a pediatric department setting, short-term and long-term outcome. Dis Esophagus. 2011;24(2):86–91.
41. Keh SM, Onyekwelu N, McManus K, McGuigan J. Corrosive injury to upper gastrointestinal tract: Still a major surgical dilemma. World J Gastroenterol. 2006;12(32):5223–8.
42. Kua K, Jonas N, O'Donnell R. The larynx and caustic soda ingestion. Arch Dis Child. 2015;100(6):570.
43. Lee M. Caustic ingestion and upper digestive tract injury. Dig Dis Sci. 2010;55(6):1547–9.
44. Landen S, Wu MH, Jeng LB, Delugelau V, Launois B. Pancreaticoduodenal necrosis due to caustic burn. Acta Chir Belg. 2000;100:205–9.
45. Lefrancois M, Gaujoux S, Resche-Rigon M, Chirica M, Munoz-Bongrand SE, Cattan P. Oesophagogastrectomy and pancreaticoduodenectomy for caustic injury. Br J Surg. 2011;98:983–90.
46. Losanoff J, Kjossef K. Multivisceral injury after liquid caustic ingestion. Surgery. 1996;119:720.
47. Mamede RCM, De Mello Filho FV. Treatment of caustic ingestion: an analysis of 239 cases. Dis Esophagus. 2002;15:210–3.
48. Munoz-Bongrand N, Cattan P, de Chaisemartin C, Bothereau H, Honigman I, Sarfati E. Extensive digestive caustic burns: what are the limits for resection? A series of 12 patients. Ann Chir. 2003;128(6):373–8.
49. Ramakrishnaiah VP, Gangavatiker R, Dash NR, Sahni P. Pancreas-sparing duodenectomy in a patient with acute corrosive injury. Updates Surg. 2013;65(4):309–11.
50. Rigo GP, Camellini L, Azzolini F, Guazzetti S, Bedogni G, Merighi A, et al. What is the utility of selected clinical and endoscopic parameters in predicting the risk of death after caustic ingestion? Endoscopy. 2002;34(4):304–10.
51. Ryu HH, Jeung KW, Lee BK, Uhm JH, Park YH, Shin MH, et al. Caustic injury: can CT scan grading system enable prediction of esophageal stricture? Clin Toxicol. 2010;48:137–42.
52. Sarfati E, Jacob L, Servant JM, d'Acremont B, Roland E, Ghidalia T, et al. Tracheobronchial necrosis after caustic ingestion. J Thorac Cardiovasc Surg. 1992;103:412–3.
53. Subasinghe D, Rathnasena BG. Early laparoscopic gastrojejunostomy for corrosive injury of upper gastrointestinal tract. Trop Gastroenterol. 2011;32(4):333–5.
54. Tohda G, Sugawa C, Gayer C, Chino A, McGuire TW, Lucas CE. Clinical evaluation and management of caustic injury in the upper gastrointestinal tract in 95 adult patients in an urban medical center. Surg Endosc. 2008;22(4):1119–25.
55. Vereczkei A, Varga G, Pótó L, Horváth OP. Management of corrosive injuries of the esophagus. Acta Chir Hung. 1999;38(1):119–22.
56. Wu MH, Lai WW, Hwang TL, Lee SC, Hsu HK, Lin TS. Surgical results of corrosive injuries involving esophagus to jejunum. Hepatogastroenterology. 1996;43:846–50.
57. Zerbib P, Voisin B, Truant S, Saulnier F, Vinet A, Chambon JP, et al. The conservative management of severe caustic gastric injuries. Ann Surg. 2011;253(4):684–8.
58. Baskin D, Urganci N, Abbasoğlu L, Alkim C, Yalçin M, Karadağ C, et al. A standardised protocol for the acute management of corrosive ingestion in children. Pediatr Surg Int. 2004;20:824–8.
59. Berger M, Ure B, Lacher M. Mitomycin C in the therapy of recurrent esophageal strictures: hype or hope? Eur J Pediatr Surg. 2012;22:109–16.
60. Betalli P, Rossi A, Bini M, Bacis G, Borrelli O, Cutrone C, et al. Update on management of caustic and foreign body ingestion in children. Diagn Ther Endosc. 2009;2009:969868. doi:10.1155/2009/969868.
61. Bueno R, Swanson SJ, Jaklitsch MT, Lukanich JM, MentzerSJ SDJ. Combined antegrade and retrogradedilation: a new endoscopic technique in the management ofcomplex esophageal obstruction. Gastrointest Endosc. 2001;54:368–72.
62. Contini S, Garatti M, Swarray-Deen A, Depetris N, Cecchini S, Scarpignato C. Corrosive oesophageal strictures in children: outcomes after timely or delayed dilatation. Dig Liver Dis. 2009;41:263–8. doi:10.1016/ j.dld.2008.07.319. PMID: 18801710.
63. Contini S, Scarpignato C, Rossi A, Strada G. Features and management of esophageal corrosive lesions in children in Sierra Leone: lessons learned from 175 consecutive patients. J Pediatr Surg. 2011;46:1739–45.
64. Contini S, Swarray-Deen A, Scarpignato C. Oesophageal corrosive injuries in children: a forgotten social and health challenge in developing countries. Bull World Health Organ. 2009;87:950–4. doi:10.2471/BLT.08. PMID: 20454486.
65. Dall'Oglio L, De Angelis P. Commentary on "Esophageal endoscopic dilations". J Pediatr Gastroenterol Nutr. 2012;54(6):716–17.

66. De Peppo F, Zaccara A, Dall'Oglio L, Federici di Abriola G, Ponticelli A, Marchetti P, et al. Stenting for caustic strictures: esophageal replacement replaced. J Pediatr Surg. 1998;33:54–7.
67. Doğan Y, Erkan T, Cokuğraş FC, Kutlu T. Caustic gastroesophageal lesions in childhood: an analysis of 473 cases. Clin Pediatr (Phila). 2006;45:435–8. doi:10.1177/0009922806289618. PMID: 16891276.
68. Foschia F, De Angelis P, Torroni F, Romeo E, Caldaro T, diAbriola GF, et al. Custom dynamic stent for esophageal strictures in children. J Pediatr Surg. 2011;46:848–53.
69. Genc A, Mutaf O. Esophageal motility changes in acute and late periods of caustic esophageal burns and their relation to prognosis in children. J Pediatr Surg. 2002;37:1526.
70. Gerçek A, Ay B, Dogan V, Kiyan G, Dagli T, Gogus Y. Esophageal balloon dilation in children: prospective analysis of hemodynamic changes and complications during general anesthesia. J Clin Anesth. 2007;19:286–9.
71. Gumaste VV, Dave PB. Ingestion of corrosive substances by adults. Am J Gastroenterol. 1992;87:1–5.
72. Gün F, Abbasoğlu L, Celik A, Salman ET. Early and late term management in caustic ingestion in children: a 16-year experience. Acta Chir Belg. 2007;107:49–52. [PMID: 17405598.
73. Gundogdu HZ, Tanyel FC, Büyükpamukçu N, Hiçsönmez A. Conservative treatment of caustic esophageal strictures in children. J Pediatr Surg. 1992;27:767–70.
74. Ham YH, Kim GH. Plastic and biodegradable stents for complex and refractory benign esophageal strictures. Clin Endosc. 2014;47:295–300.
75. Karnak I, Tanyel FC, Büyükpamukçu N, Hiçsönmez A. Combined use of steroid, antibiotics and early bougienage against stricture formation following caustic esophageal burns. J Cardiovasc Surg. 1999;40(2):307–10.
76. Makharia GK, Kochhar R. Usefulness of intralesional triamcinolone in treatment of benign esophageal strictures. Gastrointest Endosc. 2002;56:829–34.
77. Kochman ML, McClave SA, Boyce HW. The refractory and the recurrent esophageal stricture: a definition. Gastrointest Endosc. 2005;62:474–5.
78. Kukkady A, Pease PW. Long-term dilatation of caustic strictures of the oesophagus. Pediatr Surg Int. 2002;18:486–90.
79. Lahoti D, Broor SL, Basu PP, Gupta A, Sharma R, Pant CS. Corrosive esophageal strictures: predictors of response to endoscopic dilation. Gastrointest Endosc. 1995;41(3):196–200.
80. Lakhdar-Idrissi M, Khabbache K, Hida M. Esophageal endoscopic dilations. J Pediatr Gastroenterol Nutr. 2012;54:744–7.
81. Lew RJ. Kochman ML A review of endoscopic methods of esophageal dilation. J Clin Gastroenterol. 2002;35:117–26.
82. Millar JW, Cox SG. Caustic injuries of the esophagus. Pediatr Surg Int. 2015;31:111–21.
83. Mutaf O, Genç A, Herek O, Demircan M, Ozcan C, Arikan A. Gastroesophageal reflux: a determinant in the outcome of caustic esophageal burns. J Pediatr Surg. 1996;31:1494–5.
84. Orive-Calzada A, Bernal-Martinez A, Navajas-Laboa M, Torres-Burgos S, Aguirresarobe M, Lorenzo-Morote M, et al. Efficacy of intralesional corticosteroid injection in endoscopic treatment of esophageal strictures. Surg Laparosc Endosc Percutan Tech. 2012;22:518–22.
85. Repici A, Hassan C, Sharma P, Conio M, Siersema P. Systematic review: the role of self-expanding plastic stents for benign oesophageal strictures. Aliment Pharmacol Ther. 2010;31:1268–75.
86. Saleem MM. Acquired oesophageal strictures in children: emphasis on the use of string-guided dilatations. Singapore Med J. 2009;50:82–6.
87. Sandgren K, Malmfors G. Balloon dilatation of oesophageal strictures in children. Eur J Pediatr Surg. 1998;8:9–11.
88. Scolapio JS, Tousif M, Gostout CJ, Mahoney DW, Zinsmeister AR, Ott BJ, et al. A randomized prospective study comparing rigid to balloon dilators for benign esophageal strictures and rings. Gastroint Endosc. 1999;50:13–7.
89. Shehata SM, Enaba ME. Endoscopic dilatation for benign oesophageal strictures in infants and toddlers: experience of an expectant protocol from North African tertiary centre. Afr J Paediatr Surg. 2012;9:187–92.
90. Spechler SJ. American gastroenterological association medical position statement on treatment of patients with dysphagia caused by benign disorders of the distal esophagus. Gastroenterology. 1999;117:229–33.
91. Temiz A, Oguzkurt P, Ezer SS, Ince E, Hicsonmez A. Long-term management of corrosive esophageal stricture with balloon dilation in children. Surg Endosc. 2010;24(9):2287–92.
92. Tiryaki T, Livanelioğlu Z, Atayurt H. Early bougienage for relief of stricture formation following caustic esophageal burns. Pediatr Surg Int. 2005;21:78–80.
93. van Halsema EE, van Hooft JE. Clinical outcomes of self-expandable stent placement for benign esophageal diseases: A pooled analysis of the literature. World J Gastrointest Endosc. 2015;7:135–53.
94. Vimalraj V, Rajendran S, Jyotibasu D, Balachandar TG, Kannan D, Jeswanth S, et al. Role of retrograde dilatation in the management of pharyngo-esophageal corrosive strictures. Dis Esophagus. 2007;20:328–32.
95. Wang RW, Zhou JH, Jiang YG, Fan SZ, Gong TQ, Zhao YPTan QY, et al. Prevention of stricture with intraluminal stenting through laparotomy after corrosive esophageal burns. Eur J Cardiothorac Surg. 2006;30:207–11.
96. Wijburg FA, Heymans HS, Urbanus NA. Caustic esophageal lesions in childhood: prevention of stricture formation. J Pediatr Surg. 1989;24(2):171–3.
97. Lerut T, Mbamendame S, Touré BM, Coulibaly Z, Kané B, Diani N, et al. Les sténoses caustiques de l'oesophage à l'hôpital du Mali. Ampleur, gravité et place de la dilatation en chirurgie. Chir Thorac Cardio-Vascul. 2014;18(4):230–6.
98. Zargar SA, Kochhar R, Mehta S, Mehta SK. The role of fiberoptic endoscopy in the management of corrosive ingestion and modified endoscopic classification of burns. Gastrointest Endosc. 1991;37:165–9.
99. Abaskharoun RD, Depew WT, Hookey LC. Nonsurgical management of severe esophageal and gastric injury following alkali ingestion. Can J Gastroenterol. 2007;21:757–60.
100. Agarwal S, Sikora SS, Kumar A, Saxena R, Kapoor VK. Surgical management of corrosive strictures of stomach. Indian J Gastroenterol. 2004;23(5):178–80.
101. Ananthakrishnan N, Parthasarathy G, Kate V. Chronic corrosive injuries of the stomach-a single unit experience of 109 patients over thirty years. World J Surg. 2010;34(4):758–64.
102. Ansari MM, Haleem S, Harris SH, Khan R, Zia I, Beg MH. Isolated corrosive pyloric stenosis without oesophageal involvement: an experience of 21 years. Arab J Gastroenterol. 2011;12(2):94–8.
103. Chaudhary A, Puri AS, Dhar P, Reddy P, Sachdev A, Lahoti D, et al. Elective surgery for corrosive-induced gastric injury. World J Surg. 1996;20(6):703–6.
104. Chibishev A, Pereska Z, Simonovska N, Chibisheva V, Glasnovic M, Chitkushev LT. Conservative therapeutic approach to corrosive poisonings in adults. J Gastrointest Surg. 2013;17(6):1044–9.
105. Tai WC, Chiu KW, Chuah SK, Chiu YC, Liang CM, Tam W, et al. The effects of endoscopic-guided balloon dilations in esophageal and gastric strictures caused by corrosive injuries. BMC Gastroenterol. 2013;13:99.
106. Gupta V, Wig JD, Kochhar R, Sinha SK, Nagi B, Doley RP, et al. Surgical management of gastric cicatrisation resulting from corrosive ingestion. Int J Surg. 2009;7(3):257–61.
107. Hogan RB, Polter DE. Non surgical management of lye-induced antral strictures with hydrostatic balloon dilation. Gastrointest Endosc. 1986;32(3):228–30.
108. Hwang TL, Chen MF. Surgical treatment of gastric outlet obstruction after corrosive injury—can early definitive operation be used instead of staged operation? Int Surg. 1996;81(2):119–21.
109. Kaushik R, Singh R, Sharma R, Attri AK, Bawa AS. Corrosive-induced gastric outlet obstruction. Yonsei Med J. 2003;44(6):991–4.
110. Kochhar R, Dutta U, Sethy PK, Singh G, Sinha SK, Nagi B, et al. Endoscopic balloon dilation in caustic-induced chronic gastric outlet obstruction. Gastrointest Endosc. 2009;69(4):800–5.
111. Kochhar R, Poornachandra KS, Dutta U, Agrawal A, Singh K. Early endoscopic balloon dilation in caustic-induced gastric injury. Gastrointest Endosc. 2010;71:737–44.
112. Kochhar R, Sethy PK, Nagi B, Wig JD. Endoscopic balloon dilatation of benign gastric outlet obstruction. J Gastroenterol Hepatol. 2004;19:418–22.
113. Lebeau R, Coulibaly A, Kountélé Gona S, Koffi Gnangoran M, Kouakou B, Yapo P, et al. Isolated gastric outlet obstruction due to corrosive ingestion. J Visc Surg. 2011;148(1):59–63.
114. Lu LS, Tai WC, Hu ML, Wu KL, Chiu YC. Predicting the progress of caustic injury to complicated gastric outlet obstruction and esophageal stricture, using modified endoscopic mucosal injury grading scale. Biomed Research International 2014:919870. doi:10.1155/2014/919870. Epub 2014 Aug 4.
115. Manta R, Conigliaro R, Bertani H, Manno M, Soliman A, Fedeli P, Bassotti G. Self-Expandable Metal Stenting of Refractory Upper Gut Corrosive Strictures: A New Role for Endoscopy? Case Reports in Gastrointestinal Medicine 2011, doi:10.1155/2011/346413
116. Rana SS, Bhasin DK, Chandail VS, Gupta R, Nada R, Kang M, et al. Endoscopic balloon dilatation without fluoroscopy for treating gastric outlet obstruction because of benign etiologies. Surg Endosc. 2011;25:1579–158.

117. Solt J, Bajor J, Szabó M, Horváth OP. Long-term results of balloon catheter dilation for benign gastric outlet stenosis. Endoscopy. 2003;35(6):490–5.
118. Tseng YL, Wu MH, Lin MY, Lai WW. Early surgical correction for isolated gastric stricture following acid corrosion injury. Dig Surg. 2002;19(4):276–80.
119. Bonavina L, Chella B, Segalin A, Luzzani S. Surgical treatment of the redundant interposed colon after retrosternal esophagoplasty. Ann Thorac Surg. 1998;65:1446–8.
120. Bothereau H, Munoz-Bongrand N, Lambert B, Montemagno S, Cattan P, Sarfati E. Esophageal reconstruction after caustic injury: is there still a place for right coloplasty? Am J Surg. 2007;193:660–4.
121. Boukerrouche A. Left colonic graft in esophageal reconstruction for caustic stricture: mortality and morbidity. Dis Esoph. 2013;26:788–93.
122. Chana JS, Chen HC, Sharma R, Gedebou TM, Feng GM. Microsurgical reconstruction of the esophagus using supercharged pedicled jejunum flaps: special indications and pitfalls. Plast Reconstr Surg. 2002;110(3):742–8.
123. Cheng YJ, Wang KU, Chen HC, Hsieh KC, Chang PC. Esophageal mucocele with compression of the right recurrent laryngeal nerve 20 years after surgical intervention for caustic esophagitis. Ann Thorac Surg. 2010;90:e28–29.
124. Chirica M, Veyrie N, Munoz-Bongrand N, Zohar S, Halimi B, Celerier M, et al. Late morbidity after colon interposition for corrosive esophageal injury. Risk factors, management and outcome. A 20-years experience. Ann Surg. 2010;252:271–80.
125. Deng B, Wang RW, Jiang YG, Gong TQ, Zhou JH, Lin YD, et al. Prevention and management of complications after colon interposition for corrosive esophageal burns. Dis Esophagus. 2008;21(1):57–62.
126. Evans KFK, Mardini S, Salgado CJ, Chen HC. Esophagus and hypopharyngeal reconstruction. Semin Plast Surg. 2010;24:219–26.
127. Ezemba N, Eze JC, Nwafor IA, Etukokwu KC, Orakwe OI. Colon interposition graft for corrosive esophageal stricture: midterm functional outcome. World J Surg. 2014;38:2352–57.
128. Gerzic ZB, Knezevic JB, Milicevic MN, Jovanovic BK. Esophagocoloplasty in the management of postcorrosive strictures of the esophagus. Ann Surg. 1990;211(3):329–36.
129. Guha G, Gupta S, Chakraborty S. Pharyngo-oesophageal strictures and its reconstruction by delto-pectoral flaps. Indian J Otolaryngol Head Neck Surg. 2005;57(3):229–34.
130. Gupta S. Surgical management of corrosive strictures following acid burns of upper gastrointestinal tract. Eur J Cardiothorac Surg. 1996;10(11):934–40.
131. Gupta NM, Gupta R. Transhiatal esophageal resection for corrosive injury. Ann Surg. 2004;239:359–63.
132. Han Y, Cheng QS, Li XF, Wang XP. Surgical management of esophageal strictures after caustic burns: A 30 years of experience. World J Gastroenterol. 2004;10(19):2846–49.
133. Harlak A, Yigit T, Coskun K, Ozer T, Mentes O, Gulec B, et al. Surgical treatment of caustic esophageal strictures in adults. Int J Surg. 2013;11:164–8.
134. Ho AC, Yeo MS, Ciudad P, Chen HC. 2-Stage free and pedicle jejunum for esophageal replacement after failed colon interposition for caustic injury in a 5 year-old child. J Plast Reconstr Aesthet Surg. 2014;67(3):417–22.
135. Javed A, Pal S, Dash NR, Sahni P, Chattopadhyay TK. Outcome following surgical management of corrosive strictures of the esophagus. Ann Surg. 2011;254:62–6.
136. Jiang YG, Lin YD, Wang RW, Zhou JH, Gong TQ, Ma Z, et al. Pharyngocolonic anastomosis for esophageal reconstruction in corrosive esophageal stricture. Ann Thorac Surg. 2005;79(6):1890–94.
137. Kane TD, Nwomeh BC, Nadler EP. Thoracoscopic-assisted esophagectomy and laparoscopic gastric pull-up for lye injury. JSLS. 2007;11:474–80.
138. Khwa-Otsyula BO, Matthews HR, Shenoi PM. Laryngectomy and coloplasty for major oesophagogastric corrosive stricture: case report and literature review. East Afr Med J. 1993;70(5):319–21.
139. Kim YT, Sung SW, Kim JH. Is it necessary to resect the diseased esophagus in performing reconstruction for corrosive esophageal stricture? Eur J Cardiothorac Surg. 2001;20:1–6.
140. Liu HP, Chang CH, Lin PJ, Chang JP. Video-assisted endoscopic esophagectomy with stapled intrathoracic esophagogastric anastomosis. World J Surg. 1995;19(5):745–7.
141. Nwomeh BC, Luketich JP, Kane TD. Minimally invasive esophagectomy for caustic esophageal stricture in children. J Pediatr Surg. 2004;39(3):276–81.
142. Park JK, Sim SB, Lee SH, Jeon HM, Kwack MS. Pharyngo-enteral anastomosis for esophageal reconstruction in diffuse corrosive esophageal stricture. Ann Thorac Surg. 2001;72(4):1141–43.
143. Popovici Z. A new philosophy in esophageal reconstruction with colon. Thirty-years experience. Dis Esophagus. 2003;16(4):323–7.
144. Radovanović N, Simić A, Kotarac M, Stojakov D, Sabljak P, Skrobić O, et al. Colon interposition for pharyngoesophageal postcorrosive strictures. Hepatogastroenterology. 2009;56(89):139–43.
145. Ribet M, Chambon JP, Pruvot FR. Oesophagectomy for severe corrosive injuries: is it always legitimate? Eur J Cardiothorac Surg. 1990;4:347–50.
146. Sa YJ, Kim YD, Kim CK, Park JK, Moon SW. Recurrent cervical esophageal stenosis after colon conduit failure: use of myocutaneous flap. World J Gastroenterol. 2013;19(2):307–10.
147. Saetti R, Silvestrini M, Cutrone C, Barion U, Mirri L, Narne S. Endoscopic treatment of upper airway and digestive tract lesions caused by caustic agents. Ann Otol Rhinol Laryngol. 2003;112(1):29–36.
148. Spitz L, Kiely E, Pierro A. Gastric transposition in children - A 21-year experience. J Pediatr Surg. 2004;39:276–81.
149. Tettey M, Edwin F, Aniteye E, Tamatey M, Entsua-Mensah K, Ofosu-Appiah E, et al. Colopharyngoplasty for intractable caustic pharyngoesophageal strictures in an indigenous African community – adverse impact of concomitant tracheostomy on outcome. Interact Cardiovasc Thorac Surg. 2011;12(2):213–7.
150. Pungpapong SA, Udomsawaengsup S, Navicharern P. Thoracoscopic approach for esophageal resection in chronic severe corrosive esophageal stricture: report of 2 cases. J Med Assoc Thai. 2010;93(9):1103–6.
151. Yannopoulos P, Lytras D, Paraskevas KI. Esophageal reconstruction with intraoperative dilatation of the hypopharynx for the management of chronic corrosive esophageal strictures. A technical tip. Eur J Cardiothorac Surg. 2006;30(6):940–2Javed A, Agarwal AK. Total laparoscopic esophageal bypass using a colonic conduit for corrosive-induced esophageal stricture. Surg Endosc. 2013;27(10):3726–32.
152. Yasuda T, Shiozaki H. Esophageal reconstruction using a pedicled jejunum with microvascular augmentation. Ann Thorac Cardiovasc Surg. 2011;17:103–9.
153. Yildirim S, Koksal H, Celayir T, Erdem L, Oner M, Baykan A. Colonic interposition vs. gastric pull-up after total esophagectomy. J Gastrointest Surg. 2004;8:675–8.
154. Wu MH, Lai WW. Esophageal reconstruction for esophageal strictures or resection after corrosive injury. Ann Thorac Surg. 1992;53:798–802.
155. Wu MH, Tseng YL, Lin MY, Lai WW. Esophageal reconstruction for hypopharyngoesophageal strictures after corrosive injury. Eur J Cardio-Thorac Surg. 2001;19:400–5.
156. Zhou JH, Jiang YG, Wang RW, Lin YD, Gong TQ, Zhao YP, et al. Management of corrosive esophageal burns in 149 cases. J Thorac Cardiovasc Surg. 2005;130(2):449–55.
157. Anderson KD, Rouse TM, Randolph JG. A controlled trial of corticosteroids in children with corrosive injury of the esophagus. N Engl J Med. 1990;323:637–40.
158. Kluger Y et al. Caustic ingestion management: World Society of Emergency Surgery preliminary survey of expert opinion. World J Emerg Surg 2015 (in press).

23

2017 WSES guidelines on colon and rectal cancer emergencies: obstruction and perforation

Michele Pisano[1*], Luigi Zorcolo[2], Cecilia Merli[3], Stefania Cimbanassi[4], Elia Poiasina[1], Marco Ceresoli[5], Ferdinando Agresta[6], Niccolò Allievi[1], Giovanni Bellanova[7], Federico Coccolini[8], Claudio Coy[9], Paola Fugazzola[1], Carlos Augusto Martinez[10], Giulia Montori[11], Ciro Paolillo[12], Thiago Josè Penachim[13], Bruno Pereira[14], Tarcisio Reis[15], Angelo Restivo[2], Joao Rezende-Neto[16], Massimo Sartelli[17], Massimo Valentino[18], Fikri M. Abu-Zidan[19], Itamar Ashkenazi[20], Miklosh Bala[21], Osvaldo Chiara[4], Nicola de' Angelis[22], Simona Deidda[2], Belinda De Simone[23], Salomone Di Saverio[24], Elena Finotti[6], Inaba Kenji[25], Ernest Moore[26], Steven Wexner[27], Walter Biffl[28], Raul Coimbra[29], Angelo Guttadauro[5], Ari Leppäniemi[30], Ron Maier[31], Stefano Magnone[1], Alain Chicom Mefire[32], Andrew Peitzmann[33], Boris Sakakushev[34], Michael Sugrue[35], Pierluigi Viale[36], Dieter Weber[37], Jeffry Kashuk[38], Gustavo P. Fraga[39], Ioran Kluger[40], Fausto Catena[41] and Luca Ansaloni[8]

Abstract

Obstruction and perforation due to colorectal cancer represent challenging matters in terms of diagnosis, life-saving strategies, obstruction resolution and oncologic challenge. The aims of the current paper are to update the previous WSES guidelines for the management of large bowel perforation and obstructive left colon carcinoma (OLCC) and to develop new guidelines on obstructive right colon carcinoma (ORCC).

Methods: The literature was extensively queried for focused publication until December 2017. Precise analysis and grading of the literature has been performed by a working group formed by a pool of experts: the statements and literature review were presented, discussed and voted at the Consensus Conference of the 4th Congress of the World Society of Emergency Surgery (WSES) held in Campinas in May 2017.

Results: CT scan is the best imaging technique to evaluate large bowel obstruction and perforation. For OLCC, self-expandable metallic stent (SEMS), when available, offers interesting advantages as compared to emergency surgery; however, the positioning of SEMS for surgically treatable causes carries some long-term oncologic disadvantages, which are still under analysis. In the context of emergency surgery, resection and primary anastomosis (RPA) is preferable to Hartmann's procedure, whenever the characteristics of the patient and the surgeon are permissive. Right-sided loop colostomy is preferable in rectal cancer, when preoperative therapies are predicted.

With regards to the treatment of ORCC, right colectomy represents the procedure of choice; alternatives, such as internal bypass and loop ileostomy, are of limited value.

Clinical scenarios in the case of perforation might be dramatic, especially in case of free faecal peritonitis. The importance of an appropriate balance between life-saving surgical procedures and respect of oncologic caveats must be stressed. In selected cases, a damage control approach may be required.

Medical treatments including appropriate fluid resuscitation, early antibiotic treatment and management of co-existing

(Continued on next page)

* Correspondence: mpisano@asst-pg23.it

[1]General Surgery Papa Giovanni XXII Hospital Bergamo, Bergamo, Italy

Full list of author information is available at the end of the article

(Continued from previous page)
medical conditions according to international guidelines must be delivered to all patients at presentation.

Conclusions: The current guidelines offer an extensive overview of available evidence and a qualitative consensus regarding management of large bowel obstruction and perforation due to colorectal cancer.

Keywords: Colon, Rectum, Cancer, Obstruction, Perforation, Emergency

Background

In 2010, the World Society of Emergency Surgery (WSES) published the guidelines for the management of obstructive left colon cancer [1]. The 2017 guidelines represent both an update and an implementation of the previous edition: the management of perforation and obstruction associated with right-sided colon cancer is also included into the current guidelines.

The relevance of the topic is evident with the help of the following statements:

- Colorectal cancer (CRC) is the third most commonly diagnosed malignancy, accounting for about 1.4 million new cases per year. It represents the third most common cancer in men (746,000 cases, 10.0% of the total) and the second in women (614,000 cases, 9.2% of the total) worldwide; it is the fourth leading cause of cancer death in the world, with almost 700,000 deaths in 2012 [2, 3].
- The incidence of CRC varies by geographic region: in Europe, the incidence is higher than in North America, followed by Oceania, Latin America and Africa. However, the trend of CRC seems to vary according to the Human Development Index (HDI), with a variability parallel to changes in diet, smoke attitude, activity patterns and screening programs. A decreasing rate is reported in North America, Oceania and Europe and in particular in the USA, New Zealand and France; on the other side, an increasing incidence is observed in Latin America, Asia and Eastern Europe [3].

A word of caution must be spent with regards to the increasing incidence of CRC in the population younger than 50 years: this could potentially encourage an update in screening programs [4, 5].

- Complications of large bowel diseases account for 47% of gastrointestinal emergencies [6].
- CRC presents as emergency in a wide range of patients (from 7 to 40% of the total), but the vast majority of reports present a figure of around 30% [6–15].
- Large bowel obstruction (LBO) represents almost 80% (15–30% of CRC) of the emergencies related to CRC, while perforation accounts for the remaining 20% (1–10% of CRC) [7, 12, 16, 17].
- The most common location of CRC obstruction is the sigmoid colon, with 75% of the tumours located distal to the splenic flexure [18].
- Perforation occurs at the tumour site in almost 70% of cases and proximal to the tumour site in around 30% of cases [6, 19, 20].

Management of obstruction and perforation of the colon and rectum secondary to CRC is challenging in terms of clinical severity, diagnostic and therapeutic options and management of septic and oncologic issues.

Focused guidelines lack of evidence and consensus is often limited to short sections within general colon and rectal cancer guidelines edited by Surgical Societies [21–23].

Materials and methods: consensus conference organisational model

In July 2016, the Scientific Board of the WSES endorsed the President of the Society and the President of the 4th World Congress of the WSES to prepare the Consensus Conference on Colon Rectal Cancer Emergencies (CRCE) focusing on obstruction and perforation.

The Presidents and the six members of the Scientific Secretariat agreed on six key questions to develop the topics for the current guidelines; according to the skills (residency program, work and scientific experience), 12 international experts, affiliates of the WSES, were chosen as Scientific Committee of the Consensus Conference. Each question was developed by members of the Scientific Committee in a variable number from 2 to 4 according to the magnitude of the topic: the Scientific Secretariat members and the Presidents supervised each group.

The documentarist of the Papa Giovanni XXIII Hospital medical library, with the support of the Scientific Secretariat, provided the electronic search in PubMed and EMBASE databases, according to specific key words for each questions, without time or language restrictions (Table 1).

The additional bibliography research was developed by each group before starting and updated to May 2017. The research presented at the CC as "in press" has been kept in consideration if published before the final revision of the present guidelines. Each working group, before the CC, developed a focused draft and a variable number of statements along with the level of evidence (LoE) and the grade of recommendation (GoR) for each statement. The

Table 1 Questions and MeSH terms

Questions	Key words
Diagnosis	diagnosis, cancer, neoplasm, colon, rectum, bowel, perforation, obstruction, physical examination, radiology, laboratory, abdominal ultrasound, CT scan, colonic enema
Perforation	perforation, cancer, neoplasm, colon, rectum, bowel, tumour perforation, diastatic perforation, faecal peritonitis, treatment, surgery, acute care surgery
Obstruction left	obstruction, left colon, rectum, cancer, neoplasm, surgery, acute care surgery, stent, SEMS, Hartmann's procedure, colostomy, resection, anastomosis, tube decompression
Obstruction right	obstruction, right colon, rectum, neoplasm, surgery, acute care surgery, stent, SEMS, loop ileostomy, intestinal bypass, resection, anastomosis, tube decompression
Unstable patients	unstable patient, haemodynamic instability, critically ill patient, sepsis, peritonitis, obstruction, cancer, neoplasm, colon, rectum, surgery, acute care surgery, damage control, open abdomen.
Antibiotics	antibiotics, therapy, prophylaxis, colon, rectum, perforation, obstruction, unstable patient, haemodynamic instability, critically ill patient obstruction, bowel, sepsis, peritonitis, surgery, acute care surgery.

2011 Oxford Classification was used to grade the LoE and GoR (available at https://www.cebm.net/category/ebm-resources/loe/).

The provisional statements and the supporting literature were reviewed by the SS and the Presidents, discussed with the members of each working groups by email and call conferences and modified if necessary.

The Consensus Conference on CRCE has been held in Campinas, Brazil, on May 18, 2017, during the 4th World Congress of the WSES.

The designated member of each working group presented the statements to the audience, along with LoE, GoR and the literature supporting each statement. The audience, represented by 45 experts, voted each statement using a red/green double face card (green, agreement; red, disagreement). The exact agreement/disagreement ratio was not calculated simultaneously to avoid waste of time: for the entire vote, it ranged from 45/0 to 38/7 (18%); despite the small percentage of disagreement, each red card comment was discussed and a final agreement reached among participants.

The agreement required some statement modification, performed by the Presidents and by the Scientific Secretariat; all the statements were eventually reviewed by the WSES board and modified accordingly (Table 6 in Appendix 1).

Further literature published between May and December 2017 was also considered. Clinicians and surgeons must be aware that the present WSES guidelines should be considered as an adjunctive tool for decision and management but they are not substitute of the clinical judgement for the individual patient.

Results

The results are hereby presented separately as O (obstruction) and P (perforation) when required; otherwise, the statements can be considered valid for both conditions.

Diagnosis

Statement 1.1: The clinical presentation is variable, except for lower rectal cancer, in which case digital examination could be diagnostic. Laboratory tests are not specific. Clinical evaluation and laboratory tests have high variability and low specificity; therefore, the escalation to further diagnostic tools, whenever available, is mandatory. LoE 3, GoR B.

Obstruction

Large bowel obstruction can present acutely, with colic-like abdominal pain, abdominal bloating and absence of bowel movement and flatus, while vomiting is less frequent than in small bowel obstruction, or subacutely, with gradual development of symptoms, changes in bowel habits and recurrent left lower quadrant abdominal pain. In a series of 150 consecutive patients suffering from acute mechanical bowel obstruction, 24% presented with large bowel obstruction. Absence of passage of flatus (90%) and/or faeces (80.6%) and abdominal distension (65.3%) were the most common symptoms and physical signs [24].

Abdominal examination shows tenderness, abdominal distension and hyperactive or absent bowel sounds.

Previous complaint of bloody stools and passage of blood per rectum, despite the absence of bowel movement, can be associated with colon cancer. A rectal cancer may be palpable as an intrinsic lesion [25, 26].

Laboratory tests are directed at evaluating the electrolyte imbalances, elevated urea nitrogen and metabolic alkalosis that may occur as a consequence of vomiting and dehydration.

Perforation

When perforation occurs at the tumour site, peritoneal contamination is usually localised; at the opposite, when perforation is located proximal to the tumour site, the faecal spread results in diffuse peritonitis and septic shock.

In this setting, physical examination reveals an acutely ill patient characterised by fever, tachypnea, tachycardia and confusion.

The abdomen may be diffusely tender or may present localised tenderness, guarding, or rebound tenderness. Bowel sounds are usually absent. The toxic symptoms of peritonitis are usually delayed, but are considered an ominous sign [27]. Leukocytosis and neutrophilia, elevated amylase levels and lactic acidosis suggest perforation or necrosis [28]. The suspicion of large bowel obstruction or perforation is based on aspecific symptoms, signs and laboratory findings: adjunctive diagnostic tests are mandatory, whenever available (Fig. 1).

Statement 1.2: (a) In case of clinical suspicion of colon obstruction, computed tomography (CT) scan achieves diagnostic confirmation better than abdominal ultrasound (US), which performs better than abdominal plain X-ray. If CT scan is not available, a water-soluble contrast enema is a valid alternative for identifying the site and the nature of obstruction. (b) In case of clinical suspicion of perforation, abdominal CT scan, which performs better than abdominal US, should achieve diagnostic confirmation. US performs better than abdominal plain X-ray. LoE 3, GoR B.

Abdominal plain X-ray and abdominal US are screening imaging tests, with the latter representing the more performing alternative. With these results, after adequate training, bedside abdominal ultrasound examination could replace abdominal plain X-ray (Table 2).

As a consequence, the clinical suspicion of bowel obstruction should be, as a first step, tested by abdominal US or by plain abdominal X-ray when the abdominal US expertise is not available or the US machine is not promptly available.

Despite contrast enema shows acceptable sensitivity and specificity, abdominal CT scan, with high sensitivity and specificity, has the absolute advantage to provide the clinician with an optimal grade of information, in particular regarding the complications of cancer-related LBO. Moreover, it is possible to stage the neoplastic disease and to identify synchronous neoplasms (Table 2). Due to this multifaceted profile, CT scan represents the imaging test of choice in current clinical practice; if CT is available, the water-soluble contrast enema can be considerate obsolete.

When the clinical scenario is suggestive of bowel perforation, abdominal US or abdominal plain X-ray should be used as first screening imaging tests. Bedside abdominal US, performed by a trained physician or surgeon, has higher sensitivity and same specificity of abdominal plain X-ray [29]; moreover, it reduces the mobilisation of a critically-ill patient. One of the limitations of the abdominal US and of the abdominal plain X-ray is the risk of false negatives of pneumoperitoneum, when a small amount of intraperitoneal free air is present, such as in the case of early perforation at the tumour site (Table 3).

When bowel perforation is suspected, screening imaging tests are represented by abdominal US or abdominal plain X-ray. The literature shows that bedside abdominal US has a higher sensitivity and same specificity with abdominal plain X-ray; moreover, it allows environmental stress reduction to an acutely ill patient [30].

Statement 1.3: In stable patients, direct visualisation of the site of colonic obstruction should be considered when colonoscopy is available. In this situation, biopsies should be obtained, especially when the deployment of an endoscopic stent is planned. LoE 3, GoR B

The role of colonoscopy in the setting of the diagnosis of LBO is limited; this is mainly due to its low availability in the emergency setting. The aim of the direct visualisation is to explore the various aetiologies of obstruction. Biopsies and histologic examination of the lesions should be performed when an emergency surgical resection has not been planned or endoscopic stent placement can be expected [18, 21, 31].

Statement 1.4: In case of diagnosis of perforation at abdominal US or abdominal X-ray in a stable patient, abdominal CT scan should be considered, in order to

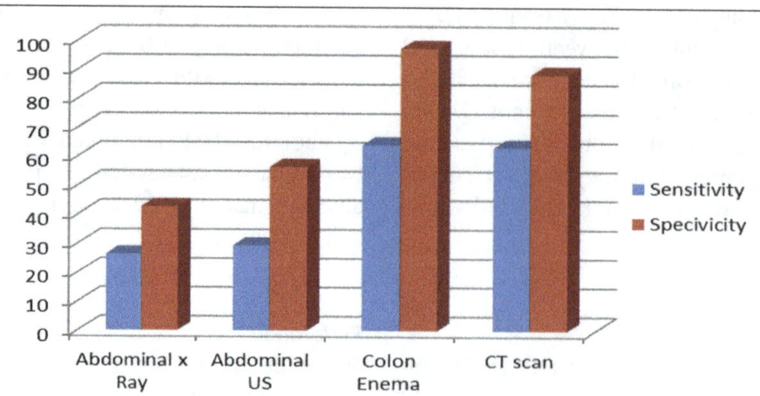

Fig. 1 Cumulative diagram for the three items (confirmation, cause, site of LBO) according to imaging study. *US* ultrasound, *CT* computerized tomography

Table 2 Comparison of imaging studies for confirmation, cause and site of LBO

	Confirmation of LBO obstruction		Cause of LBO		Site of LBO	
	Sensitivity	Specificity	Sensitivity	Specificity	Sensitivity	Specificity
Plain X-ray	74–84% [26]	50–72% [26, 211, 212]	0	7% [212]	0	60% [212]
Abdominal US	88% [211]	76% [211]	0	23% [212]	0	70% [212]
Colonic enema	96% [26]	98% [26]	0	96% [26]	96% [26]	98% [26]
CT scan	93–96% [212, 213]	93–100% [212, 213]	0	66–87% [212, 214]	95% [213]	90–94% [29, 213]

define the cause and the site of perforation. If there are clear signs of diffuse peritonitis, CT scan should not delay the appropriate treatment. Early involvement of the surgeon is required. LoE 3, GoR B

Although free air in the peritoneal cavity leads, in the vast majority of cases, to surgical exploration, CT scan examination is suggested if available.

In fact, in few cases of pneumoperitoneum, a conservative management could be attempted, depending on the gastrointestinal perforation site; moreover, there are some cases of pneumoperitoneum which are unrelated to intestinal perforation [32, 33].

Furthermore, CT scan can help the surgeon to foresee the operative scenario, with a better prediction of the resources needed for the intervention [34].

Despite its utility, it must be stressed that CT scan, even when readily available, should never expose the patient to unsafe delays in the appropriate treatment.

Statement 1.5: There is no specific data regarding staging pathways of CRC presenting as an emergency. CT scan performs better than US in the abdomen and should be suggested for staging in the suspicion of cancer-related colorectal emergencies. CT scan of the thorax is not strictly recommended. LoE 3, GoR B

The 2017 NCCN guidelines on colon cancer recommend CT scanning for staging of liver metastases from a colorectal primary tumour, given its best accuracy among the available preoperative tests [35].

Evidence to support the indication for routine CT of the thorax is weak: a resolving power of 2–3 mm for lung nodules leads to a sensitivity of 100%, but the specificity is low, with a false positive rate of 34%. On the other side, chest X-ray has a low sensitivity (30–64%), but has a specificity as high as 90% [36].

This data should be kept into consideration also when approaching CRCE: if available, preoperative CT scan of the abdomen should be obtained for staging, while X-ray of the chest may be appropriate for staging of the chest. As previously stated, CT scan for staging should never expose the patient to a safety risk, in terms of time and actions subtracted to the patient's care.

2. Management of perforation

Statement 2.1: When diffuse peritonitis occurs in cancer-related colon perforation, the priority is the control of the source of sepsis. Prompt combined medical treatment is advised. LoE 2, GoR B

While keeping in mind the caveats of oncologic treatment for patients with perforated CRC, the priority must be directed to immediate patient safety and therefore to treatment of the septic status and to control of the source of sepsis (see Appendix 2).

When free peritonitis, usually related to perforation proximal to tumour site, occurs, patients are at a higher risk of development of septic shock, as compared to patients with a contained collection, which is usually related to perforation at the tumour site for necrosis [6, 19, 20, 37–39].

In cases of contained intra-abdominal collections from perforated CRC, the mortality rate is between 0 and 24%, with an increase to 19–65% in the case of diffuse faecal peritonitis: this difference reaches statistical significance. Despite this finding, the severity of peritonitis, at multivariate analysis, is not an independent factor influencing the in-hospital mortality [6, 20].

Moreover, the in-hospital mortality is related to the site of perforation, varying from 37 to 60% for perforation at the tumour site or proximal to the tumour site, respectively [20].

Table 3 Comparison of imaging studies for confirmation and site of perforation

	Confirmation of perforation		Site of perforation	
	Sensitivity	Specificity	Sensitivity	Specificity
Abdominal plain X-ray	53% [30]	53% [30]	NS	NS
Abdominal US	92% [30]	53% [30]	NS	NS
Colonic enema	NS	NS	NS	NS
CT scan	95% [29]	90% [29]	NS	90% [29]

NS not stated

The treatment of patients with septic shock due to intra-abdominal infection (IAI) is time-dependent; the medical treatment and the source control should be started as soon as possible. The details of the treatment of complicated IAI lie outside the intent of the present study; a number of guidelines are available on this topic [40, 41].

Statement 2.2: Oncologic resection should be performed in order to obtain better oncologic outcomes.

- *Perforation at the tumour site: formal resection with or without anastomosis, with or without stoma.*
- *Perforation proximal to tumour site (diastasic): simultaneous tumour resection and management of proximal perforation is indicated. Depending on the colonic wall conditions, a subtotal colectomy may be required. LoE 3, GoR B*

The surgeon should consider that only a small proportion of patients undergo reversal of a terminal stoma.

In CRCE, the long-term oncologic outcome can be influenced by an advanced disease and by the higher rate of incomplete preoperative workup. However, in case of perforation, the presence of undiagnosed metastases has a small impact in the treatment strategy.

Keeping in mind that immediate patient safety takes priority, the performance of a standard oncologic resection can lead to similar results, as compared to elective cases.

In the series of Zielinski et al., oncologic features in perforated CRC were obtained: patients were matched comparing free peritonitis versus contained collection; a third group of CRC without perforation was used as a control group (all groups were balanced for demographics and tumour staging). Authors observed a progressive increase in the lymph node harvesting rate across the three groups (free peritonitis, contained collection and no perforation cases); statistical significance was reached only when comparing all perforations versus no perforation (11 versus 16; $p < 0.001$). This significance, however, was not evident when comparing the positive nodes only. For other outcomes, such as completeness of resection, rate of adjuvant therapy and time to adjuvant therapy, the comparison showed no significant difference [6].

Biondo et al., interestingly, observed similar results when comparing patients undergoing emergency surgery for occluded CRC to patients with perforated CRC [19].

Long-term oncologic outcomes were analysed in the same studies: Zielinski and colleagues showed that, when adjusted by excluding the perioperative mortality, overall survival (OS) was similar for free faecal peritonitis, as compared to contained collection and in all perforated compared with non-perforated cases. At the opposite, the inclusion of the perioperative mortality dramatically increases the difference in terms of OS in case of free faecal peritonitis; however, at the multivariate analysis, perforation is not an independent factor for OS [6]. Similar results were obtained by Biondo et al. [19].

As a consequence, in case of perforation at the tumour site:

- For right-sided perforation, a right colectomy should be performed. In case of poor general or adverse local conditions, a resection without anastomosis and terminal ileostomy should be performed.
- For transverse/left-sided perforation: resection with anastomosis, with or without ileostomy, should be attempted. Hartmann's procedure might be considered, keeping in mind the low rate of stoma reversal. In case of perforation at a distant site from the tumour (generally the neoplasm is in the left colon and the perforation is found in the caecum), a subtotal colectomy should be attempted. The literature reports a better control of postoperative diarrhoea with resection of less than 10 cm of terminal ileum and a distant colon remnant above the peritoneal reflection of at least 10 cm of length [42, 43].

The surgeon managing CRC perforation should decide whether to perform the intestinal anastomosis or to carry out a derivative stoma. There is no evidence of sound quality to guide evidence-based decisions, as specific studies mostly consider heterogeneous groups of perforated and obstructed cancer-related LBO. The rate of anastomotic leak (AL) in right colon resections varies from 0.5 to 4.6% in perforated emergency cases and should be compared with 0.5–1.4% reported for elective surgery; the AL rate after left colonic resection ranges from 3.5 to 30% in emergency versus 5–10% in elective cases [30, 44].

As a general rule, principles of oncologic resection should be followed, always considering the importance of the medical comorbidities and of the septic status on the one side and the aim of a shortened uncomplicated postoperative course in order to allow oncologic staging completion and the start of chemotherapy programs, on the other side.

A word of caution should be spent on the risk of peritoneal carcinomatosis in perforated CRC: a single prospective series is available in the literature. All other series included a small number of patients, with a long data collection time and inclusion criteria, seldom explicated, were heterogeneous (inclusion or exclusion of patients with perforation proximal the tumour site etc.). In 2013, Honoréet al. published a systematic review, concluding that the rate of peritoneal carcinomatosis in perforated CRC ranges between 14 and 54%,with a level of evidence 3b to 4 [45].

Management of obstruction: left colon (from the distal transverse colon to the anus)

Several options to manage obstructive left colon cancer (OLCC) are available (see Table 4 and Appendix 3).

Statement 3.1: Loop colostomy (C) versus Hartmann's procedure (HP)

Hartmann's procedure should be preferred to simple colostomy, since colostomy appears to be associated with longer overall hospital stay and need for multiple operations, without a reduction in perioperative morbidity LoE 2, GoR B.

Loop colostomy should be reserved to unresectable tumours (if SEMS is not feasible), for severely ill patients who are too unfit for major surgical procedures or general anaesthesia.

A stoma provides colonic decompression with minimal surgical trauma, reduces the risk of contamination from an unprepared bowel and allows an intensive resuscitation of the patient and a better staging prior to the definitive treatment.

However, Fielding et al. [46] did not find any differences in the mortality rate between 47 patients treated with loop colostomy and 90 patients who received a primary resection.

A RCT [47] between Hartmann's procedure (63 patients) and colostomy (58 patients) found no difference in terms of mortality and morbidity rate, recurrence rate and cancer-specific survival between the two surgical approaches. On the other hand, the overall length of hospital stay was shorter in the primary resection (35 days) than in the staged resection group (49 days) ($p = 0.01$).

A Cochrane systematic review [48] considered only other four retrospective cases series and no RCT; therefore, a meta-analysis could not be performed.

Since then, another RCT was published [49]; the authors found a similar impact on mortality and hospitalisation with both surgical techniques.

Statement 3.2: Hartmann's procedure (HP) versus resection and primary anastomosis (RPA)

RPA should be the preferred option for uncomplicated malignant left-sided large bowel obstruction in absence of other risk factors.

Patients with high surgical risk are better managed with HP. LoE 3-GoR B.

HP remains one of the most common procedures in emergency surgery of the left colon [50–52]. However, the historical concept that a completely clear colon is necessary to avoid AL [53] has been questioned by others [54, 55], and there is now good evidence supporting that the presence of faeces in the large bowel does not influence the rate of anastomotic dehiscence, [56, 57] nor its severity [58].

In recent years, there has been an increasing trend toward a one-stage resection for left-sided obstruction, but unfortunately, no RCTs were conducted comparing HP and RPA; therefore, neither grade A nor B evidence are available, and the choice generally depends on the individual surgeon's judgement.

The first major report regarding RPA for obstructive cancer came from the Large Bowel Cancer Project (LBCP). The authors reported a mortality of 35% for staged resections and of only 14% for primary resection [46].

Since then, many prospective and retrospective series on RPA in OLCC reported rates of anastomotic dehiscence ranging from 2.2 to 12% [59–65]; these results are almost comparable to the 2–8% rate after elective surgery [56, 57, 66, 67].

Meyer et al. [51] reached different conclusions: they compared HP and RPA performed for OLCC both with curative and palliative intent. Despite the significantly higher preoperative risk within the HP group, postoperative mortality rate was lower as compared to the RPA group, both for curative (7.5 versus 9.2%; p value reported as not significant) and palliative procedures (33 versus 39%; p value reported as not significant). The limit of this study was the high number of participating institutions (309), which were also very heterogeneous in terms of intensity of care, spanning from regional to university hospitals.

Table 4 Treatment options for OLCC

Main options	Choices among main options	Ancillary manoeuvres among main option and choices
Loop colostomy (C) (bridge to resection or palliation)		
Primary resection with end colostomy: Hartmann's procedure (HP)		
Resection and primary anastomosis (RPA)	Total/subtotal colectomy (TC) Segmental colectomy (SC)	Intraoperative colonic irrigation (ICI) Manual decompression (MD) Covering stoma
Tube decompression		
Endoscopic colonic stenting by self-expanding metallic stents (SEMS)	Bridge to surgery Palliation	

The main advantage of RPA is to avoid a second major operation, which is associated to a morbidity rate of 20–50% and a dehiscence rate of 2–7% [68–72].

Furthermore, it should be considered that the majority of stomas (up to 90%) created during HP for CRC do not get reversed, due to necessity of adjuvant treatment and/or disease progression [62, 73].

In favour of RPA, it has also been postulated that this choice may result in long-term survival benefits, although evidence on this aspect is weak [65].

These unquestionable advantages of RPA must be counterbalanced by the potentially catastrophic situation resulting from AL in a fragile patient. For this reason, many parameters, related to both the surgeon and the patient, should be taken into account before deciding to perform a colo-colonic or colo-rectal anastomosis [63, 64, 74]. Historically, two main elements prevent anastomotic dehiscence: a tension-free anastomosis and good blood supply to the anastomotic rim; despite the single surgeon's experience may play a pivotal role in the evaluation of these parameters, evidence exists regarding the validity of the assessment of the anastomotic blood supply using intraoperative near-infrared indocyanine green [75, 76]. Risk stratification is the cornerstone of patient's selection. The Association of Coloproctology of Great Britain and Ireland (ACPGBI) identified four important predictors of outcome—age, ASA grade, operative urgency, and Dukes' stage [64]; others showed similar results [63, 74].

The experience and subspecialty of the surgeon also seem to be important factors in surgical decision. It has been demonstrated that primary anastomosis is more likely to be performed by colorectal rather than general surgeons, and by consultants rather than unsupervised trainees, with lower rate of anastomotic dehiscence and mortality [46, 74, 77–80].

Keeping in mind these considerations, HP could be more appropriate for patients deemed to be at high risk and when they are managed in an emergency setting by unspecialised surgeons.

Statement 3.3: RPA: the role of diverting stoma

There is no evidence supporting that a covering stoma can reduce the risk of anastomotic leak and its severity. LoE 4-GoR C

Unfortunately, there are very few data and no RCT comparing the use of diverting stoma versus no use of diverting stoma after surgery for OLCC; therefore, very weak recommendations can be drawn.

Kube et al. [81] analysed the results of 743 patients who underwent emergency radical surgery for OLCC. Of these, 30% had HP, 58% RPA and 12% RPA and covering stoma.

The morbidity and hospital mortality did not differ significantly between the groups, and the addition of a protective stoma did not affect the rate of anastomotic dehiscence (7 and 8% respectively), or the rate of re-operation (5.6 versus 5.7%).

We may postulate that a protective stoma does not reduce the rate of AL, but the rate of AL requiring re-operation [82]. A leak originating from an intraperitoneal anastomosis is likely to cause diffuse peritonitis and therefore mandates a reoperation. For this reason, the role of diverting stoma after resection and primary anastomosis for OLCC seems limited.

Statement 3.4: Total colectomy versus segmental colectomy

In absence of caecal tears/perforation, evidence of bowel ischemia or synchronous right colonic cancers, total colectomy should not be preferred to segmental colectomy, since it does not reduce morbidity and mortality and is associated with higher rates of impaired bowel function. LoE 2, GoR B.

Total colectomy (TC) with ileo-rectal anastomosis was proposed as an alternative procedure to avoid a stoma and at the same time to overcome the problems related to a distended unprepared colon [83–85]. This operation has an absolute indication when obstruction has determined a right colonic ischemia, caecal tears or perforation, or when synchronous proximal malignant tumours are present [21].

Major disadvantages of TC are represented by a technically challenging procedure, prolonged operative time and poor functional results, with many patients complaining of diarrhoea and possibly developing electrolyte disturbances [84, 86].

A single RCT, the SCOTIA (Subtotal Colectomy versus On-Table Irrigation and Anastomosis) trial was published [86]; 91 patients from 12 different centres were randomised to total/subtotal colectomy (47 patients) versus segmental colectomy with on-table lavage (44 patients). The authors found no differences in terms of morbidity and mortality, but significantly worse functional results after TC.

Statement 3.5: Intraoperative colonic irrigation (ICI) versus *manual decompression (MD)*

ICI and MD are associated with similar mortality/morbidity rate. The only significant difference is that MD is a shorter and simpler procedure. Either procedure could be performed, depending on the experience/preference of the surgeon. LoE 2-GoR B

There was only a RCT that compared ICI (24 patients) with MD (25 patients) in OLCC [87]. They concluded that MD is shorter and simpler than ICI and offers similar results in terms of mortality, morbidity and AL rates. However, the power of this study was low.

A systematic review published in 2009, which included the above-mentioned RCT, one prospective comparative trial and 5 prospective descriptive case series, concluded that, although the power of the studies was poor and a large-scale prospective randomised trial is desirable, no statistical significance could be shown between the two procedures [88].

Statement 3.6: RPA: the role of laparoscopy

The use of laparoscopy in the emergency treatment of OLCC cannot be recommended and should be reserved to selected favourable cases and in specialised centers.

LoE 4-GoR C

Traditionally, CO has been considered an absolute contraindication to laparoscopy, because of the high-risk patient profile and the level of operative technical difficulties due to dilated and vulnerable bowel [89].

However, with the diffusion of colo-rectal laparoscopy and increasing experience, some limited series became available with favourable results [90, 91], but no randomised trials have been produced.

Ballian et al. [92] evaluated the role of laparoscopy for emergency restorative colectomy using the American College of Surgeons National Surgical Quality Improvement Program (ACS NSQIP) database. They found that less than 10% of patients with OLCC were managed laparoscopically with colon resection and primary anastomosis, with comparable rates of morbidity and mortality, but faster recovery.

A systematic review published in 2014 analysed the results of 47 studies on laparoscopy in emergency colorectal surgery, but most of them regarded acute presentation of IBD or diverticular disease, while only a small number presented data on OLCC [93].

Statement 3.7: Tube decompression (TD)

TD can be a valid alternative option as BTS for high-risk OLCC. LoE 4-GoR C

Transanal TD is a minimally invasive endoscopic procedure that may allow the decompression of an obstructed colon in order to safely delay elective surgery with RPA. Despite the appeal for this bridge to surgery technique, unfortunately only few data is available.

Efficacy and safety of TD have been reported [94–102], with 80 to 100% rate of technical success and 72.5 to 100% rate of clinical success. Complications, such as perforation, are infrequent (incidence ranging from 0 to 10%) and may be caused by the pressure of the tip of the tube against the colonic wall.

However, there is lack of trial-based evidence to confirm the usefulness of TD and its efficacy in terms of short- and long-term outcomes.

Theoretically, TD has some advantages over self-expandable metallic stent (SEMS): the colon can be cleaned by lavage through the tube; tumour manipulation is minor and costs are contained. However, there are no randomised trials but only one retrospective study that compared these two techniques and did not show significant differences [103].

Despite these results appear promising, the available level of evidence is suboptimal, and therefore, no conclusions can be drawn.

Statement 3.8: Palliation: SEMS versus *colostomy*

In facilities with capability for stent placement, SEMS should be preferred to colostomy for palliation of OLCC since it is associated with similar mortality/morbidity rates and shorter hospital stay. LoE 1-GoR A

Alternative treatments to SEMS should be considered in patients eligible to a bevacizumab-based therapy. Involvement of the oncologist in the decision is strongly recommended. LoE 3-GoR B

Endoscopic stent placement was initially introduced in the palliative treatment of obstructive rectal [104] or recto-sigmoid cancer [105].

The development of SEMS, which can be introduced through a colonoscope, allowed to extend their use to a range of scenarios of CO [106, 107], not only with palliative intent to avoid a stoma, but also with the aim of transforming an emergency surgical operation into an elective procedure, and od reducing morbidity, mortality and stoma rate [108].

Several RCTs, case-matched studies and retrospective series have been published, but results are controversial.

We found five RCT comparing colostomy versus SEMS for palliation of malignant CO [109–112]; one of them was an update of a previous RCT [113].

Xinopoulos et al. [109] randomised 30 patients. A stent was successfully placed in 14/15 (93.3%) randomised to stenting, and CO was permanently resolved in eight of them (57%). There was no mortality related to the procedure in both groups. Mean survival was 21.4 months in SEMS group and 20.9 months in C group. Mean hospital stay was significantly higher in C group, and costs were comparable. The authors concluded that SEMS placement represents a good alternative to colostomy, providing a better quality of life for the patient, without the psychological repercussions of a colostomy, and it appears to be cost-effective.

Fiori et al. [110] randomised 22 patients: in both groups, the mortality was 0% and the morbidity was similar. SEMS group had shorter time to oral intake, restoration of bowel function, and hospital stay.

Some years later, the same group published the long-term results [113]: mean survival was 297 days (125–612) with SEMS and 280 days (135–591) in patients with stomas (p = n.s.). There was no mortality related to the procedures. Patients with stomas found them unacceptable, and the same feelings were present in their family members. On the contrary, none of the patients with stents or their family members reported any inconveniences related to the procedure.

The Dutch Stent-in I multicenter RCT [111] was terminated prematurely after enrolling 21 patients; the decision was taken after the incidence of four stent-related perforations among 10 patients enrolled for SEMS (in particular occurring12, 12, 44 and 106 days after stent placement), resulting in three fatal events.

No clear explanation for such a high perforation rate was retrieved; the authors suggested that changes made in the design of the stents (WallFlex, Boston Scientific Natick, MA), which have a larger diameter of the proximal end (30 mm) and are made of braided nitinol instead of stainless steel, might have had a role in the aetiology of the perforation. However, other subsequent series in which the Wallflex stent was used reported a perforation rate of around 5% [114–116], which is in line with commonly observed figures with other SEMS [116].

A more recent RCT [112] enrolled 26 patients in the SEMS group and 26 in the surgery group, with the primary aim to assess the quality of life through a validated questionnaire. Stent insertion was successful in 19 cases (73%), while the remaining patients required a stoma. There were no stent-related perforations. The SEMS group had significantly reduced procedure time ($p = 0.014$) and post-procedure stay ($p = 0.027$). Thirty-day mortality was 8% in the SEMS group and 15% in the surgery group ($p = 0.668$). There was no difference in median survival (5.2 versus 5.5 months), but the surgery group had significantly reduced quality of life.

Several meta-analyses [117–120], pooling data from RCT and from prospective non-randomised or retrospective studies, showed results in favour of stent placement.

According to the available RCTs [109, 112, 113], palliation with the use of SEMS could affect the OS indirectly, by increasing the risk of local complications, such as tumour site perforation, and therefore requiring the interruption of chemotherapy [118, 119].

A correlation between chemotherapy with bevacizumab and stent-related perforation has been noticed [116, 121].

A recent meta-analysis, including 4086 patients from 86 studies, confirmed an increased risk of perforation in patients with bevacizumab treatment, as compared to absence of concomitant chemotherapy (12.5 versus 9.0%) [122].

For this specific reason, the recently published European Society of Gastrointestinal Endoscopy (ESGE) Clinical Guidelines do not recommend the use of SEMS in patients who are being treated with or are expected to be commenced on antiangiogenic drugs [123].

Statement 3.9: Bridge to surgery: SEMS and planned surgery versus *emergency surgery.*

SEMS as bridge to elective surgery offers a better short-term outcome than direct emergency surgery. The complications are comparable, but the stoma rate is significantly smaller. LoE 1-GoR A

Long-term outcomes appear comparable, but evidence remains suboptimal; further studies are necessary.

For these reasons, SEMS as BTS cannot be considered the treatment of choice in the management of OLCC, whilst it may represent a valid option in selected cases and in tertiary referral hospitals. LoE 1-GoR B

SEMS as BTS allows timely resolution of the obstruction before definitive surgical treatment, giving the possibility of an elective surgical procedure.

For this reason, soon after the introduction of the new devices [105, 124], BTS with SEMS has been considered a pivotal change in the management of colonic obstruction [106] and has been rapidly implemented in clinical practice, although solid scientific evidences were still missing.

In 2012, Zhang et al. [125] performed a meta-analysis of eight studies, including six retrospective studies. Pooled data showed impressive results in favour of stent placement.

These extremely favourable results, however, were not confirmed by other studies, which reported a worrisome trend towards a stent-driven enhanced risk of oncologic recurrence [126–128].

When adjunctive results from randomised controlled trials became available, the overall efficacy of BTS with SEMS appeared to be less definite than previously reported.

Considering a total of seven trials [111, 129–134], three were prematurely terminated for the following reasons: very high morbidity rate in the SEMS BTS group [111], very high morbidity rate in the ES group[130] and high technical failure rate with SEMS [131], respectively.

Summarising the results of these trials, the following main findings arise.

Firstly, the rate of clinical success, which was originally reported to be over 90%, dropped to a mean of around 70%. Secondly, short-term results (in particular postoperative morbidity and mortality, length of hospital stay) appeared comparable between ES and BTS with SEMS. This was also confirmed by the most recently published RCT [134]. The trial was designed to recognise a 20% decrease in morbidity in the stent group as compared to the ES group, but in fact, complications occurred in 51.8% of SEMS group patients and 57.6% of direct surgery group ($p = 0.5$).

On the other hand, all the RCTs have shown that the use of SEMS is related to a reduction in the rate of stomas.

Moreover, the use of SEMS increments the odds of laparoscopic resection. The so-called endo-laparoscopic approach consists in endoscopic stent followed by laparoscopic elective surgery [129, 135, 136].

In the RCT by Cheung et al. [129], all patients undergoing direct surgery had an open approach, while 60% of patients in the SEMS group were managed laparoscopically.

All these considerations have been confirmed by comprehensive data from different meta-analyses [137–143] it can therefore be affirmed that SEMS as BTS provides better short-term outcomes than direct ES.

The oncologic issues related to this approach remain uncertain, and this represents a relevant field of future research.

Analysis of available data from RCT considering long-term outcomes [130, 133, 134, 144, 145] does not show significant harmful effects in OS with SEMS use; however, three of them [130, 133, 145] have reported a tendency towards a diminished disease-free survival (DFS). In particular, Alcantara et al. [130]reported a rate of recurrence as high as 53.3% (8/15) after SEMS versus 15.4% (2/13) after ES.

Moreover, a recent case-control study suggested that SEMS placement might have a critical negative impact on the tumour anatomical site; the authors noticed a significantly higher percentage of tumour ulceration, perineural invasion and lymph node invasion in the SEMS group as compared to the surgery-only group [126].

The main problem related to a potential augmented risk of recurrence after SEMS is the risk of perforation, which is reported in up to 13% of cases. In addition, Pirlet et al. described a peculiar analysis on postoperative pathology, showing that an undetected perforation was present in almost 27% of SEMS [131]. Risk of perforation constitutes a major concern, as underlined by a post hoc analysis of one RCT, in which the 4-year DFS rate was 0% in patients with a stent-related perforation, versus 45% in patients without perforation [145].

Although worrisome to a certain extent, these results come from studies with small number of patients and with an overall short follow-up time to guide definitive conclusions.

Matsuda et al. performed a meta-analysis to specifically investigate the long-term outcomes of SEMS [142]: 11 studies were included, with a total of 1136 patients, but only two of them were RCT, while two were prospective series and seven retrospective.

OS was reported in all studies (3-year OS in 3 of them), while DFS and recurrence in six and eight studies, respectively. Pooled data showed no significant difference between SEMS as a BTS and ES groups neither in OS (RR = 0.95; 95% CI 0.75–1.21; $p = 0.66$), nor in DFS (RR = 1.06; 95% CI = 0.91–1.24; $p = 0.43$) and recurrence rate (RR = 1.13; 95% CI 0.82–1.54; $p = 0.46$).

Similar results were presented in the meta-analysis from Ceresoli et al. [146]. Seventeen studies (5 RCTs, 3 prospective and 9 retrospective comparative cohort studies), for a total of 1333 patients, were included in the analysis. No significant differences were noticed in recurrence rate (RR = 1.11 95% CI 0.84–1.47, $p = 0.47$), 3-year mortality (RR = 0.90 95% CI 0.73–1.12, $p = 0.34$) and 5-year mortality (RR = 1.00 95% CI 0.82–1.22, $p = 0.99$). No differences were found among randomised and observational studies.

As stated by the authors, both these meta-analyses have a great limitation related to the quality of the considered studies: none of the included studies was designed for long-term follow-up, median follow-up times were generally short and heterogeneous and survival rates were estimated with the Kaplan–Meier method rather than with observed events.

For these reasons, although encouraging, these results must be considered with extreme caution. A "non-inferiority" RCT with survival as primary end point would be the appropriate method to correctly investigate long-term outcomes after SEMS as BTS versus ES.

Statement 3.10: Extraperitoneal rectal cancer.

Locally advanced rectal cancers are better treated with a multimodal approach including neoadjuvant chemoradiotherapy. LoE 1-GoR A

In case of acute obstruction, resection of the primary tumour should be avoided and a stoma should be fashioned, in order to permit a correct staging and a more appropriate oncologic treatment.

Transverse colostomy seems to be the best option, but other modalities can be considered. SEMS is not indicated.

Extraperitoneal rectal cancers have particular features, which deeply influence the management of obstructive disease.

It has to be considered that a rectal cancer producing an obstruction invariably represents a locally advanced disease. For this reason, if curative resection is judged to be possible, elective surgery should be preceded by neoadjuvant chemotherapeutic treatment [147–150]. The direct consequence of this consideration is that, in case of obstructive emergency, the surgical procedure of choice has to be restricted to techniques aiming to solve the obstruction and to permit a timely initiation of multimodal therapies. Furthermore, the surgical procedure should provide a long-term solution, allowing to conduct the patient through the entire duration of neoadjuvant treatment, until the execution of definitive surgery, and avoiding interferences with the therapeutic schedules and final oncologic result.

- Decompressive stoma versus SEMS

No comparative studies between endoscopic stenting and faecal diversion are available.

However, use of SEMS in low rectal cancer has been linked to chronic pain and tenesmus [102] and a consequential worsening of quality of life. Radiation and chemotherapy, determining tumour necrosis and shrinkage, may favour the development of complications such as migration and perforation that might compromise the final oncologic results.

Moreover, it should be considered that a stoma will be fashioned in any case at the time of surgical resection, either in the case of abdominal-perineal resection or in the case of low anterior resection, where a diverting temporary stoma is highly recommended [151–153].

All these being considered, it is always preferable to manage rectal obstruction with a stoma; the surgeon should plan the future surgical resection and choose the stoma type and location accordingly.

- Loop ileostomy versus loop colostomy versus end colostomy

In essence, and in an ideal situation, the type and location of the emergency stomas should correspond to the type and location of future diverting or definitive stoma.

Previous studies [151, 154, 155] and a recent meta-analysis [156] of trials comparing loop ileostomy versus loop colostomy after elective anterior resection showed better results after loop ileostomy.

Despite this, in case of an emergency rectal obstruction and a planned future anastomosis, a loop ileostomy is a viable option only if the obstruction is incomplete or the ileocaecal valve is patent; otherwise, colonic distension would not be solved. In presence of a complete obstruction and a competent ileocaecal valve, a colostomy is mandatory. Scientific evidence to guide the choice of type a location of the emergency colostomy is limited.

As stated above, the choice of type (end or loop) and site (transverse versus sigmoid colon) of colostomy should be tailored on the individual patient considering the planned definitive treatment.

Limited to patients at high risk for general anaesthesia, a loop left side colostomy could be fashioned under local anaesthesia and intravenous sedation via left side skin incision (the so-called trephine stoma) [157].

A widely used practical approach consists in a right-sided loop transverse colostomy. This is preferred over a sigmoid colostomy because it can be left in place to protect the anastomosis after the planned surgical resection, it is easier to be fashioned due to the mobility of the transverse colon, it avoids the risk of damage to the marginal arcade and it does not alter the left abdominal region in case a permanent end colostomy becomes necessary at the time of definitive surgical resection. When an abdominal-perineal resection is predictable, an end sigmoid colostomy could be a valid alternative [158].

Management of obstruction: right colon

Different surgical and non-surgical procedures could be offered in the case of obstructive right colon cancer (ORCC) (Table 5); however, right colectomy with anastomosis has been considered safe, and the literature is poor or absent in comparing theoretical options.

Statement 4.1.

In case of right-sided colon cancer causing acute obstruction, right colectomy with primary anastomosis is the preferred option. A terminal ileostomy associated with colonic fistula represents a valid alternative if a primary anastomosis is considered unsafe. LoE 2-GOR B

The literature regarding ORCC is definitely less extensive than for OLCC, and this may be related to favourable anatomical reasons and limitation of alternatives to surgery, which lead to the predominance of RC with primary anastomosis as the treatment of choice. Several anatomical reasons can explain this phenomenon: firstly, the hepatic flexure is easier to mobilise as compared to the splenic flexure; secondly, the mobility of the small bowel allows the surgeon to perform the ileo-colic anastomosis without adjunctive surgical manoeuvres; thirdly, the ileo-colic anastomosis benefits from an optimal blood supply, as compared to some critical zones of the left colon and rectum, whose blood supply is dependent on the patency of the marginal arcade and the hypogastric vessels. Segmental right colon resection is extremely rare, due to the reduced length of the right colon and to the common compromise of the caecum [102].

Ileostomy creation should be balanced with the risk of electrolyte imbalance; moreover, alternatives to surgery are scarce and this is related to the considerable technical difficulty of performing operative manoeuvres, stenting or tube decompression, once reached the right colon.

For these reasons, RC with primary ileo-colic anastomosis reprsents the option of choice in ORCC, despite the fact that patients are usually older and with a more advanced locoregional disease than patients with OLCC [159].

Table 5 Treatment option for ORCC

Main options	Choices among main options
Resection and anastomosis	
Resection and anastomosis with proximal stoma creation	
Resection and stoma creation	
Stoma creation	
Intestinal internal bypass	
Endoscopic stent placement	Palliative/definitive
	Bridge to surgery

As previously mentioned, results from the literature are often mixed inside the broader class of colon emergencies. The rate of AL in the emergency RC is considered to be acceptable, especially when compared to left colon resection with primary anastomosis and to elective cases. However, retrospective studies reached heterogeneous results: Lee et al. reported no differences in the mortality or leak rate between patients with right-sided and left-sided lesions (mortality: 7.3 versus 8.9%; leakage: 5.2 versus 6.9%) [160, 161]; furthermore, in other reports, the AL rate in RC ranges from 0.5 to 4.6% in perforated emergency cases and it should be compared to 0.5–1.4% reported for elective surgery. The interpretation of the comparison of AL risk between ORCC and OLCC may be cryptic: the high heterogeneity of results in several studies, in which the AL rates range for OLCC from 3.5 to 30% for emergency cases and from 5 to 10% for elective cases, underlines this issue [27, 30, 44, 162].

No relevant reports exist comparing the AL rate, the overall complications and the surgery-related mortality between RC and ileo-colic anastomosis with or without proximal loop ileostomy.

Statement 4.2: For unresectable right-sided colon cancer, a side-to-side anastomosis between the terminal ileum and the transverse colon (the internal bypass) can be performed; alternatively, a loop ileostomy can be fashioned. Decompressive caecostomy should be abandoned. LoE 2-GOR B

No relevant studies compare the possible options to manage ORCC with unresectable right colon cancer: internal bypass should be preferred to loop ileostomy. Surgical caecostomy should be abandoned for the high rate of malfunction and complications: the role of caecostomy could be reserved, via percutaneous technique, to an extremely small group of fragile patients [23, 163–167]; the use of covered expandable stent over previous malfunctioning percutaneous catheter has been reported [168].

Statement 4.3:

SEMS as bridge to elective surgery for ORCC is not recommended. It may represent an option in high-risk patients. LoE 2-GOR B

We already fully analysed SEMS as BTS in the OLCC section.

The experience for ORCC especially looks into feasibility and safety. In a recent multicenter retrospective study [169], the most appropriate treatment approach for patients with ORCC was evaluated, by comparing short-term postoperative outcomes and long-term oncologic outcomes after ES (emergency surgery), and BTS short-term and long-term outcomes in the BTS group were not inferior to those in the ES group. Right colon stenting is considered technically challenging and future comparative studies are needed for the development of an evidence-based recommendation for clinical decision-making [170].

Statement 4.4:

In a palliative setting, SEMS can be an alternative to emergency surgery (ES) for obstruction due to right colon cancer. LoE 3, GOR B

The use of stents in patients with incurable large-bowel obstruction presents a number of advantages and some benefits in terms of quality of life, such as faster return to oral diet, decreased stoma rates and reduced post-procedure stay [112].

Shim et al. evaluated the use of a new self-expanding through-the-scope (TTS) double colonic stent in the palliative management of patients with inoperable proximal malignant CO. He concluded that placement of these new self-expanding through-the-scope double colonic stents for the management of inoperable proximal malignant CO is a feasible, effective, and safe form of palliative treatment for the prevention of stent migration and tumour ingrowth [171].

Unstable patients

Statement 5.1: A patient with perforation/obstruction due to colorectal cancer should be considered unstable and therefore amenable for damage control treatment, if at least one of the following items is present:

- *pH < 7.2*
- *Core temperature < 35 °C*
- *BE < − 8*
- *Laboratory/clinical evidence of coagulopathy*
- *Any signs of sepsis/septic shock, including the necessity of inotropic support*

LoE 2-GoR C

Obstruction or perforation for CRC could lead to instability of the clinical conditions: some reasons can be recognised in fluid and electrolyte imbalance, bacterial overgrowth with translocation across the intestinal wall, peritonitis and pre-existing comorbidities.

When facing this scenario, the emergency physician, the surgeon, and the anesthesiologist should keep in mind the appropriateness of the damage control philosophy. Correct patient selection is crucial to maximise the benefit of damage control surgery (DCS), avoiding at the same time its overuse. Suboptimal evidence is available for non-trauma patients; however, as in trauma setting, the clinical picture may be represented by a mix of patient's factors (comorbidities, medical therapies), physiologic parameters (hypothermia, acidosis, coagulopathy, early organ dysfunction) and treatment/iatrogenic factors (magnitude and quality of resuscitation, time spent in surgery); when these items are present simultaneously, they could depict a patient with a severe physiological derangement and thus an "unstable patient" in the setting of non-traumatic acute care surgery [172–174].

A new definition of septic shock has been recently proposed [175], as a persisting hypotension requiring vasopressors to maintain MAP over 65 and a persistent lactate level > 2 despite adequate volume resuscitation. Several scores have been developed: the APACHE score is validated for use within an ICU setting [176], the MEDS allows to stratify septic patients presenting to the ED [177], the SOFA score allows a calculation of both the number and the severity of organ dysfunctions [178], PIRO is a staging system [179] and the quick SOFA (qSOFA) is validated to identify adult patient with suspected infection who are likely to have poor outcomes [180]. WSES Sepsis Severity Score [181] has been recently validated as a practical clinical score for patients having complicated intra-abdominal infections. A score of 5.5 is predictive of mortality with a sensitivity of 89.2% and a specificity of 83.5% [181]. Each of these scores can be successfully applied, depending on the experience and preference of the clinician involved: the adoption of an institutional score, among the validated ones, should be encouraged in order to allow early recognition of unstable patients.

Statement 5.2: Damage control should be started as soon as possible, in rapid sequence after resuscitation. LoE 2-GoR C

The damage control (DC) concept has been extended from trauma surgery to non-trauma surgical emergencies taking into account that, despite different aetiologies, the physiological derangements experienced by the patient are comparable. Often, in emergency general surgery, the physiologic exhaustion is driven by sepsis or septic shock, as in perforated patients or in patients with a closed loop colonic obstruction induced by cancer determining a bacterial overgrowth in the obstructed segment, with mucosal barrier breakdown and subsequent bacterial translocation. In a retrospective analysis on 291 non-trauma patients, Person et al. [172] demonstrated that peritonitis was the most common indication for abbreviated laparotomy in accordance to DC philosophy and that 29% of subjects who underwent DC was unstable on admission to the emergency department.

The key in the preoperative phase is to correctly identify patients who can benefit from DC and thus to consider early and expedite surgery.

Some trigger points to dictate DC in emergency general surgery may be borrowed from the trauma setting, such as hypothermia (core temperature below 35 °C), metabolic acidosis (pH < 7.2; BD > 8) and clinical or laboratory evidence of coagulopathy [173]. In a recent retrospective review of non-trauma emergencies, Becher et al. [174] confirmed that the aforementioned conditions, in association with signs of sepsis or septic shock, age ≥ 70 years and multiple comorbidities identify a profile of decompensated patient who benefits from the DC approach. This evidence supports previous results, published by Subramanian et al. [182], which demonstrated that DC is safe and effective if applied in elderly non-trauma patients with diminished physiological reserve due to intra-abdominal catastrophes.

Differently from a trauma setting, the application of DC in non-trauma surgical emergency requires an initial period of resuscitation, before surgical intervention, in order to prevent haemodynamic instability on induction of anaesthesia. Few hours are necessary to re-establish adequate—and not necessarily optimal—organ perfusion and to start broad-spectrum antibiotic therapy [183].

Azuhata and coworkers [184], in a prospective observational study, demonstrated that the time from admission to initiation of surgery for source control is a critical determinant of 60-day survival in patient with GI perforation with associated septic shock, showing a survival rate of 0% when time to initiation of surgery was greater than 6 h.

Trying to achieve the aims of central venous pressure (CVP) of 8–12 mmHg, mean arterial pressure (MAP) ≥ 65 mmHg and central venous oxygen saturation ($ScvO_2$) ≥ 70% within 6 h from the admission, the resuscitation phase should utilise goal-directed methods to guide treatments [185–187].

In addition to volume resuscitation, vasoactive medications may be required, being noradrenaline the first-line agents and adrenaline the second-line agent, while the use of dopamine should be restricted. The administration of solutions containing bicarbonate is not recommended to correct hypoperfusion-induced lactic acidosis, unless pH < 7.15. The alkalinizing agents may be needed in patients with severe acidosis (pH < 7.15) secondary to catecholamine receptor resistance-induced hypotension [183].

Once in the operating theatre, the aim of DC is to obtain source control, while the anatomical reconstruction and abdominal closure must be considered as secondary goals, to be deferred to a secondary procedure after physiological normalization. The precise technical procedure used to achieve source control of sepsis will vary depending on the local situation, the pathology encountered and the degree of physiological derangement.

Statement 5.3: If the patient is unstable, definitive treatment can be delayed. LoE 2-GoR C

Right-sided obstruction

Right colectomy with terminal ileostomy should be considered the procedure of choice.

Severely unstable patients should be treated with a loop ileostomy.

Right-sided perforation

Right colectomy with terminal ileostomy should be considered the procedure of choice.

If an open abdomen has to be considered, the stoma creation should be delayed.

Right colectomy with ileo-colic anastomosis could be performed if no significant increase in operative time is required and good bowel vascularisation is present and expected in the perioperative time.

Left-sided obstruction

Hartmann's procedure should be considered the procedure of choice. Severe unstable patients should be treated with a loop transverse colostomy.

Left-sided perforation

Hartmann's procedure should be considered the procedure of choice. If an open abdomen has to be considered, the stoma creation should be delayed.

For patient presenting acutely, the prognosis is poorer as compared to patients presenting under elective admission. Emergency patients are older and have more advanced tumours. Colon obstruction causes volume depletion and electrolyte disorders, while perforation may induce generalized peritonitis. These coexisting factors may lead to patient instability, represented by metabolic impairment, coagulopathy and signs of sepsis/septic shock. All these factors contribute to the alteration of the upstream of the intestinal wall that explain the high risk of AL in the emergency setting, ranging from 4 to 13% [30, 161].

Literature data regarding outcomes after emergency abdominal surgery in patients with advanced cancer suggests that patients experience a high burden of complications and high postoperative mortality after these interventions [188, 189].

As a general principle, all efforts should be made to resect the tumour at the index operation, but this concept has to be balanced with caveats of Damage Control Surgey: exhausted patients should undergo only the procedures they can tolerate, and usually this corresponds to technically easy and rapidly performed interventions, representing life-saving procedures.

Therefore, surgical options for complicated colorectal cancer depend primarily on the location of the tumour, comorbidities of the patient and degree of their clinical status derangement at presentation.

For right-sided lesions, a definitive treatment RC and ileocolic anastomosis can be considered, on the basis of a non-significant increase in operative time as compared to staged procedures; however, surgeon should remember that the AL rate and the mortality for resection in emergency is higher than in elective cases (0.5–4.6 versus 0.5–1.4%; 7 versus 5.3%): although no specific data is available, a higher rate of AL is reasonably expected in the critical scenarios.

If the clinical condition suggests to avoid the creation of an anastomosis, a terminal ileostomy is recommended. The transverse colon can be stapled or a mucous fistula can be occasionally created.

If an open abdomen (OA) has to be considered, stoma creation should be avoided and the bowel should be left stapled inside the abdominal cavity.

Loop ileostomy should be reserved for obstruction when the tumour is not easily resectable or in case a very abbreviated laparotomy is required. For left-sided lesions in unstable patients, a single-stage procedure represents a time-consuming intervention, at high risk of AL, due to faecal loading and impaired microcirculation induced by sepsis and by the premorbid status of the patient.

Effectiveness of staged procedures (two- or three-step) have been compared in recently published guidelines [1]. In an emergency setting, HP seems suitable for patients who are too unwell to tolerate time-consuming procedures, such as an anastomosis. In fact, HP is a rapid intervention, it minimises surgical trauma it achieves cancer resection, and it eliminates the risk of anastomotic failure. If compared with loop colostomy, HP appears to be associated with shorter overall hospital stay, while perioperative morbidity appears to be the same. Loop colostomy should be reserved for unresectable disease or if neoadjuvant therapy is be planned.

Statement 5.4: In patient with perforation/obstruction due to colorectal lesions, open abdomen (OA) should be considered if abdominal compartment syndrome is expected; bowel viability should be reassessed after resection. LoE 2-GoRC

There is no clear indication to OA in patients with peritonitis. LoE 1-GoR B

OA should be closed within 7 days. LoE 1-GoR B

The OA is defined as the intentional creation of a controlled laparostomy, by leaving the fascial edges of the abdominal wall unapproximated. When used appropriately, this approach is useful in the management of patients at risk of development of abdominal compartment syndrome, or in case the viability of the resected bowel must be reassessed, after an abbreviated laparotomy, before performing an anastomosis. On the contrary, when misused, OA may potentially expose the patient to serious complications, among which the onset of entero-atmospheric fistula is the most worrisome. The inability to re-approximate fascial edges is another drawback of prolonged OA.

In a 1-year series of non-trauma OA described by Bruns et al. [190], the most common preoperative indications for index laparotomy leading to OA were perforated viscus and/or the presence of extra luminal gas on abdominal imaging. Fifty-eight patients received bowel resection at initial operation, and 86% of them were left with intestinal discontinuity at the index operation. DC surgery mandated OA in 37% of cases, while the need for a second look was the indication in 27%; the excessive contamination represented the indication for OA only in 10% of patients. The use of OA in the management of patients with peritonitis is still controversial. Several authors [191, 192] reported no significant differences in morbidity and mortality between on-demand re-laparotomy and planned re-laparotomy groups but showed that on-demand group had shorter ICU and hospital stay. Therefore, peritoneal contamination per se does not represent a strict indication to OA. Aggressive source control followed by abdomen closure should be attempted, and on-demand re-laparotomy should be used instead [193].

In cases when planned re-laparotomy represents a necessity, this should be performed 24–48 h after the initial operation. An abdominal exploration delayed over this period increases the risk of iatrogenic enteric injury, related to intraperitoneal adhesions. The goal to be achieved after OA is the early and definitive closure of the abdominal wall, in order to reduce complications associated to OA. In a systematic review [194], it has been demonstrated that early fascial closure, within 4–7 days of the initial laparotomy, compared to delayed closure was associated with reduced mortality (12.3 versus 24.8%, RR 0.53, $p < .0001$) and complications (RR 0.68, $p < .0001$). In a retrospective review of 42 non-trauma patients, Khan et al. [195]achieved fascial closure within 7 days in 57% of patients, while observing the onset of entero-atmospheric fistula in 4 of 18 patients of the delayed closure group.

Statement 5.5: A close intraoperative communication between surgeon and anesthesiologist is essential to assess the effectiveness of resuscitation, in order to decide the best treatment option. LoE 2-GoR C

A uniform approach for critically ill non-trauma patients is crucial to achieve satisfactory outcomes. In terms of decision-making, it is vital to recognise and solve pitfalls in DC or in clinical decision-making. Effective communication and the expression of non-technical skills among anesthesiologists, nurses and surgeons are essential to manage this typology of patients [196]. It has been demonstrated that failure to communicate critical information in the operating room occurs in approximately 30% of team exchanges [197] and this could lead to inefficiency, emotional tension, delays, resource waste, patient inconvenience, and procedural error, all of which can be detrimental. Similarly, failure to communicate critical information by the anesthesiologist during non-trauma resuscitation of the non-trauma critically ill patient, such as the impairment of metabolic parameters or their improvement achieved by goal-directed resuscitation strategy, may leave the surgeon unaware of the degree of the patient physiologic exhaustion, leading him/her towards wrong surgical decisions. Effective and prompt communication allow the anesthesiologist and the surgeon to recognise potential issues or dangerous circumstances and to adjust their strategies accordingly [198], considering an early DC approach during the multi-faced management of critically ill surgical patients.

Antibiotic therapy

Statement 6.1: In patients with colorectal carcinoma obstruction and no systemic signs of infection, antibiotic prophylaxis mainly targeting Gram-negative bacilli and anaerobic bacteria is recommended, because of the potential ongoing bacterial translocation. LoE 1, GoR A

To establish the effectiveness of antimicrobial prophylaxis for the prevention of surgical wound infection in patients undergoing colorectal surgery, a Cochrane review was published in 2014 including 260 trials and 68 different antibiotics [199].

The review found high-quality evidence, showing that prophylaxis with antibiotics covering aerobic and anaerobic bacteria prior to elective colorectal surgery reduces the risk of surgical wound infection.

Generally, patients with intestinal obstruction with no systemic signs of infections present a risk of surgical site infections similar to patients undergoing elective surgery; in general, antibiotic prophylaxis is sufficient.

A dense population of microorganisms, referred to as the bacterial flora, colonizes the human gastrointestinal tract. Although the gut provides a functional barrier between these organisms and the host, bacterial translocation is a possible event.

Gut translocation of bacteria is defined as the passage of gastrointestinal microflora across the lamina propria to local mesenteric lymph nodes and from there to extranodal sites [200].

Major conditions can contribute to bacterial translocation including a breakdown of the intestinal barrier, an impairment of host immune defense and a loss of the colonisation resistance with bacterial overgrowth in the intestinal tract [201].

Several studies support the concept considering the gut as the source of septic complications; in this sense, bacterial translocation may be an important intermediary mechanism in the development of sepsis [202].

When the mucosa is injured and the intestinal barrier is compromised, a translocation of intestinal microorganisms can occur.

Obstruction cause mucosal injury with a subsequent increase of mucosal permeability and thus bacterial translocation [203, 204].

Statement 6.2: Prophylactic antibiotics should be discontinued after 24 h (or 3 doses). LoE 1-GoR A. In these patients, in the light of the need to reduce infections from opportunistic microorganisms—such as *C. difficile*—and to minimise the evolution of multidrug-resistant bacteria, such as ESBL, VRE or KPC, prophylactic antibiotics should be discontinued after 24 h (3 doses) [199].

In 2015, a retrospective review of prospectively collected data on 143 patients with AL after colorectal cancer surgery was published [205]. Of the 143 enrolled patients, 46 (32.2%) were classified in the multidrug-resistant (MDR) group. The use of antibiotics for more than 5 days before diagnosis of AL and diabetes mellitus were identified as independent risk factors of MDR acquisition by multivariate analysis.

Statement 6.3: In patients with colon carcinoma perforation, antibiotic therapy mainly targeting Gram-negative bacilli and anaerobic bacteria is always suggested. Furthermore, in critically ill patients with sepsis early, use of broader-spectrum antimicrobials is suggested. LoE 1-GoR A

Antimicrobial therapy, typically empiric antibiotic treatment, plays an important role in the management of colon cancer perforation. Initial antimicrobial therapy for patients with IAI is empiric in nature because patients need immediate treatment and microbiological data (culture and susceptibility results) usually requires ≥ 24–48 h for the identification of pathogens and patterns of antibiotic susceptibility [206].

The empirically designed antimicrobial regimen depends on the pathogens presumed to be involved, the risk factors indicative of major resistance patterns and the underlying severity of infection.

Considering the intestinal microbiota of the large bowel, patients with colon cancer perforations require antibiotic coverage for Gram-negative bacteria, as well as for anaerobes.

The virulent microorganisms in colorectal procedures are derived from the bowel lumen, where there are high concentrations of bacteria, such as *B. fragilis* and other obligate anaerobes and *Enterobacteriaceae* including *E. coli* [207].

The choice of the antimicrobial regimen poses serious problems for the management of unstable patients with sepsis. In these patients, an early and appropriate empirical antimicrobial therapy has a significant impact on the outcome [208]. Therefore, in these patients, early use of broad-spectrum intravenous antimicrobials is always suggested.

Statement 6.4: In patients with perforated colorectal cancer, antibiotic therapy should consider bacterial resistance and should be refined according to the microbiological findings, once available. LoE 1-GoR B

The vast majority of colon cancer perforations represent community-acquired infections. The main resistance threat in these IAI is posed by extended-spectrum beta-lactamase (ESBL) producing *Enterobacteriaceae*, which are becoming increasingly common in community-acquired infections worldwide [209].

The results of microbiological testing may have great importance for the choice of therapeutic strategy of every patient, in particular in the rationalisation of targeted antimicrobial treatment [206].

The duration of antibiotic therapy is a matter of debate, usually ranging from 4 to 7 days according to clinical features (source control, fever, leukocytosis, C-reactive protein, procalcitonin) [207, 210].

Conclusions: grey areas and opportunities for improvements

We found some limitations within the present guidelines:

- They fail to cover all the possible abdominal scenarios when colon cancer occurs as an emergency: for example, associated resections were not taken into considerations, neither we discussed about therapeutic strategies in case of evidence of peritoneal carcinomatosis.
- Despite our attempts to underline suggestions in case of low technical resources, the present guidelines are generally oriented toward hospitals with high level of resources.

On the other side, in our opinion, the current guidelines suggest some stimuli for doctors involved in this field:

- To review the approach to patient suffering from abdominal pain by introducing and promoting the use of bedside abdominal US.
- To bear in mind that the emergency surgeon should have a strong oncologic background or that the specialised colorectal surgeon should have a strong background of surgical pathophysiology, emergency surgery and damage control philosophy.
- To promote the use of clinical pathways within singular Hospitals.

All the considerations mentioned above, and further by readers, will be an incentive for further revisions and improvements.

Appendix 1

Table 6 Table of statements

Topic	No.	LoE	GoR	
1. Diagnosis	1.1	3	B	The clinical presentation is variable, except for lower rectal cancer, in which case digital examination could be diagnostic. Laboratory tests are not specific. Clinical evaluation and laboratory tests have high variability and low specificity; therefore, the escalation to further diagnostic tools, whenever available, is mandatory.
	1.2	3	B	(a) In case of clinical suspicion of colon obstruction, computed tomography (CT) scan achieves the confirmation of diagnosis better than abdominal ultrasound (US), which performs better than abdominal plain X-ray. If CT scan is not available, a water-soluble colonic contrast enema is a valid alternative in for identifying the site and the nature of obstruction. (b) In case of clinical suspicion of perforation, abdominal CT scan, which performs better than abdominal US, should achieve diagnostic confirmation. US performs better than abdominal plain X-ray. LoE 3, GoR B.
	1.3	3	B	In stable patients, direct visualisation of the site of colonic obstruction should be considered when colonoscopy is available. In this situation, biopsies should be obtained, especially when the deployment of an endoscopic stent is planned. LoE 3, GoR B.
	1.4	3	B	In case of clinical suspicion of perforation, abdominal CT scan, which performs better than abdominal US, should achieve diagnostic confirmation. US performs better than abdominal plain X-ray.
	1.5	3	B	There is no specific data regarding staging pathways of CRC presenting as an emergency. CT scan performs better than US in the abdomen and should be suggested for staging in the suspicion of cancer-related colorectal emergencies. CT scan of the thorax is not strictly recommended. LoE 3, GoR B
	1.6	3	B	There is no specific data regarding staging pathways of CRC presenting as emergency. CT scan performs better than US in the abdomen and should be suggested for staging in the suspicion of cancer-related colorectal emergencies. CT scan of the thorax is not strictly recommended.
2. Perforation	2.1	2	B	When diffuse peritonitis occurs in cancer-related colon perforation, the priority is the control of the sepsis source of sepsis. Prompt combined medical treatment is advised. LoE 2, GoR B
	2.2	3	B	Oncologic resection should be performed in order to obtain better oncologic outcomes. • Perforation at the tumour site: formal resection with or without anastomosis, with or without stoma • Perforation proximal to tumour site (diastasic): simultaneous tumour resection and management of proximal perforation is indicated. Depending on the colonic wall conditions, a subtotal colectomy may be required. The surgeon should consider that only a small proportion of patients undergo reversal of terminal stoma.
3. Left colon obstruction	3.1	2	B	Loop colostomy (C) versus Hartmann's procedure (HP). Hartmann's procedure should be preferred to simple colostomy, since colostomy appears to be associated with longer overall hospital stay and need for multiple operations, without a reduction in perioperative morbidity LoE 2, GoR B. Loop colostomy should be reserved for to unresectable tumours (if SEMS is not feasible), for severely ill patients who are too unfit for major surgical procedures or general anaesthesia.
	3.2	3	B	Hartmann's procedure (HP) versus resection and primary anastomosis (RPA) RPA should be the preferred option for uncomplicated malignant left-sided large bowel obstruction in absence of other risk factors. Patients with high surgical risk are better managed with HP.
	3.3	4	C	RPA: the role of diverting stoma There is no evidence supporting that a covering stoma can reduce the risk of anastomotic leak and its severity.
	3.4	2	B	Total colectomy versus segmental colectomy. In absence of caecal tears/perforation or, evidence of bowel ischemia or synchronous right colonic cancers, total colectomy should not be preferred to segmental colectomy, since it does not reduce morbidity and mortality and is associated with higher rates of impaired bowel function. LoE 2, GoR B.
	3.5	2	B	Intraoperative colonic irrigation (ICI) versus manual decompression (MD) ICI and MD are associated with same mortality/morbidity rate. The only significant difference is that MD is a shorter and simpler procedure. Either procedure could be performed, depending on the experience/preference of the surgeon.
	3.6	4	C	RPA: the role of laparoscopy. The role use of laparoscopy in the emergency treatment of OLCC cannot be recommended and should be reserved to selected favourable cases and in specialised centers.
	3.7	4	C	Tube decompression (TD) TD can be a valid alternative option as BTS for high-risk OLCC.
	3.8	3	B	Palliation: SEMS versus colostomy. In facilities with capability for stent placement, SEMS should be preferred to colostomy for palliation of OLCC since it is associated with similar mortality/morbidity rates and shorter hospital stay. LoE 1-GoR A. Alternative treatments to SEMS should be considered in patients eligible for to a bevacizumab-based therapy. Involvement of the oncologist in the decision is strongly recommended. LoE 3-GoR B
	3.9	1	B	Bridge to surgery (BTS): SEMS and planned surgery versus emergency surgery SEMS as bridge to elective surgery offers a better short-term outcome than direct emergency surgery. The complications are comparable, but the stoma rate is significantly smaller. Long-term outcomes appear comparable as well, but evidence remains suboptimal; further studies are necessary. For these reasons, SEMS as BTS cannot be considered the treatment of choice in the management of OLCC, whilst it may represent a valid option in selected cases and in tertiary referral hospitals.

Table 6 Table of statements *(Continued)*

Topic	No.	LoE	GoR	
	3.10	1	A	Extraperitoneal rectal cancer. Locally advanced rectal cancers are better cured treated with a multimodal approach including neoadjuvant chemoradiotherapy. LoE 1-GoR A. In case of acute obstruction, resection of the primary tumour should be avoided and a stoma should be fashioned, in order to permit a correct staging and a more appropriate oncologic treatment. Transverse colostomy seems to be the best option, but other modalities can be considered. SEMS is not indicated.
4. Right occlusion	4.1	2	B	In case of right-sided colon cancer causing acute obstruction, right colectomy with primary anastomosis is the preferred option. A terminal ileostomy associated with colonic fistula represents a valid alternative when if a primary anastomosis is considered unsafe. LoE 2-GOR B
	4.2	2	B	For unresectable right-sided colon cancer, a side-to-side anastomosis between the terminal ileum and the transverse colon (the internal bypass) can be performed; alternatively, a loop ileostomy can be fashioned. Decompressive caecostomy should be abandoned.
	4.3	4	B	SEMS as bridge to elective surgery for ORCC is not recommended. It may represent an option in high-risk patients.
	4.4	3	B	In a palliative setting, SEMS can be an alternative to emergency surgery (ES) in for obstruction due to right colon cancer obstruction. LoE 3, GOR B
5. Unstable patients	5.1	2	C	A patient with perforation/obstruction due to colorectal cancer should be considered unstable and therefore amenable for damage control treatment, if at least one of the following items is present: • pH < 7.2 • Core temperature < 35 °C • BE < -8 • Laboratory/clinical evidence of coagulopathy • Any signs of sepsis/septic shock, including the necessity of inotropic support.
	5.2	2	C	Damage control should be started as soon as possible, in rapid sequence after resuscitation.
	5.3	2	C	If the patient is unstable, definitive treatment can be delayed. Right-sided obstruction: Right colectomy with terminal ileostomy should be considered the procedure of choice. Severely unstable patients should be treated with a loop ileostomy. Right-sided perforation: Right colectomy with terminal ileostomy should be considered the procedure of choice. If an open abdomen has to be considered, the stoma creation should be delayed. Right colectomy with ileo-colic anastomosis could be performed if no significant increase in operative time is required and good bowel vascularisation is present and expected in the perioperative time. Left-sided obstruction: Hartmann's procedure should be considered the procedure of choice. Severe unstable patients should be treated with a loop transverse colostomy. Left-sided perforation: Hartmann's procedure should be considered the procedure of choice. If an open abdomen has to be considered, the stoma creation should be delayed.
	5.4	2	C	In patient with perforation/obstruction due to colorectal lesions, open abdomen (OA) should be considered if abdominal compartment syndrome is expected; bowel viability should be reassessed after resection. There is no clear indication to OA in patients with peritonitis. OA should be closed within 7 days.
	5.5	2	C	A close intraoperative communication between surgeon and anesthesiologist is essential to assess the effectiveness of resuscitation, in order to decide the best treatment option.
6. Antibiotic therapy	6.1	1	A	In patients with colorectal carcinoma obstruction with no systemic signs of infection, antibiotic prophylaxis is recommended.
	6.2	1	A	Prophylactic antibiotics should be discontinued after 24 h (or 3 doses).
	6.3	1	B	In patients with intestinal obstruction, even without systemic signs of infections, antibiotic prophylaxis mainly targeting Gram-negative bacilli and anaerobic bacteria is suggested, because of the potential ongoing bacterial translocation.
	6.4	1	A	In patients with colon carcinoma perforation, antibiotic therapy mainly targeting Gram-negative bacilli and anaerobic bacteria is always suggested. Furthermore, in critically ill patients with sepsis early, use of broader-spectrum antimicrobials is suggested.
	6.5	1	B	In patients with perforated colorectal cancer, antibiotic therapy should consider bacterial resistance, and should be refined according to the microbiological findings, once available.

Appendix 2

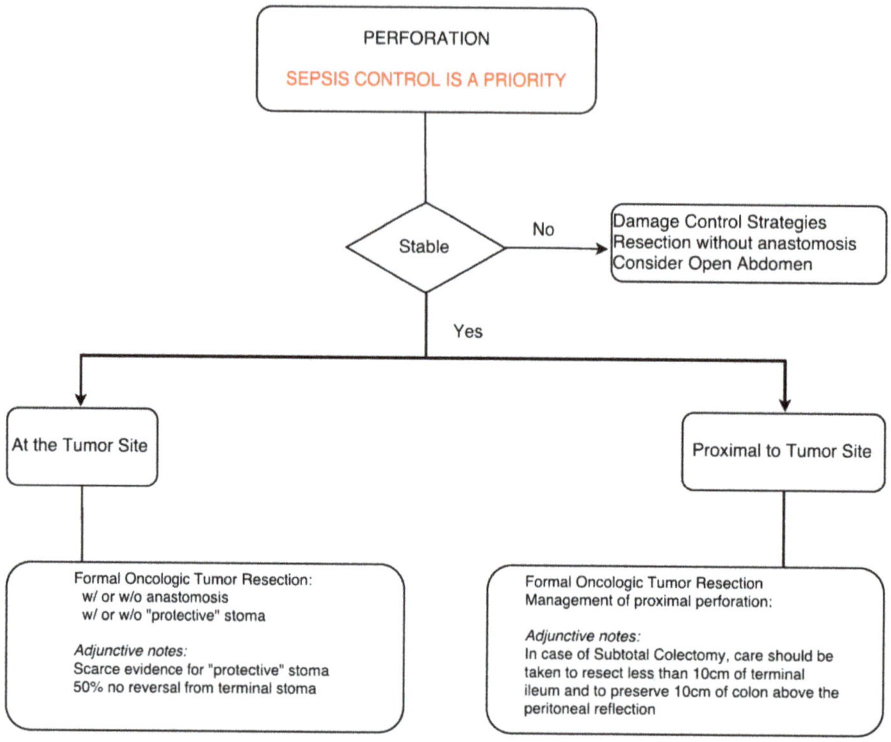

Fig. 2 Flowchart for the management of colonic perforation due to colorectal cancer

Appendix 3

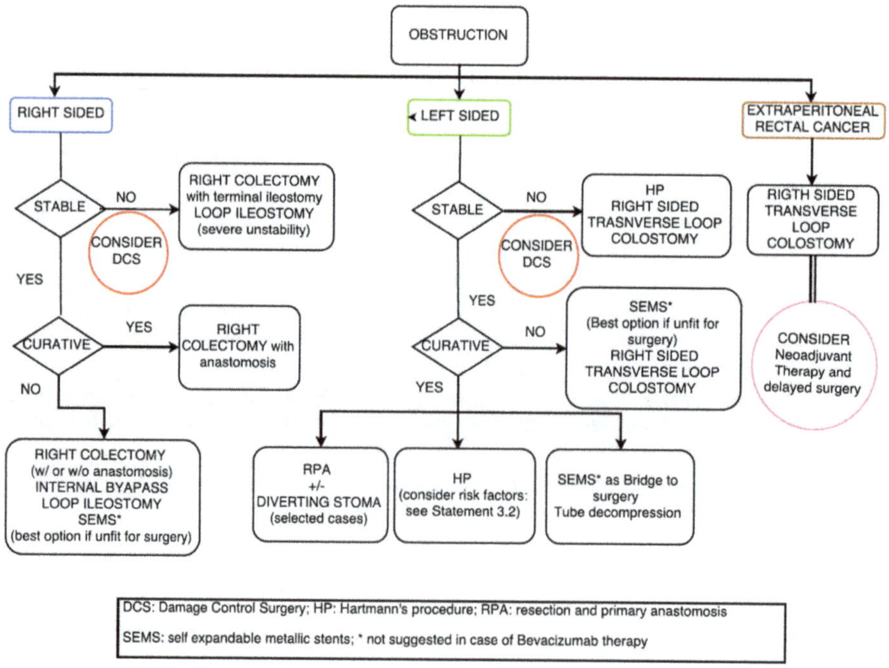

Fig. 3 Flowchart for the management of colonic obstruction due to colorectal cancer

Abbreviations

AL: Anastomotic leak; BTS: Bridge to surgery; CRCE: Colon Rectal Cancer Emergencies; CT scan : Computed Tomography; DC: Damage control; DFS: Disease-free survival; ES: Emergency surgery; GoR: Grade of recommendation; HP: Hartmann's procedure; IAI: Intra-abdominal infection; ICI: Intraoperative colonic irrigation; LBO: Large bowel obstruction; LoE: Level of evidence; MD: Manual decompression; OLCC: Obstructed left colon cancer; ORCC: Obstructed right colon cancer; OS: Overall survival; RCT: Randomised clinical trial; RPA: Resection and primary anastomosis; SEMS: Self-expanding metallic stent; US: Ultrasound; WSES: World Society of Emergency Surgery

Acknowledgements

The authors would like to acknowledge Miss Franca Boschini (Librarian at the Papa Giovanni Hospital, Bergamo, Italy) for the initial references search.

Funding

No authors received funding or resources in relation to this article. The authors received a WSES institutional waiver for this publication.

Authors' contributions

MP, LA, FC (10) and FC (50) focused on the topic of the paper. MP, CM, CP, MV, EP, LZ, AR, SD, FA, EF, SC, MS and TR wrote the preliminary drafts. MP, LA, LZ, EP, MC, NA, SC and SW reviewed all preliminary draft sections. The vast majority of authors discussed the statements at the Consensus Conference, strongly contributing to the final version of statements. MP, LZ, MS, MC and SC reviewed the statements after the Consensus Conference. All the authors contributed to the final version of the paper, and final approval was obtained.

Competing interests

The authors declare that they have no competing interests.

Author details

[1]General Surgery Papa Giovanni XXII Hospital Bergamo, Bergamo, Italy. [2]Colorectal Unit, Department of Surgery, University of Cagliari, Cagliari, Italy. [3]Unit of Emergency Medicine Ospedale Bufalini Cesena, AUSL Romagna, Romagna, Italy. [4]Trauma TeamGOM Niguarda, Milan, Italy. [5]Department of General Surgery, School of Medicine, University of Milano, Milan, Italy. [6]Department of General Surgery ULSS5 del Veneto, Adria, (RO), Italy. [7]S.S. Annunziata Hospital, Taranto, Italy. [8]Unit of General and Emergency Surgery, Ospedale Bufalini Cesena, AUSL Romagna, Romagna, Italy. [9]Colorectal Unit, Campinas State University, Campinas, SP, Brazil. [10]Division of Colorectal Surgery, University of Campinas, Campinas, SP, Brazil. [11]General Surgery ASST, Bergamo, Italy. [12]Emergency Department Udine Healthcare and University Integrated Trust, Udine, Italy. [13]Centro Radiológico Campinas, Vera Cruz Hospital, São Paulo, Brazil. [14]Department of Surgery, University of Campinas, Campinas, Brazil. [15]Oncology Surgery and Intensive Care, Oswaldo Cruz Hospital, Recife, Brazil. [16]Department of Surgery Division of General Surgery, University of Toronto, Toronto, Canada. [17]Surgical Department, University of Macerata, Macerata, Italy. [18]Radiology Unit Emergency Department, S. Antonio Abate Hospital, Tolmezzo, UD, Italy. [19]Department of Surgery, College of Medicine and Health Sciences, UAE University, Al-Ain, United Arab Emirates. [20]Hillel Yaffe Medical Center Hadera, Hadera, Israel. [21]Trauma and Acute Care Surgery Unit Hadassah, Hebrew University Medical Center, Jerusalem, Israel. [22]Unit of Digestive Surgery, HPB Surgery and Liver Transplant Henri Mondor Hospital, Créteil, France. [23]Department of General and Emergency Surgery Cannes' Hospital Cannes, Cedex, Cannes, France. [24]Cambridge Colorectal Unit, Cambridge University Hospitals, Cambridge, UK. [25]Division of Trauma & Critical Care University of Southern California, Los Angeles, USA. [26]Department of Surgery, Denver Health Medical Center, University of Colorado, Denver, CO, USA. [27]Digestive Disease Center, Department of Colorectal Surgery Cleveland Clinic Florida, Tallahassee, USA. [28]Acute Care Surgery The Queen's Medical Center, Honolulu, HI, USA. [29]Division of Trauma, Surgical Critical Care, Burns, and Acute Care Surgery, University of California San Diego Health Sciences, San Diego, USA. [30]Second Department of Surgery, Meilahti Hospital, Helsinki, Finland. [31]Department of Surgery, Harborview Medical Centre, Seattle, USA. [32]Department of Surgery and Obs/Gyn, Faculty of Health Sciences, University of Buea, Buea, Cameroon. [33]Department of Surgery, Trauma and Surgical Services, University of Pittsburgh School of Medicine, Pittsburgh, USA. [34]General Surgery Department, Medical University, University Hospital St George, Plovdiv, Bulgaria. [35]General Surgery Department, Letterkenny Hospital, Letterkenny, Ireland. [36]Infectious Diseases Unit, Department of Medical and Surgical Sciences, Sant'Orsola Hospital, University of Bologna, Bologna, Italy. [37]Trauma and General Surgeon, Royal Perth Hospital, Perth, Australia. [38]Surgery and Critical Care Assuta Medical Centers, Tel Aviv, Israel. [39]Division of Trauma Surgery, Department of Surgery, School of Medical Sciences, University of Campinas (Unicamp), Campinas, SP, Brazil. [40]Department of General Surgery, Division of Surgery, Rambam Health Care Campus, Haifa, Israel. [41]Department of Emergency Surgery, Parma Maggiore Hospital, Parma, Italy.

References

1. Ansaloni L, Andersson RE, Bazzoli F, Catena F, Cennamo V, Di Saverio S, Fuccio L, Jeekel H, Leppaniemi A, Moore E, Pinna AD, Pisano M, Repici A, Sugarbaker PH, Tuech JJ. Guidelines in the management of obstructing cancer of the left colon: consensus conference of the world society of emergency surgery (WSES) and peritoneum and surgery (PnS) society. World J Emerg Surg. 2010;5:29.
2. Arnold M, Sierra MS, Laversanne M, Soerjomataram I, Jemal A, Bray F. Global patterns and trends in colorectal cancer incidence and mortality. Gut. 2017;66(4):683–91.
3. Torre LA, Siegel RL, Ward EM, Jemal A. Global cancer incidence and mortality rates and trends—an update. Cancer Epidemiol Biomarkers Prev. 2016;25(1):16–27.
4. Benson AB 3rd, Venook AP, Cederquist L, Chan E, Chen YJ, Cooper HS, Deming D, Engstrom PF, Enzinger PC, Fichera A, Grem JL, Grothey A, Hochster HS, Hoffe S, Hunt S, Kamel A, Kirilcuk N, Krishnamurthi S, Messersmith WA, Mulcahy MF, Murphy JD, Nurkin S, Saltz L, Sharma S, Shibata D, Skibber JM, Sofocleous CT, Stoffel EM, Stotsky-Himelfarb E, Willett CG, Wu CS, Gregory KM, Freedman-Cass D. Colon cancer, version 1.2017, NCCN Clinical Practice Guidelines in Oncology. J Natl Compr Canc Netw. 2017;15(3):370–98.
5. Bailey CE, Hu CY, You YN, Bednarski BK, Rodriguez-Bigas MA, Skibber JM, Cantor SB, Chang GJ. Increasing disparities in the age-related incidences of colon and rectal cancers in the United States, 1975-2010. JAMA Surg. 2015;150(1):17–22.
6. Zielinski MD, Merchea A, Heller SF, You YN. Emergency management of perforated colon cancers: how aggressive should we be? J Gastrointest Surg. 2011;15(12):2232–8.
7. Alvarez JA, Baldonedo RF, Bear IG, Truan N, Pire G, Alvarez P. Presentation, treatment, and multivariate analysis of risk factors for obstructive and perforative colorectal carcinoma. Am J Surg. 2005;190(3):376–82.
8. Runkel NS, Hinz U, Lehnert T, Buhr HJ, Herfarth C. Improved outcome after emergency surgery for cancer of the large intestine. Br J Surg. 1998;85(9):1260–5.
9. Umpleby HC, Williamson RC. Survival in acute obstructing colorectal carcinoma. Dis Colon Rectum. 1984;27(5):299–304.
10. Ohman U. Prognosis in patients with obstructing colorectal carcinoma. Am J Surg. 1982;143(6):742–7.
11. Kyllonen LE. Obstruction and perforation complicating colorectal carcinoma. An epidemiologic and clinical study with special reference to incidence and survival. Acta Chir Scand. 1987;153(10):607–14.
12. Gunnarsson H, Holm T, Ekholm A, Olsson LI. Emergency presentation of colon cancer is most frequent during summer. Colorectal Dis. 2011;13(6):663–8.
13. Bass G, Fleming C, Conneely J, Martin Z, Mealy K. Emergency first presentation of colorectal cancer predicts significantly poorer outcomes: a review of 356 consecutive Irish patients. Dis Colon Rectum. 2009;52(4):678–84.

14. Smothers L, Hynan L, Fleming J, Turnage R, Simmang C, Anthony T. Emergency surgery for colon carcinoma. Dis Colon Rectum. 2003; 46(1):24–30.
15. Kelley WE Jr, Brown PW, Lawrence W Jr, Terz JJ. Penetrating, obstructing, and perforating carcinomas of the colon and rectum. Arch Surg. 1981;116(4):381–4.
16. Barnett A, Cedar A, Siddiqui F, Herzig D, Fowlkes E, Thomas CR Jr. Colorectal cancer emergencies. J Gastrointest Cancer. 2013;44(2):132–42.
17. Laine L, Yang H, Chang SC, Datto C. Trends for incidence of hospitalization and death due to GI complications in the United States from 2001 to 2009. Am J Gastroenterol. 2012;107(8):1190–5. quiz 1196
18. Frago R, Ramirez E, Millan M, Kreisler E, del Valle E, Biondo S. Current management of acute malignant large bowel obstruction: a systematic review. Am J Surg. 2014;207(1):127–38.
19. Biondo S, Kreisler E, Millan M, Fraccalvieri D, Golda T, Marti Rague J, Salazar R. Differences in patient postoperative and long-term outcomes between obstructive and perforated colonic cancer. Am J Surg. 2008;195(4):427–32.
20. Anwar MA, D'Souza F, Coulter R, Memon B, Khan IM, Memon MA. Outcome of acutely perforated colorectal cancers: experience of a single district general hospital. Surg Oncol. 2006;15(2):91–6.
21. Finan PJ, Verma SCR, MacFie J, Gatt M, Parker MC, Bhardwaj R, Hall NR. The management of malignant large bowel obstruction: ACPGBI position statement. Colorectal Dis. 2007;9(Supp 4):17.
22. van de Velde CJ, Boelens PG, Tanis PJ, Espin E, Mroczkowski P, Naredi P, Pahlman L, Ortiz H, Rutten HJ, Breugom AJ, Smith JJ, Wibe A, Wiggers T, Valentini V. Experts reviews of the multidisciplinary consensus conference colon and rectal cancer 2012: science, opinions and experiences from the experts of surgery. Eur J Surg Oncol. 2014;40(4):454–68.
23. Chang GJ, Kaiser AM, Mills S, Rafferty JF, Buie WD, Standards Practice C, Task Force of the American Society of Colon and Rectal Surgeons. Practice parameters for the management of colon cancer. Dis Colon Rectum. 2012;55(8):831–43.
24. Markogiannakis H, Messaris E, Dardamanis D, Pararas N, Tzertzemelis D, Giannopoulos P, Larentzakis A, Lagoudianakis E, Manouras A, Bramis I. Acute mechanical bowel obstruction: clinical presentation, etiology, management and outcome. World J Gastroenterol. 2007;13(3):432–7.
25. Cappell MS, Batke M. Mechanical obstruction of the small bowel and colon. Med Clin North Am. 2008;92(3):575–97. viii.
26. Lopez-Kostner F, Hool GR, Lavery IC. Management and causes of acute large-bowel obstruction. Surg Clin North Am. 1997;77(6):1265–90.
27. Yang XF, Pan K. Diagnosis and management of acute complications in patients with colon cancer: bleeding, obstruction, and perforation. Chin J Cancer Res. 2014;26(3):331–40.
28. Kahi CJ, Rex DK. Bowel obstruction and pseudo-obstruction. Gastroenterol Clin North Am. 2003;32(4):1229–47.
29. Imuta MK, Awai Y, Nakayama YM, Asao C, Matsukawa T, Yamashita Y. Multidetector CT findings suggesting a perforation site in the gastrointestinal tract: analysis in surgically confirmed 155 patients. Radiat Med. 2007;25(3):113–8.
30. Chen SC, Yen ZS, Wang HP, Lin FY, Hsu CY, Chen WJ. Ultrasonography is superior to plain radiography in the diagnosis of pneumoperitoneum. Br J Surg. 2002;89(3):351–4.
31. Gainant A. Emergency management of acute colonic cancer obstruction. J Visc Surg. 2012;149(1):e3–e10.
32. Mularski RA, Sippel JM, Osborne ML. Pneumoperitoneum: a review of nonsurgical causes. Crit Care Med. 2000;28(7):2638–44.
33. Tang A, Huddleston P, Attaluri P, Cruz A, Joseph S, Lavy D. Clinical cases of nonsurgical pneumoperitoneum: categorizing the disease and treatment options. Am Surg. 2015;81(5):E206–8.
34. Lay PL, Huang HH, Chang WK, Hsieh TY, Huang TY, Lin HH. Outcome of nonsurgical intervention in patients with perforated peptic ulcers. Am J Emerg Med. 2016;34(8):1556–60.
35. Network, N.C.C. Clinical Practice Guideline on Colon Cancer NCCN Available from: https://www.nccn.org/professionals/physician_gls/pdf/colon.pdf.
36. Grossmann I, Avenarius JK, Mastboom WJ, Klaase JM. Preoperative staging with chest CT in patients with colorectal carcinoma: not as a routine procedure. Ann Surg Oncol. 2010;17(8):2045–50.
37. Mandava N, Kumar S, Pizzi WF, Aprile IJ. Perforated colorectal carcinomas. Am J Surg. 1996;172(3):236–8.
38. Kriwanek S, Armbruster C, Dittrich K, Beckerhinn P. Perforated colorectal cancer. Dis Colon Rectum. 1996;39(12):1409–14.
39. Carraro PG, Segala M, Orlotti C, Tiberio G. Outcome of large-bowel perforation in patients with colorectal cancer. Dis Colon Rectum. 1998; 41(11):1421–6.
40. Mazuski JE, Tessier JM, May AK, Sawyer RG, Nadler EP, Rosengart MR, Chang PK, O'Neill PJ, Mollen KP, Huston JM, Diaz JJ Jr, Prince JM. The Surgical Infection Society Revised Guidelines on the Management of Intra-Abdominal Infection. Surg Infect (Larchmt). 2017;18(1):1–76.
41. Sartelli M, Catena F, Abu-Zidan FM, Ansaloni L, Biffl WL, Boermeester MA, Ceresoli M, Chiara O, Coccolini F, De Waele JJ, Di Saverio S, Eckmann C, Fraga GP, Giannella M, Girardis M, Griffiths EA, Kashuk J, Kirkpatrick AW, Khokha V, Kluger Y, Labricciosa FM, Leppaniemi A, Maier RV, May AK, Malangoni M, Martin-Loeches I, Mazuski J, Montravers P, Peitzman A, Pereira BM, Reis T, Sakakushev B, Sganga G, Soreide K, Sugrue M, Ulrych J, Vincent JL, Viale P, Moore EE. Management of intra-abdominal infections: recommendations by the WSES 2016 consensus conference. World J Emerg Surg. 2017;12:22.
42. Cuffy M, Abir F, Audisio RA, Longo WE. Colorectal cancer presenting as surgical emergencies. Surg Oncol. 2004;13(2–3):149–57.
43. Papa MZ, Karni T, Koller M, Klein E, Scott D, Bersuk D, Sareli M, Ben Ari G. Avoiding diarrhea after subtotal colectomy with primary anastomosis in the treatment of colon cancer. J Am Coll Surg. 1997;184(3):269–72.
44. Veyrie N, Ata T, Muscari F, Couchard AC, Msika S, Hay JM, Fingerhut A, Dziri C, French Associations for Surgical Research. Anastomotic leakage after elective right versus left colectomy for cancer: prevalence and independent risk factors. J Am Coll Surg. 2007;205(6):785–93.
45. Honore C, Goere D, Souadka A, Dumont F, Elias D. Definition of patients presenting a high risk of developing peritoneal carcinomatosis after curative surgery for colorectal cancer: a systematic review. Ann Surg Oncol. 2013;20(1):183–92.
46. Fielding LP, Stewart-Brown S, Blesovsky L. Large-bowel obstruction caused by cancer: a prospective study. Br Med J. 1979;2(6189):515–7.
47. Kronborg O. Acute obstruction from tumour in the left colon without spread. Int J Colorect Dis. 1995;10:5.
48. De Salvo GL, Gava C, Lise M, Pucciarelli S. Curative surgery for obstruction from primary left colorectal carcinoma: primary or staged resection? Cochrane Database of Systematic Reviews. 2004;(2):CD002101. https://doi.org/10.1002/14651858.CD002101.pub2.
49. Krstic S, Resanovic V, Alempijevic T, Resanovic A, Sijacki A, Djukic V, Loncar Z, Karamarkovic A. Hartmann's procedure vs loop colostomy in the treatment of obstructive rectosigmoid cancer. World J Emerg Surg. 2014;9(1):52.
50. Trompetas V. Emergency management of malignant acute left-sided colonic obstruction. Ann R Coll Surg Engl. 2008;90(3):181–6.
51. Meyer F, Marusch F, Koch A, Meyer L, Fuhrer S, Kockerling F, Lippert H, Gastinger I, C. German Study Group "Colorectal. Emergency operation in carcinomas of the left colon: value of Hartmann's procedure. Tech Coloproctol. 2004;(8 Suppl 1):s226–9.
52. Alves A, Panis Y, Mathieu P, Mantion G, Kwiatkowski F, Slim K, C. Association Francaise de. Postoperative mortality and morbidity in French patients undergoing colorectal surgery: results of a prospective multicenter study. Arch Surg. 2005;140(3):278–83. discussion 284.
53. Irvin TT, Goligher JC. Aetiology of disruption of intestinal anastomoses. Br J Surg. 1973;60(6):461–4.
54. Duthie GS, Foster ME, Price-Thomas JM, Leaper DJ. Bowel preparation or not for elective colorectal surgery. J R Coll Surg Edinb. 1990;**35**(3):169–71.
55. Schein M, Assalia A, Eldar S, Wittmann DH. Is mechanical bowel preparation necessary before primary colonic anastomosis? An experimental study. Dis Colon Rectum. 1995;38(7):749–52. discussion 752–4.
56. Guenaga KF, Matos D, Wille-Jorgensen P. Mechanical bowel preparation for elective colorectal surgery. Cochrane Database Syst Rev. 2011;9:CD001544.
57. Zmora O, Mahajna A, Bar-Zakai B, Hershko D, Shabtai M, Krausz MM, Ayalon A. Is mechanical bowel preparation mandatory for left-sided colonic anastomosis? Results of a prospective randomized trial. Tech Coloproctol. 2006;10(2):131–5.
58. Ji WB, Hahn KY, Kwak JM, Kang DW, Baek SJ, Kim J, Kim SH. Mechanical bowel preparation does not affect clinical severity of anastomotic leakage in rectal cancer surgery. World J Surg. 2017;41(5):1366-74. https://doi.org/10.1007/s00268-016-3839-9.
59. Poon RT, Law WL, Chu KW, Wong J. Emergency resection and primary anastomosis for left-sided obstructing colorectal carcinoma in the elderly. Br J Surg. 1998;85(11):1539–42.

60. Deen KI, Madoff RD, Goldberg SM, Rothenberger DA. Surgical management of left colon obstruction: the University of Minnesota experience. J Am Coll Surg. 1998;187(6):573–6.
61. Fazio VW. Restorative colectomy for large bowel obstruction: a new paradigm? J Am Coll Surg. 1998;187(6):631.
62. Zorcolo L, Covotta L, Carlomagno N, Bartolo DC. Safety of primary anastomosis in emergency colo-rectal surgery. Colorectal Dis. 2003;5(3):262–9.
63. Biondo S, Pares D, Frago R, Marti-Rague J, Kreisler E, De Oca J, Jaurrieta E. Large bowel obstruction: predictive factors for postoperative mortality. Dis Colon Rectum. 2004;47(11):1889–97.
64. Tekkis PP, Kinsman R, Thompson MR, Stamatakis JD. The Association of Coloproctology of Great Britain and Ireland study of large bowel obstruction caused by colorectal cancer. Annals of Surgery. 2004;240(1):76–81.
65. Villar JM, Martinez AP, Villegas MT, Muffak K, Mansilla A, Garrote D, Ferron JA. Surgical options for malignant left-sided colonic obstruction. Surg Today. 2005;35(4):275–81.
66. Kim J, Mittal R, Konyalian V, King J, Stamos MJ, Kumar RR. Outcome analysis of patients undergoing colorectal resection for emergent and elective indications. Am Surg. 2007;73(10):991–3.
67. Bellows CF, Webber LS, Albo D, Awad S, Berger DH. Early predictors of anastomotic leaks after colectomy. Tech Coloproctol. 2009;13(1):41–7.
68. Isbister WH, Prasad J. Hartmann's operation: a personal experience. Aust N Z J Surg. 1995;65(2):98–100.
69. Aydin HN, Tekkis PP, Remzi FH, Constantinides V, Fazio VW. Evaluation of the risk of a nonrestorative resection for the treatment of diverticular disease: the Cleveland Clinic diverticular disease propensity score. Dis Colon Rectum. 2006;49(5):629–39.
70. Regenet N, Pessaux P, Hennekinne S, Lermite E, Tuech JJ, Brehant O, Arnaud JP. Primary anastomosis after intraoperative colonic lavage vs. Hartmann's procedure in generalized peritonitis complicating diverticular disease of the colon. Int J Colorectal Dis. 2003;18(6):503–7.
71. Lin FL, Boutros M, Da Silva GM, Weiss EG, Lu XR, Wexner SD. Hartmann reversal: obesity adversely impacts outcome. Dis Colon Rectum. 2013;56(1):83–90.
72. Aydin HN, Remzi FH, Tekkis PP, Fazio VW. Hartmann's reversal is associated with high postoperative adverse events. Dis Colon Rectum. 2005;48(11):2117–26.
73. Desai DC, Brennan EJ Jr, Reilly JF, Smink RD Jr. The utility of the Hartmann procedure. Am J Surg. 1998;175(2):152–4.
74. Zorcolo L, Covotta L, Carlomagno N, Bartolo DC. Toward lowering morbidity, mortality, and stoma formation in emergency colorectal surgery: the role of specialization. Dis Colon Rectum. 2003;46(11):1461–7. discussion 1467–8
75. Jafari MD, Wexner SD, Martz JE, McLemore EC, Margolin DA, Sherwinter DA, Lee SW, Senagore AJ, Phelan MJ, Stamos MJ. Perfusion assessment in laparoscopic left-sided/anterior resection (PILLAR II): a multi-institutional study. J Am Coll Surg. 2015;220(1):82–92. e1.
76. Blanco-Colino R, Espin-Basany E. Intraoperative use of ICG fluorescence imaging to reduce the risk of anastomotic leakage in colorectal surgery: a systematic review and meta-analysis. Tech Coloproctol. 2018;22(1):15–23.
77. Phillips RK, Hittinger R, Fry JS, Fielding LP. Malignant large bowel obstruction. Br J Surg. 1985;72(4):296–302.
78. Darby CR, Berry AR, Mortensen N. Management variability in surgery for colorectal emergencies. Br J Surg. 1992;79(3):206–10.
79. Biondo S, Kreisler E, Millan M, Fraccalvieri D, Golda T, Frago R, Miguel B. Impact of surgical specialization on emergency colorectal surgery outcomes. Arch Surg. 2010;145(1):79–86.
80. Archampong D, Borowski D, Wille-Jorgensen P, Iversen LH. Workload and surgeon's specialty for outcome after colorectal cancer surgery. Cochrane Database Syst Rev. 2012;3:CD005391.
81. Kube R, Granowski D, Stubs P, Mroczkowski P, Ptok H, Schmidt U, Gastinger I, Lippert H, K.R.-K. Study group Qualitatssicherung. Surgical practices for malignant left colonic obstruction in Germany. Eur J Surg Oncol. 2010;36(1):65–71.
82. Gastinger I, Marusch F, Steinert R, Wolff S, Koeckerling F, Lippert H, C. Working Group 'Colon/Rectum. Protective defunctioning stoma in low anterior resection for rectal carcinoma. Br J Surg. 2005;92(9):1137–42.
83. Arnaud JP, Bergamaschi R. Emergency subtotal/total colectomy with anastomosis for acutely obstructed carcinoma of the left colon. Dis Colon Rectum. 1994;37(7):685–8.
84. Torralba JA, Robles R, Parrilla P, Lujan JA, Liron R, Pinero A, Fernandez JA. Subtotal colectomy vs. intraoperative colonic irrigation in the management of obstructed left colon carcinoma. Dis Colon Rectum. 1998;41(1):18–22.
85. Hennekinne-Mucci S, Tuech JJ, Brehant O, Lermite E, Bergamaschi R, Pessaux P, Arnaud JP. Emergency subtotal/total colectomy in the management of obstructed left colon carcinoma. Int J Colorectal Dis. 2006;21(6):538–41.
86. Group, T.S.S. Single-stage treatment for malignant left-sided colonic obstruction: a prospective randomized clinical trial comparing subtotal colectomy with segmental resection following intraoperative irrigation. The SCOTIA Study Group. Subtotal Colectomy versus On-table Irrigation and Anastomosis. Br J Surg. 1995;82(12):1622–7.
87. Lim JF, Tang CL, Seow-Choen F, Heah SM. Prospective, randomized trial comparing intraoperative colonic irrigation with manual decompression only for obstructed left-sided colorectal cancer. Dis Colon Rectum. 2005;48(2):205–9.
88. Kam MH, Tang CL, Chan E, Lim JF, Eu KW. Systematic review of intraoperative colonic irrigation vs. manual decompression in obstructed left-sided colorectal emergencies. Int J Colorectal Dis. 2009;24(9):1031–7.
89. Marcello PW, Milsom JW, Wong SK, Brady K, Goormastic M, Fazio VW. Laparoscopic total colectomy for acute colitis: a case-control study. Dis Colon Rectum. 2001;44(10):1441–5.
90. Gash K, Chambers W, Ghosh A, Dixon AR. The role of laparoscopic surgery for the management of acute large bowel obstruction. Colorectal Dis. 2011;13(3):263–6.
91. Odermatt M, Miskovic D, Siddiqi N, Khan J, Parvaiz A. Short- and long-term outcomes after laparoscopic versus open emergency resection for colon cancer: an observational propensity score-matched study. World J Surg. 2013;37(10):2458–67.
92. Ballian N, Weisensel N, Rajamanickam V, Foley EF, Heise CP, Harms BA, Kennedy GD. Comparable postoperative morbidity and mortality after laparoscopic and open emergent restorative colectomy: outcomes from the ACS NSQIP. World J Surg. 2012;36(10):2488–96.
93. Chand M, Siddiqui MR, Gupta A, Rasheed S, Tekkis P, Parvaiz A, Mirnezami AH, Qureshi T. Systematic review of emergent laparoscopic colorectal surgery for benign and malignant disease. World J Gastroenterol. 2014;20(45):16956–63.
94. Araki Y, Isomoto H, Matsumoto A, Kaibara A, Yasunaga M, Hayashi K, Yatsugi H, Yamauchi K. Endoscopic decompression procedure in acute obstructing colorectal cancer. Endoscopy. 2000;32(8):641–3.
95. Horiuchi A, Maeyama H, Ochi Y, Morikawa A, Miyazawa K. Usefulness of Dennis colorectal tube in endoscopic decompression of acute, malignant colonic obstruction. Gastrointest Endosc. 2001;54(2):229–32.
96. Tanaka T, Furukawa A, Murata K, Sakamoto T. Endoscopic transanal decompression with a drainage tube for acute colonic obstruction: clinical aspects of preoperative treatment. Dis Colon Rectum. 2001; 44(3):418–22.
97. Horiuchi A, Nakayama Y, Tanaka N, Kajiyama M, Fujii H, Yokoyama T, Hayashi K. Acute colorectal obstruction treated by means of transanal drainage tube: effectiveness before surgery and stenting. Am J Gastroenterol. 2005;100(12):2765–70.
98. Yokohata K, Sumiyoshi K, Hirakawa K. Merits and faults of transanal ileus tube for obstructing colorectal cancer. Asian J Surg. 2006;29(3):125–7.
99. Xu M, Zhong Y, Yao L, Xu J, Zhou P, Wang P, Wang H. Endoscopic decompression using a transanal drainage tube for acute obstruction of the rectum and left colon as a bridge to curative surgery. Colorectal Dis. 2009;11(4):405–9.
100. Yamada T, Shimura T, Sakamoto E, Kurumiya Y, Komatsu S, Iwasaki H, Nomura S, Kanie H, Hasegawa H, Orito E, Joh T. Preoperative drainage using a transanal tube enables elective laparoscopic colectomy for obstructive distal colorectal cancer. Endoscopy. 2013;45(4):265–71.
101. Shigeta K, Baba H, Yamafuji K, Kaneda H, Katsura H, Kubochi K. Outcomes for patients with obstructing colorectal cancers treated with one-stage surgery using transanal drainage tubes. J Gastrointest Surg. 2014;18(8):1507–13.
102. Shimura T, Joh T. Evidence-based clinical management of acute malignant colorectal obstruction. J Clin Gastroenterol. 2016;**50**(4):273–85.
103. Li CY, Guo SB, Wang NF. Decompression of acute left-sided malignant colorectal obstruction: comparing transanal drainage tube with metallic stent. J Clin Gastroenterol. 2014;48(5):e37–42.
104. Rupp KD, Dohmoto M, Meffert R, Holzgreve A, Hohlbach G. Cancer of the rectum—palliative endoscopic treatment. Eur J Surg Oncol. 1995; 21(6):644–7.

105. Itabashi M, Hamano K, Kameoka S, Asahina K. Self-expanding stainless steel stent application in rectosigmoid stricture. Dis Colon Rectum. 1993;36(5):508–11.
106. Tejero E, Mainar A, Fernandez L, Tieso A, Cuezva JF, San Jose A. New procedure for relief of malignant obstruction of the left colon. Br J Surg. 1995;82(1):34–5.
107. Baron TH, Dean PA, Yates MR 3rd, Canon C, Koehler RE. Expandable metal stents for the treatment of colonic obstruction: techniques and outcomes. Gastrointest Endosc. 1998;47(3):277–86.
108. Harris GJ, Senagore AJ, Lavery IC, Fazio VW. The management of neoplastic colorectal obstruction with colonic endolumenal stenting devices. Am J Surg. 2001;181(6):499–506.
109. Xinopoulos D, Dimitroulopoulos D, Theodosopoulos T, Tsamakidis K, Bitsakou G, Plataniotis G, Gontikakis M, Kontis M, Paraskevas I, Vassilobpoulos P, Paraskevas E. Stenting or stoma creation for patients with inoperable malignant colonic obstructions? Results of a study and cost-effectiveness analysis. Surg Endosc. 2004;18(3):421–6.
110. Fiori E, Lamazza A, De Cesare A, Bononi M, Volpino P, Schillaci A, Cavallaro A, Cangemi V. Palliative management of malignant rectosigmoidal obstruction. Colostomy vs. endoscopic stenting. A randomized prospective trial. Anticancer Res. 2004;24(1):265–8.
111. van Hooft JE, Fockens P, Marinelli AW, Timmer R, van Berkel AM, Bossuyt PM, Bemelman WA, G. Dutch Colorectal Stent. Early closure of a multicenter randomized clinical trial of endoscopic stenting versus surgery for stage IV left-sided colorectal cancer. Endoscopy. 2008;40(3):184–91.
112. Young CJ, De-Loyde KJ, Young JM, Solomon MJ, Chew EH, Byrne CM, Salkeld G, Faragher IG. Improving quality of life for people with incurable large-bowel obstruction: randomized control trial of colonic stent insertion. Dis Colon Rectum. 2015;58(9):838–49.
113. Fiori E, Lamazza A, Schillaci A, Femia S, Demasi E, Decesare A, Sterpetti AV. Palliative management for patients with subacute obstruction and stage IV unresectable rectosigmoid cancer: colostomy versus endoscopic stenting: final results of a prospective randomized trial. Am J Surg. 2012;204(3):321–6.
114. Repici A, De Caro G, Luigiano C, Fabbri C, Pagano N, Preatoni P, Danese S, Fuccio L, Consolo P, Malesci A, D'Imperio N, Cennamo V. WallFlex colonic stent placement for management of malignant colonic obstruction: a prospective study at two centers. Gastrointest Endosc. 2008;67(1):77–84.
115. Brehant O, Fuks D, Bartoli E, Yzet T, Verhaeghe P, Regimbeau JM. Elective (planned) colectomy in patients with colorectal obstruction after placement of a self-expanding metallic stent as a bridge to surgery: the results of a prospective study. Colorectal Dis. 2009;11(2):178–83.
116. Cennamo V, Fuccio L, Mutri V, Minardi ME, Eusebi LH, Ceroni L, Laterza L, Ansaloni L, Pinna AD, Salfi N, Martoni AA, Bazzoli F. Does stent placement for advanced colon cancer increase the risk of perforation during bevacizumab-based therapy? Clin Gastroenterol Hepatol. 2009;7(11):1174–6.
117. Sebastian S, Johnston S, Geoghegan T, Torreggiani W, Buckley M. Pooled analysis of the efficacy and safety of self-expanding metal stenting in malignant colorectal obstruction. Am J Gastroenterol. 2004;99(10):2051–7.
118. Zhao XD, Cai BB, Cao RS, Shi RH. Palliative treatment for incurable malignant colorectal obstructions: a meta-analysis. World J Gastroenterol. 2013;19(33):5565–74.
119. Liang TW, Sun Y, Wei YC, Yang DX. Palliative treatment of malignant colorectal obstruction caused by advanced malignancy: a self-expanding metallic stent or surgery? A system review and meta-analysis. Surg Today. 2014;44(1):22–33.
120. Takahashi H, Okabayashi K, Tsuruta M, Hasegawa H, Yahagi M, Kitagawa Y. Self-expanding metallic stents versus surgical intervention as palliative therapy for obstructive colorectal cancer: a meta-analysis. World J Surg. 2015;39(8):2037–44.
121. Manes G, de Bellis M, Fuccio L, Repici A, Masci E, Ardizzone S, Mangiavillano B, Carlino A, Rossi GB, Occhipinti P, Cennamo V. Endoscopic palliation in patients with incurable malignant colorectal obstruction by means of self-expanding metal stent: analysis of results and predictors of outcomes in a large multicenter series. Arch Surg. 2011;146(10):1157–62.
122. van Halsema, E.E., J.E. van Hooft, A.J. Small, T.H. Baron, J. Garcia-Cano, J.H. Cheon, M.S. Lee, S.H. Kwon, S. Mucci-Hennekinne, P. Fockens, M.G. Dijkgraaf, and A. Repici, Perforation in colorectal stenting: a meta-analysis and a search for risk factors. Gastrointest Endosc, 2014. 79(6): p. 970–982 e7; quiz 983 e2, 983 e5.
123. van Hooft JE, van Halsema EE, Vanbiervliet G, Beets-Tan RG, DeWitt JM, Donnellan F, Dumonceau JM, Glynne-Jones RG, Hassan C, Jimenez-Perez J, Meisner S, Muthusamy VR, Parker MC, Regimbeau JM, Sabbagh C, Sagar J, Tanis PJ, Vandervoort J, Webster GJ, Manes G, Barthet MA, Repicii A, E, European Society of Gastrointestinal. Self-expandable metal stents for obstructing colonic and extracolonic cancer: European Society of Gastrointestinal Endoscopy (ESGE) Clinical Guideline. Endoscopy. 2014; 46(11):990–1053.
124. Yoshimoto R, Dohmoto H, Yamada K, Goto A. Prolonged inhibition of vascular contraction and calcium influx by the novel 1,4-dihydropyridine calcium antagonist cinaldipine (FRC-8653). Jpn J Pharmacol. 1991;56(2):225–9.
125. Zhang Y, Shi J, Shi B, Song CY, Xie WF, Chen YX. Self-expanding metallic stent as a bridge to surgery versus emergency surgery for obstructive colorectal cancer: a meta-analysis. Surg Endosc. 2012;26(1):110–9.
126. Sabbagh C, Browet F, Diouf M, Cosse C, Brehant O, Bartoli E, Mauvais F, Chauffert B, Dupas JL, Nguyen-Khac E, Regimbeau JM. Is stenting as "a bridge to surgery" an oncologically safe strategy for the management of acute, left-sided, malignant, colonic obstruction? A comparative study with a propensity score analysis. Ann Surg. 2013;258(1):107–15.
127. Kim JS, Hur H, Min BS, Sohn SK, Cho CH, Kim NK. Oncologic outcomes of self-expanding metallic stent insertion as a bridge to surgery in the management of left-sided colon cancer obstruction: comparison with nonobstructing elective surgery. World J Surg. 2009;33(6):1281–6.
128. Gorissen KJ, Tuynman JB, Fryer E, Wang L, Uberoi R, Jones OM, Cunningham C, Lindsey I. Local recurrence after stenting for obstructing left-sided colonic cancer. Br J Surg. 2013;100(13):1805–9.
129. Cheung HY, Chung CC, Tsang WW, Wong JC, Yau KK, Li MK. Endolaparoscopic approach vs conventional open surgery in the treatment of obstructing left-sided colon cancer: a randomized controlled trial. Arch Surg. 2009;144(12):1127–32.
130. Alcantara M, Serra-Aracil X, Falco J, Mora L, Bombardo J, Navarro S. Prospective, controlled, randomized study of intraoperative colonic lavage versus stent placement in obstructive left-sided colonic cancer. World J Surg. 2011;35(8):1904–10.
131. Pirlet IA, Slim K, Kwiatkowski F, Michot F, Millat BL. Emergency preoperative stenting versus surgery for acute left-sided malignant colonic obstruction: a multicenter randomized controlled trial. Surg Endosc. 2011;25(6):1814–21.
132. Ho KS, Quah HM, Lim JF, Tang CL, Eu KW. Endoscopic stenting and elective surgery versus emergency surgery for left-sided malignant colonic obstruction: a prospective randomized trial. Int J Colorectal Dis. 2012;27(3):355–62.
133. Ghazal AH, El-Shazly WG, Bessa SS, El-Riwini MT, Hussein AM. Colonic endolumenal stenting devices and elective surgery versus emergency subtotal/total colectomy in the management of malignant obstructed left colon carcinoma. J Gastrointest Surg. 2013;17(6):1123–9.
134. Arezzo A, Balague C, Targarona E, Borghi F, Giraudo G, Ghezzo L, Arroyo A, Sola-Vera J, De Paolis P, Bossotti M, Bannone E, Forcignano E, Bonino MA, Passera R, Morino M. Colonic stenting as a bridge to surgery versus emergency surgery for malignant colonic obstruction: results of a multicentre randomised controlled trial (ESCO trial). Surg Endosc. 2017;31(8): 3297-305. https://doi.org/10.1007/s00464-016-5362-3.
135. Stipa F, Pigazzi A, Bascone B, Cimitan A, Villotti G, Burza A, Vitale A. Management of obstructive colorectal cancer with endoscopic stenting followed by single-stage surgery: open or laparoscopic resection? Surg Endosc. 2008;22(6):1477–81.
136. Targownik LE, Spiegel BM, Sack J, Hines OJ, Dulai GS, Gralnek IM, Farrell JJ. Colonic stent vs. emergency surgery for management of acute left-sided malignant colonic obstruction: a decision analysis. Gastrointest Endosc. 2004;60(6):865–74.
137. Cirocchi R, Farinella E, Trastulli S, Desiderio J, Listorti C, Boselli C, Parisi A, Noya G, Sagar J. Safety and efficacy of endoscopic colonic stenting as a bridge to surgery in the management of intestinal obstruction due to left colon and rectal cancer: a systematic review and meta-analysis. Surg Oncol. 2013;22(1):14–21.
138. De Ceglie A, Filiberti R, Baron TH, Ceppi M, Conio M. A meta-analysis of endoscopic stenting as bridge to surgery versus emergency surgery for left-sided colorectal cancer obstruction. Crit Rev Oncol Hematol. 2013; 88(2):387–403.
139. Liu Z, Kang L, Li C, Huang M, Zhang X, Wang J. Meta-analysis of complications of colonic stenting versus emergency surgery for acute left-sided malignant colonic obstruction. Surg Laparosc Endosc Percutan Tech. 2014;24(1):73–9.

140. Zhao X, Liu B, Zhao E, Wang J, Cai M, Xia Z, Xia Q, Shuai X, Tao K, Wang G, Cai K. The safety and efficiency of surgery with colonic stents in left-sided malignant colonic obstruction: a meta-analysis. Gastroenterol Res Pract. 2014;2014:407325.
141. Huang X, Lv B, Zhang S, Meng L. Preoperative colonic stents versus emergency surgery for acute left-sided malignant colonic obstruction: a meta-analysis. J Gastrointest Surg. 2014;18(3):584–91.
142. Matsuda A, Miyashita M, Matsumoto S, Matsutani T, Sakurazawa N, Takahashi G, Kishi T, Uchida E. Comparison of long-term outcomes of colonic stent as "bridge to surgery" and emergency surgery for malignant large-bowel obstruction: a meta-analysis. Ann Surg Oncol. 2015;22(2):497–504.
143. Allievi N, Ceresoli M, Fugazzola P, Montori G, Coccolini F, Ansaloni L. Endoscopic stenting as bridge to surgery versus emergency resection for left-sided malignant colorectal obstruction: an updated meta-analysis. Int J Surg Oncol. 2017;2017:2863272.
144. Tung KL, Cheung HY, Ng LW, Chung CC, Li MK. Endo-laparoscopic approach versus conventional open surgery in the treatment of obstructing left-sided colon cancer: long-term follow-up of a randomized trial. Asian J Endosc Surg. 2013;6(2):78–81.
145. Sloothaak DA, van den Berg MW, Dijkgraaf MG, Fockens P, Tanis PJ, van Hooft JE, Bemelman WA, Collaborative Dutch Stent-In study group. Oncological outcome of malignant colonic obstruction in the Dutch Stent-In 2 trial. Br J Surg. 2014;101(13):1751–7.
146. Ceresoli M, Allievi N, Coccolini F, Montori G, Fugazzola P, Pisano M, Sartelli M, Catena F, Ansaloni L. Long term oncologic outcomes of stents as a bridge to surgery vs. emergency surgery in malignant left side colonic obstruction: a meta-analysis. Journal of Surgical Oncology. 2017;8:867–76.
147. Pahlman L, Glimelius B. Pre- or postoperative radiotherapy in rectal and rectosigmoid carcinoma. Report from a randomized multicenter trial. Ann Surg. 1990;211(2):187–95.
148. Kapiteijn E, Marijnen CA, Nagtegaal ID, Putter H, Steup WH, Wiggers T, Rutten HJ, Pahlman L, Glimelius B, van Krieken JH, Leer JW, van de Velde CJ. Preoperative radiotherapy combined with total mesorectal excision for resectable rectal cancer. N Engl J Med. 2001;345(9):638–46.
149. Sauer R, Becker H, Hohenberger W, Rodel C, Wittekind C, Fietkau R, Martus P, Tschmelitsch J, Hager E, Hess CF, Karstens JH, Liersch T, Schmidberger H, Raab R. Preoperative versus postoperative chemoradiotherapy for rectal cancer. N Engl J Med. 2004;351(17):1731–40.
150. Bosset JF, Collette L, Calais G, Mineur L, Maingon P, Radosevic-Jelic L, Daban A, Bardet E, Beny A, Ollier JC. Chemotherapy with preoperative radiotherapy in rectal cancer. N Engl J Med. 2006;355(11):1114–23.
151. Huser N, Michalski CW, Erkan M, Schuster T, Rosenberg R, Kleeff J, Friess H. Systematic review and meta-analysis of the role of defunctioning stoma in low rectal cancer surgery. Ann Surg. 2008;248(1):52–60.
152. Tan WS, Tang CL, Shi L, Eu KW. Meta-analysis of defunctioning stomas in low anterior resection for rectal cancer. Br J Surg. 2009;96(5):462–72.
153. Montedori A, Cirocchi R, Farinella E, Sciannameo F, Abraha I. Covering ileo- or colostomy in anterior resection for rectal carcinoma. Cochrane Database Syst Rev. 2010;5:CD006878.
154. Guenaga KF, Lustosa SA, Saad SS, Saconato H, Matos D. Ileostomy or colostomy for temporary decompression of colorectal anastomosis. Cochrane Database Syst Rev. 2007;1:CD004647.
155. Rondelli F, Reboldi P, Rulli A, Barberini F, Guerrisi A, Izzo L, Bolognese A, Covarelli P, Boselli C, Becattini C, Noya G. Loop ileostomy versus loop colostomy for fecal diversion after colorectal or coloanal anastomosis: a meta-analysis. Int J Colorectal Dis. 2009;24(5):479–88.
156. Geng HZ, Nasier D, Liu B, Gao H, Xu YK. Meta-analysis of elective surgical complications related to defunctioning loop ileostomy compared with loop colostomy after low anterior resection for rectal carcinoma. Ann R Coll Surg Engl. 2015;97(7):494–501.
157. Nylund G, Oresland T, Hulten L. The trephine stoma: formation of a stoma without laparotomy. Eur J Surg. 1997;163(8):627–9.
158. Vermeer TA, Orsini RG, Nieuwenhuijzen GA, Rutten HJ, Daams F. Stoma placement in obstructive rectal cancer prior to neo-adjuvant treatment and definitive surgery: a practical guideline. Eur J Surg Oncol. 2016;42(2):273–80.
159. Faucheron JL, Paquette B, Trilling B, Heyd B, Koch S, Mantion G. Emergency surgery for obstructing colonic cancer: a comparison between right-sided and left-sided lesions. Eur J Trauma Emerg Surg. 2018;44(1):71–7.
160. Hsu TC. Comparison of one-stage resection and anastomosis of acute complete obstruction of left and right colon. Am J Surg. 2005;189(4):384–7.
161. Lee YM, Law WL, Chu KW, Poon RT. Emergency surgery for obstructing colorectal cancers: a comparison between right-sided and left-sided lesions. J Am Coll Surg. 2001;192(6):719–25.
162. Yeo HL, Lee SW. Colorectal emergencies: review and controversies in the management of large bowel obstruction. J Gastrointest Surg. 2013; 17(11):2007–12.
163. Lynch CR, Jones RG, Hilden K, Wills JC, Fang JC. Percutaneous endoscopic cecostomy in adults: a case series. Gastrointest Endosc. 2006;64(2):279–82.
164. Marker DR, Perosi N, Ul Haq F, Morefield W, Mitchell S. Percutaneous cecostomy in adult patients: safety and quality-of-life results. J Vasc Interv Radiol. 2015;26(10):1526–32. e1.
165. Chait PG, Shlomovitz E, Connolly BL, Temple MJ, Restrepo R, Amaral JG, Muraca S, Richards HF, Ein SH. Percutaneous cecostomy: updates in technique and patient care. Radiology. 2003;227(1):246–50.
166. Donkol RH, Al-Nammi A. Percutaneous cecostomy in the management of organic fecal incontinence in children. World J Radiol. 2010;2(12):463–7.
167. Tewari SO, Getrajdman GI, Petre EN, Sofocleous CT, Siegelbaum RH, Erinjeri JP, Weiser MR, Thornton RH. Safety and efficacy of percutaneous cecostomy/colostomy for treatment of large bowel obstruction in adults with cancer. J Vasc Interv Radiol. 2015;26(2):182–8.
168. Lim CH, McDonald NM, Freeman ML, Amateau SK. Percutaneous cecostomy with fully covered self-expandable metal stent for initial management of severe malignant colon obstruction. Endoscopy. 2017;49(12):E313–5.
169. Kye BH, Lee YS, Cho HM, Kim JG, Oh ST, Lee IK, Kang WK, Ahn CH, Lee SC, Park JK, Kim HJ. Comparison of long-term outcomes between emergency surgery and bridge to surgery for malignant obstruction in right-sided colon cancer: a multicenter retrospective study. Ann Surg Oncol. 2016;23(6):1867–74.
170. Amelung FJ, de Beaufort HW, Siersema PD, Verheijen PM, Consten EC. Emergency resection versus bridge to surgery with stenting in patients with acute right-sided colonic obstruction: a systematic review focusing on mortality and morbidity rates. Int J Colorectal Dis. 2015;**30**(9):1147–55.
171. Shim CS, Cho JY, Jung IS, Ryu CB, Hong SJ, Kim JO, Lee JS, Lee MS, Kim BS. Through-the-scope double colonic stenting in the management of inoperable proximal malignant colonic obstruction: a pilot study. Endoscopy. 2004;36(5):426–31.
172. Person B, Dorfman T, Bahouth H, Osman A, Assalia A, Kluger Y. Abbreviated emergency laparotomy in the non-trauma setting. World J Emerg Surg. 2009;4:41.
173. Weber DG, Bendinelli C, Balogh ZJ. Damage control surgery for abdominal emergencies. Br J Surg. 2014;101(1):e109–18.
174. Becher RD, Peitzman AB, Sperry JL, Gallaher JR, Neff LP, Sun Y, Miller PR, Chang MC. Damage control operations in non-trauma patients: defining criteria for the staged rapid source control laparotomy in emergency general surgery. World J Emerg Surg. 2016;11:10.
175. Shankar-Hari M, Phillips GS, Levy ML, Seymour CW, Liu VX, Deutschman CS, Angus DC, Rubenfeld GD, Singer M, F. Sepsis Definitions Task. Developing a new definition and assessing new clinical criteria for septic shock: for the Third International Consensus Definitions for Sepsis and Septic Shock (Sepsis-3). JAMA. 2016;315(8):775–87.
176. Knaus WA, Draper EA, Wagner DP, Zimmerman JE. APACHE II: a severity of disease classification system. Crit Care Med. 1985;13(10):818–29.
177. Shapiro NI, Wolfe RE, Moore RB, Smith E, Burdick E, Bates DW. Mortality in Emergency Department Sepsis (MEDS) score: a prospectively derived and validated clinical prediction rule. Crit Care Med. 2003;31(3):670–5.
178. Vincent JL, Moreno R, Takala J, Willatts S, De Mendonca A, Bruining H, Reinhart CK, Suter PM, Thijs LG. The SOFA (Sepsis-related Organ Failure Assessment) score to describe organ dysfunction/failure. On behalf of the Working Group on Sepsis-Related Problems of the European Society of Intensive Care Medicine. Intensive Care Med. 1996;22(7):707–10.
179. Rubulotta F, Marshall JC, Ramsay G, Nelson D, Levy M, Williams M. Predisposition, insult/infection, response, and organ dysfunction: A new model for staging severe sepsis. Crit Care Med. 2009;37(4):1329–35.
180. Finkelsztein EJ, Jones DS, Ma KC, Pabon MA, Delgado T, Nakahira K, Arbo JE, Berlin DA, Schenck EJ, Choi AM, Siempos II. Comparison of qSOFA and SIRS for predicting adverse outcomes of patients with suspicion of sepsis outside the intensive care unit. Crit Care. 2017;21(1):73.
181. Sartelli M, Abu-Zidan FM, Catena F, Griffiths EA, Di Saverio S, Coimbra R, Ordonez CA, Leppaniemi A, Fraga GP, Coccolini F, Agresta F, Abbas A, Abdel Kader S, Agboola J, Amhed A, Ajibade A, Akkucuk S, Alharthi B, Anyfantakis D, Augustin G, Baiocchi G, Bala M, Baraket O, Bayrak S, Bellanova

G, Beltran MA, Bini R, Boal M, Borodach AV, Bouliaris K, Branger F, Brunelli D, Catani M, Che Jusoh A, Chichom-Mefire A, Cocorullo G, Colak E, Costa D, Costa S, Cui Y, Curca GL, Curry T, Das K, Delibegovic S, Demetrashvili Z, Di Carlo I, Drozdova N, El Zalabany T, Enani MA, Faro M, Gachabayov M, Gimenez Maurel T, Gkiokas G, Gomes CA, Gonsaga RA, Guercioni G, Guner A, Gupta S, Gutierrez S, Hutan M, Ioannidis O, Isik A, Izawa Y, Jain SA, Jokubauskas M, Karamarkovic A, Kauhanen S, Kaushik R, Kenig J, Khokha V, Kim JI, Kong V, Koshy R, Krasniqi A, Kshirsagar A, Kuliesius Z, Lasithiotakis K, Leao P, Lee JG, Leon M, Lizarazu Perez A, Lohsiriwat V, Lopez-Tomassetti Fernandez E, Lostoridis E, Mn R, major P, Marinis A, Marrelli D, Martinez-Perez A, Marwah S, McFarlane M, Melo RB, Mesina C, Michalopoulos N, Moldovanu R, Mouaqit O, Munyika A, Negoi I, Nikolopoulos I, Nita GE, Olaoye I, Omari A, Ossa PR, Ozkan Z, Padmakumar R, Pata F, Pereira Junior GA, Pereira J, Pintar T, Pouggouras K, Prabhu V, Rausei S, Rems M, Rios-Cruz D, Sakakushev B, Sanchez de Molina ML, Seretis C, Shelat V, Simoes RL, Sinibaldi G, Skrovina M, Smirnov D, Spyropoulos C, Tepp J, Tezcaner T, Tolonen M, Torba M, Ulrych J, Uzunoglu MY, van Dellen D, van Ramshorst GH, Vasquez G, Venara A, Vereczkei A, Vettoretto N, Vlad N, Yadav SK, Yilmaz TU, Yuan KC, Zachariah SK, Zida M, Zilinskas J, Ansaloni L. Global validation of the WSES Sepsis Severity Score for patients with complicated intra-abdominal infections: a prospective multicentre study (WISS study). World J Emerg Surg. 2015;10:61.

182. Subramanian A, Balentine C, Palacio CH, Sansgiry S, Berger DH, Awad SS. Outcomes of damage-control celiotomy in elderly nontrauma patients with intra-abdominal catastrophes. Am J Surg. 2010;200(6):783–8. discussion 788–9
183. Waibel BH, Rotondo MF. Damage control for intra-abdominal sepsis. Surg Clin North Am. 2012;92(2):243–57. viii
184. Azuhata T, Kinoshita K, Kawano D, Komatsu T, Sakurai A, Chiba Y, Tanjho K. Time from admission to initiation of surgery for source control is a critical determinant of survival in patients with gastrointestinal perforation with associated septic shock. Crit Care. 2014;18(3):R87.
185. Rivers E, Nguyen B, Havstad S, Ressler J, Muzzin A, Knoblich B, Peterson E, Tomlanovich M, Early Goal-Directed G. Therapy collaborative, early goal-directed therapy in the treatment of severe sepsis and septic shock. N Engl J Med. 2001;345(19):1368–77.
186. Park SK, Shin SR, Hur M, Kim WH, Oh EA, Lee SH. The effect of early goal-directed therapy for treatment of severe sepsis or septic shock: a systemic review and meta-analysis. J Crit Care. 2017;38:115–22.
187. Jiang LB, Zhang M, Jiang SY, Ma YF. Early goal-directed resuscitation for patients with severe sepsis and septic shock: a meta-analysis and trial sequential analysis. Scand J Trauma Resusc Emerg Med. 2016;24:23.
188. Cauley CE, Panizales MT, Reznor G, Haynes AB, Havens JM, Kelley E, Mosenthal AC, Cooper Z. Outcomes after emergency abdominal surgery in patients with advanced cancer: opportunities to reduce complications and improve palliative care. J Trauma Acute Care Surg. 2015;79(3):399–406.
189. Hsu CW, Wang JH, Kung YH, Chang MC. What is the predictor of surgical mortality in adult colorectal perforation? The clinical characteristics and results of a multivariate logistic regression analysis. Surg Today. 2017;47(6):683–9.
190. Bruns BR, Ahmad SA, O'Meara L, Tesoriero R, Lauerman M, Klyushnenkova E, Kozar R, Scalea TM, Diaz JJ. Nontrauma open abdomens: a prospective observational study. J Trauma Acute Care Surg. 2016;80(4):631–6.
191. van Ruler O, Mahler CW, Boer KR, Reuland EA, Gooszen HG, Opmeer BC, de Graaf PW, Lamme B, Gerhards MF, Steller EP, van Till JW, de Borgie CJ, Gouma DJ, Reitsma JB, Boermeester MA, Dutch Peritonitis Study G. Comparison of on-demand vs planned relaparotomy strategy in patients with severe peritonitis: a randomized trial. JAMA. 2007;298(8):865–72.
192. Lamme B, Boermeester MA, Reitsma JB, Mahler CW, Obertop H, Gouma DJ. Meta-analysis of relaparotomy for secondary peritonitis. Br J Surg. 2002;89(12):1516–24.
193. Sartelli M, Abu-Zidan FM, Ansaloni L, Bala M, Beltran MA, Biffl WL, Catena F, Chiara O, Coccolini F, Coimbra R, Demetrashvili Z, Demetriades D, Diaz JJ, Di Saverio S, Fraga GP, Ghnnam W, Griffiths EA, Gupta S, Hecker A, Karamarkovic A, Kong VY, Kafka-Ritsch R, Kluger Y, Latifi R, Leppaniemi A, Lee JG, McFarlane M, Marwah S, Moore FA, Ordonez CA, Pereira GA, Plaudis H, Shelat VG, Ulrych J, Zachariah SK, Zielinski MD, Garcia MP, Moore EE. The role of the open abdomen procedure in managing severe abdominal sepsis: WSES position paper. World J Emerg Surg. 2015;10:35.
194. Chen Y, Ye J, Song W, Chen J, Yuan Y, Ren J. Comparison of outcomes between early fascial closure and delayed abdominal closure in patients with open abdomen: a systematic review and meta-analysis. Gastroenterol Res Pract. 2014;2014:784056.
195. Khan A, Hsee L, Mathur S, Civil I. Damage-control laparotomy in nontrauma patients: review of indications and outcomes. J Trauma Acute Care Surg. 2013;75(3):365–8.
196. Stawicki SP, Brooks A, Bilski T, Scaff D, Gupta R, Schwab CW, Gracias VH. The concept of damage control: extending the paradigm to emergency general surgery. Injury. 2008;39(1):93–101.
197. Awad SS, Fagan SP, Bellows C, Albo D, Green-Rashad B, De la Garza M, Berger DH. Bridging the communication gap in the operating room with medical team training. Am J Surg. 2005;190(5):770–4.
198. Salas E, Cannon-Bowers JA, Weaver J. Command and control teams; principles for training and assessment. In: Flin R, Arbuthnot K, editors. Incident Command: Tales from the Hot Seat; 2002.
199. Nelson RL, Gladman E, Barbateskovic M. Antimicrobial prophylaxis for colorectal surgery. Cochrane Database Syst Rev. 2014;5:CD001181.
200. O'Boyle CJ, MacFie J, Mitchell CJ, Johnstone D, Sagar PM, Sedman PC. Microbiology of bacterial translocation in humans. Gut. 1998;42(1):29–35.
201. Samel S, Keese M, Kleczka M, Lanig S, Gretz N, Hafner M, Sturm J, Post S. Microscopy of bacterial translocation during small bowel obstruction and ischemia in vivo—a new animal model. BMC Surg. 2002;2:6.
202. Marshall JC, Christou NV, Meakins JL. The gastrointestinal tract. The "undrained abscess" of multiple organ failure. Ann Surg. 1993;218(2):111–9.
203. Deitch EA, Bridges WM, Ma JW, Ma L, Berg RD, Specian RD. Obstructed intestine as a reservoir for systemic infection. Am J Surg. 1990;159(4):394–401.
204. Sagar PM, MacFie J, Sedman P, May J, Mancey-Jones B, Johnstone D. Intestinal obstruction promotes gut translocation of bacteria. Dis Colon Rectum. 1995;38(6):640–4.
205. Lee DS, Ryu JA, Chung CR, Yang J, Jeon K, Suh GY, Lee WY, Park CM. Risk factors for acquisition of multidrug-resistant bacteria in patients with anastomotic leakage after colorectal cancer surgery. Int J Colorectal Dis. 2015;30(4):497–504.
206. Sartelli M, Weber DG, Ruppe E, Bassetti M, Wright BJ, Ansaloni L, Catena F, Coccolini F, Abu-Zidan FM, Coimbra R, Moore EE, Moore FA, Maier RV, De Waele JJ, Kirkpatrick AW, Griffiths EA, Eckmann C, Brink AJ, Mazuski JE, May AK, Sawyer RG, Mertz D, Montravers P, Kumar A, Roberts JA, Vincent JL, Watkins RR, Lowman W, Spellberg B, Abbott IJ, Adesunkanmi AK, Al-Dahir S, Al-Hasan MN, Agresta F, Althani AA, Ansari S, Ansumana R, Augustin G, Bala M, Balogh ZJ, Baraket O, Bhangu A, Beltran MA, Bernhard M, Biffl WL, Boermeester MA, Brecher SM, Cherry-Bukowiec JR, Buyne OR, Cainzos MA, Cairns KA, Camacho-Ortiz A, Chandy SJ, Che Jusoh A, Chichom-Mefire A, Colijn C, Corcione F, Cui Y, Curcio D, Delibegovic S, Demetrashvili Z, De Simone B, Dhingra S, Diaz JJ, Di Carlo I, Dillip A, Di Saverio S, Doyle MP, Dorj G, Dogjani A, Dupont H, Eachempati SR, Enani MA, Egiev VN, Elmangory MM, Ferrada P, Fitchett JR, Fraga GP, Guessennd N, Giamarellou H, Ghnnam W, Gkiokas G, Goldberg SR, Gomes CA, Gomi H, Guzman-Blanco M, Haque M, Hansen S, Hecker A, Heizmann WR, Herzog T, Hodonou AM, Hong SK, Kafka-Ritsch R, Kaplan LJ, Kapoor G, Karamarkovic A, Kees MG, Kenig J, Kiguba R, Kim PK, Kluger Y, Khokha V, Koike K, Kok KY, Kong V, Knox MC, Inaba K, Isik A, Iskandar K, Ivatury RR, Labbate M, Labricciosa FM, Laterre PF, Latifi R, Lee JG, Lee YR, Leone M, Leppaniemi A, Li Y, Liang SY, Loho T, Maegele M, Malama S, Marei HE, Martin-Loeches I, Marwah S, Massele A, McFarlane M, Melo RB, Negoi I, Nicolau DP, Nord CE, Ofori-Asenso R, Omari AH, Ordonez CA, Ouadii M, Pereira Junior GA, Piazza D, Pupelis G, Rawson TM, Rems M, Rizoli S, Rocha C, Sakakhushev B, Sanchez-Garcia M, Sato N, Segovia Lohse HA, Sganga G, Siribumrungwong B, Shelat VG, Soreide K, Soto R, Talving P, Tilsed JV, Timsit JF, Trueba G, Trung NT, Ulrych J, van Goor H, Vereczkei A, Vohra RS, Wani I, Uhl W, Xiao Y, Yuan KC, Zachariah SK, Zahar JR, Zakrison TL, Corcione A, Melotti RM, Viscoli C, Viale P. Antimicrobials: a global alliance for optimizing their rational use in intra-abdominal infections (AGORA). World J Emerg Surg. 2016;11:33.
207. Sartelli M, Viale P, Catena F, Ansaloni L, Moore E, Malangoni M, Moore FA, Velmahos G, Coimbra R, Ivatury R, Peitzman A, Koike K, Leppaniemi A, Biffl W, Burlew CC, Balogh ZJ, Boffard K, Bendinelli C, Gupta S, Kluger Y, Agresta F, Di Saverio S, Wani I, Escalona A, Ordonez C, Fraga GP, Junior GA, Bala M, Cui Y, Marwah S, Sakakushev B, Kong V, Naidoo N, Ahmed A, Abbas A, Guercioni G, Vettoretto N, Diaz-Nieto R, Gerych I, Trana C, Faro MP, Yuan KC, Kok KY, Mefire AC, Lee JG, Hong SK, Ghnnam W, Siribumrungwong B, Sato N, Murata K, Irahara T, Coccolini F, Segovia Lohse HA, Verni A, Shoko T. 2013 WSES guidelines for management of intra-abdominal infections. World J Emerg Surg. 2013;8(1):3.
208. Paul M, Shani V, Muchtar E, Kariv G, Robenshtok E, Leibovici L. Systematic review and meta-analysis of the efficacy of appropriate empiric antibiotic therapy for sepsis. Antimicrob Agents Chemother. 2010;54(11):4851–63.

209. Sartelli M, Catena F, Ansaloni L, Coccolini F, Corbella D, Moore EE, Malangoni M, Velmahos G, Coimbra R, Koike K, Leppaniemi A, Biffl W, Balogh Z, Bendinelli C, Gupta S, Kluger Y, Agresta F, Di Saverio S, Tugnoli G, Jovine E, Ordonez CA, Whelan JF, Fraga GP, Gomes CA, Pereira GA, Yuan KC, Bala M, Peev MP, Ben-Ishay O, Cui Y, Marwah S, Zachariah S, Wani I, Rangarajan M, Sakakushev B, Kong V, Ahmed A, Abbas A, Gonsaga RA, Guercioni G, Vettoretto N, Poiasina E, Diaz-Nieto R, Massalou D, Skrovina M, Gerych I, Augustin G, Kenig J, Khokha V, Trana C, Kok KY, Mefire AC, Lee JG, Hong SK, Lohse HA, Ghnnam W, Verni A, Lohsiriwat V, Siribumrungwong B, El Zalabany T, Tavares A, Baiocchi G, Das K, Jarry J, Zida M, Sato N, Murata K, Shoko T, Irahara T, Hamedelneel AO, Naidoo N, Adesunkanmi AR, Kobe Y, Ishii W, Oka K, Izawa Y, Hamid H, Khan I, Attri A, Sharma R, Sanjuan J, Badiel M, Barnabe R. Complicated intra-abdominal infections worldwide: the definitive data of the CIAOW study. World J Emerg Surg. 2014;9:37.
210. Mazuski JE, Tessier JM, May AK, Sawyer RG, Nadler EP, Rosengart MR, Chang PK, O'Neill PJ, Mollen KP, Huston JM, Diaz JJ Jr, Prince JM. The Surgical Infection Society Revised Guidelines on the Management of Intra-Abdominal Infection. Surg Infect (Larchmt). 2017;18(1):1–76.
211. Shelton BK. Intestinal obstruction. AACN Clin Issues. 1999;10(4):478–91.
212. Suri S, Gupta S, Sudhakar PJ, Venkataramu NK, Sood B, Wig JD. Comparative evaluation of plain films, ultrasound and CT in the diagnosis of intestinal obstruction. Acta Radiol. 1999;40(4):422–8.
213. Frager D, Rovno HD, Baer JW, Bashist B, Friedman M. Prospective evaluation of colonic obstruction with computed tomography. Abdom Imaging. 1998;23(2):141–6.
214. Oistamo E, Hjern F, Blomqvist L, Von Heijne A, Abraham-Nordling M. Cancer and diverticulitis of the sigmoid colon. Differentiation with computed tomography versus magnetic resonance imaging: preliminary experiences. Acta Radiol. 2013;54(3):237–41.

24

Acute care surgery: a means for providing cost-effective, quality care for gallstone pancreatitis

Patrick B. Murphy[1*], Dave Paskar[2], Richard Hilsden[1], Jennifer Koichopolos[1], Tina S. Mele[1,3]
and on behalf of Western Ontario Research Collaborative on Acute Care Surgery

Abstract

Background: Modern practice guidelines recommend index cholecystectomy (IC) for patients admitted with gallstone pancreatitis (GSP). However, this benchmark has been difficult to widely achieve. Previous work has demonstrated that dedicated acute care surgery (ACS) services can facilitate IC. However, the associated financial costs and economic effectiveness of this intervention are unknown and represent potential barriers to ACS adoption. We investigated the impact of an ACS service at two hospitals before and after implementation on cost effectiveness, patient quality-adjusted life years (QALY) and impact on rates of IC.

Methods: All patients admitted with non-severe GSP to two tertiary care teaching hospitals from January 2008–May 2015 were reviewed. The diagnosis of GSP was confirmed upon review of clinical, biochemical and radiographic criteria. Patients were divided into three time periods based on the presence of ACS (none, at one hospital, at both hospitals). Data were collected regarding demographics, cholecystectomy timing, resource utilization, and associated costs. QALY analyses were performed and incremental cost effectiveness ratios were calculated comparing pre-ACS to post-ACS periods.

Results: In 435 patients admitted for GSP, IC increased from 16 to 76% after implementing an ACS service at both hospitals. There was a significant reduction in admissions and emergency room visits for GSP after introduction of ACS services ($p < 0.001$). There was no difference in length of stay or conversion to an open operation. The implementation of the ACS service was associated with a decrease in cost of $1162 per patient undergoing cholecystectomy, representing a 12.6% savings.
The time period with both hospitals having established ACS services resulted in a highly favorable cost to quality-adjusted life year ratio (QALY gained and financial costs decreased).

Conclusions: ACS services facilitate cost-effective management of GSP. The result is improved and timelier patient care with decreased healthcare costs. Hospitals without a dedicated ACS service should strongly consider adopting this model of care.

Keywords: Acute care surgery, Quality, Cost effectiveness, Gallstone pancreatitis, Cholecystectomy

* Correspondence: pbatesmurphy@gmail.com;
patrick.murphy@londonhospitals.ca
Poster presentation of preliminary work at the 2015 Canadian Association of General Surgery Conference, Quebec City, Quebec, Canada on September 17-20, 2015.Work performed at the London Health Sciences Centre and Western University
[1]Division of General Surgery, Department of Surgery, Schulich School of Medicine and Dentistry, Western University, London, Canada
Full list of author information is available at the end of the article

Background

Dedicated ACS services continue to be implemented in North America and around the globe. Increasingly comparable to trauma systems, ACS is a growing field with developing fellowships [1], centralization of care, and on-going research particularly with respect to appendicitis [2] and acute biliary disease [3, 4]. The benefits of ACS services are many, and include the optimization of health care delivery from the perspectives of surgeons, patients, and hospitals; these positive changes have been summarized and reported in two systematic reviews to date [5, 6].

GSP is one of the most common gallstone-related emergency general surgery (EGS) conditions, the definitive management of which is index cholecystectomy (IC) [7–13]. IC is recommended as the burden of recurrence requiring additional emergency room visits and re-admissions to hospital is high if definitive management (cholecystectomy) is not provided on the index admission [14–21]. A recent randomized trial, the PONCHO trial, has confirmed the safety and efficacy of index cholecystectomy for non-severe gallstone pancreatitis [22]. A Cochrane meta-analysis further suggests that early IC (<72h) for GSP is safe [23]. However, the facilitation of IC remains a challenge in many centers [15–19]. Lack of emergency general surgical resources, specifically dedicated operating room (OR) time, is the most significant barrier to the provision of early definitive care (IC) [24]. Additional challenges include surgeon acceptance of index (vs. delayed) cholecystectomy and competition with elective practice demands. As such, significant variation persists with respect to the management of acute biliary disease, gallstone pancreatitis in particular [25].

Our previous work has demonstrated an ACS service that can facilitate IC for GSP, leading to decreased GSP recurrence and subsequently reduced emergency room (ER) visits and re-admissions [4]. The cost of ACS provision has been described for acute cholecystitis, and in general, results in cost savings [24–26]. However, no study, to our knowledge, has reported on the impact of patient quality of life, nor performed a formal health economic analysis, following the implementation of an ACS service.

It is well established that delay of definitive management confers an approximately 25% risk of re-admission for gallstone-related illness prior to elective cholecystectomy [14–23]. This potentially impacts patient quality of life with respect to pain, anxiety, and lost days of work and other forms of social functioning. A model-based cost-utility analysis using data from the recent Cochrane review has suggested IC, particularly within 72 h, is cost effective for mild acute gallstone pancreatitis [26].

In our first study, a notable increase in IC rate for GSP at a single center was noted following the initiation of an ACS service (with a non-ACS center serving as a time-control). This second institution has since added an ACS service, allowing us to examine whether the improved outcomes for GSP can be replicated. In addition, we sought to assess the sustainability of a high IC rate within a mature ACS service over time, by continuing to track performance at the first site. Moreover, we investigated the fiscal and quality of life impacts associated with implementing an ACS service by performing a formal health economic analysis from the perspective of the GSP population. We hypothesize a sustainable rate of IC in keeping with our previous results after implementing ACS as well as cost savings and improved quality of life for patients compared to non-index cholecystectomy.

Methods

Ethics approval was obtained from the Health Sciences Research Ethics Board at Western University (HSREB# 104525). The study was conducted at London Health Sciences Centre, a tertiary care, academic institution comprised of two hospital campuses (site A and site B for the purposes of this study) in London, Ontario, Canada. In July 2010, one campus (site A) implemented an ACS service and in July 2014, site B implemented a similar service. A complete description of our ACS model is available [4]. Briefly, in our model, a surgeon suspends his or her elective practice to cover emergency surgical consults, admissions, and surgeries, both through the emergency department and via other in-hospital services, for 1 week. Site A has dedicated daily emergency operative time while site B shares time with other surgical services.

We retrospectively reviewed the charts of all patients admitted to general surgery at both hospitals for the period of January 2008 to May 2015 with an initial diagnosis of pancreatitis. This group of patients was then further refined to include only those with GSP. Our inclusion criteria were as follows: age 18 years old or older, a lipase greater than 300 U/L, had not undergone ERCP within 7 days prior to presentation, and the presence of gallstones on imaging. In order to identify all potential candidates for IC, patients were excluded only if they were pregnant and/or had an intensive care unit (ICU) admission within 48 h of admission to a hospital. ICU admission was used to exclude patients with probable severe pancreatitis and/or had significant comorbidities, and thus likely not suitable candidates for IC. All patient health records were complete for all parameters of interest, and thus, no patient had missing data. In addition, our network of partner community hospitals shares an electronic health record with our institution, so we were able to detect if patients sought surgical care at these sites.

We divided this population into three time periods. Period 1 (January 1, 2008, to June 30, 2010; 2.5 years) represents when neither hospital had an ACS service. During period 2 (July 1, 2010, to June 30, 2014; 4 years), an ACS service was only present at site A. Finally, period 3 (July 1, 2014, to May 15, 2015; 10.5 months) represents the era when both sites had an ACS service.

Descriptive statistics including demographics, use of ERCP (index or not), time to OR from ER presentation, OR duration, conversion to open cholecystectomy, and site of index admission were collected. Re-admission and repeat ER visits rates for GSP, gallstone-related complaints or postoperative concerns were also tracked.

Cost analysis

The cost effectiveness was evaluated from the perspective of a single government payer, which is consistent with the public healthcare systems employed in Canada. The time horizon for the cost effectiveness analysis was either 1 year or the actual duration of illness related to gallstone pancreatitis, for patients whose disease experience in the study extended beyond 1 year. No patients in this study were awaiting management beyond 2 years. A discount rate of 3.5% per year was applied to both health effects and costs, in line with the National Institute for Health and Care Excellence (NICE) guidelines for health economic analysis [27]. Patients who presented with GSP but did not ultimately receive surgical management were excluded from the cost analysis. These patients were excluded as it cannot be assumed that non-surgical management restored these patients to their pre-morbid health state.

Costs for providing management to each individual patient were estimated using financial data available from the Ontario Case Costing Program which contains publicly available data, maintained by the Province of Ontario, Table 1 [28]. This database contains both direct and indirect costs of managing patients with particular diagnoses and of performing certain procedures, as reported by participating hospitals. Using the database, the cost of each component of care for a patient with GSP was estimated, and then was applied to each individual patient in this study, Table 1.

Quality analysis

Quality-adjusted life years (QALY) were used to evaluate health effects. All patients were assigned a QALY of 1 (full health) to represent their health condition prior to developing gallstone pancreatitis. The health multipliers for health states associated with GSP were as follows: no biliary disease—1.0, laparoscopic cholecystectomy—0.91 [29], recurrent biliary colic—0.80 [29], open cholecystectomy—0.77 [30], and acute pancreatitis—0.44 [29]. While admitted to hospital, patients were assigned the acute pancreatitis multiplier. Patients that were discharged from hospital, but who did not have IC, were assigned the recurrent biliary colic QALY multiplier to represent failure to return to normal health. Finally, patients treated surgically were assigned the QALY multiplier that represents the surgery they received for the remaining study time horizon. An incremental cost effectiveness ratio (ICER) comparing the study time periods was calculated. As per health economic analysis convention, it was predetermined that only positive ICERs would be reported in the final analysis. Outcomes that both save money and improve clinical outcomes are "dominant strategies" whose magnitude of effect cannot be described by the ICER, nor are the "dominated strategies" that result in greater economic expenditures and lead to worse outcomes. Both of these situations result in negative ICERs whose magnitude offers no practical relevance in terms of decision-aiding.

Table 1 Cost and QALY data

Cost	Value	Source
Outpatient laparoscopic cholecystectomy	$1389	Avg direct cost (OCCP)
Inpatient open cholecystectomy	$10,423	Avg direct cost (OCCP)
Inpatient laparoscopic cholecystectomy	$4349	Avg direct cost (OCCP)
ERCP	$839	Avg direct cost (OCCP)
Ultrasound abdomen	$356	Avg direct cost (OCCP)
CT abdomen	$491	Avg direct cost (OCCP)
ER visit acute cholecystitis	$286	Avg direct cost (OCCP)
Hospital admission cost per day[a]	$776	Derived from OCCP data
Surgeon fee	$478	2011 OMA SOB
Anesthesia unit fee	$15.01	2011 OMA SOB
Cholecystectomy units	7 + time units	2011 OMA SOB
QALY—health states	Value	Source
No biliary disease	1	
Laparoscopic cholecystectomy	0.91	Bass, et. al. 1993 [30]
Recurrent biliary colic	0.8	Cook, et. al. 1993 [29]
Open cholecystectomy	0.77	Bass, et. al. 1993 [30]
Acute pancreatitis	0.44	Cook, et. al. 1993 [29]
Death	0	

OCCP Ontario Case Costing Program 2011 values, *OMA SOB* Ontario Medical Association Schedule of Benefits
[a]Includes indirect costs related to hospital admission

Statistical analysis

Continuous parameters were expressed as mean with standard deviation and nonparametric data were expressed as median and interquartile range. Categorical data were expressed as proportions. We performed one-way ANOVA analysis of variance, Pearson Chi-squared or Mann-Whitney U tests to determine statistical significance, with an alpha of 0.05, depending on the nature of the variable. Multivariate logistic regression was used to determine factors influencing IC performance. The primary clinical outcome was IC rate, and the primary cost end-point was an incremental cost effectiveness ratio (ICER). The student's t test was used to compare each time period (periods 2 and 3) to the reference period of neither site having ACS (period 1). Secondary end-points included length of stay, OR duration, number of ER visits, and re-admissions for gallstone pancreatitis. SPSS Version 20 (IBM Inc., 2011) was used as a statistical platform.

Results

There were a total of 435 patients admitted to general surgery with GSP during the study periods, Table 2. There was no difference with respect to the sex and age of patients in any of the periods. The implementation of an ACS service drastically increased the rate of IC from 16% in period 1 to 76% in period 3 when both sites had an ACS service; Table 3, Fig. 1. When examining the sites separately, there was an increase in IC rate from 19 to 70% ($p < 0.001$) and 25 to 83% ($p < 0.001$) following ACS implementation at sites A and B, respectively. The median ER to OR time for IC was 3.3 days (2.4–4.6) and for elective operation was 53.6 days (18.6–101.4) ($p < 0.001$). In a multivariate model of predicting IC that included age, sex, site of admission, and presence of an ACS service, only age (OR 0.97; 95% CI 0.95–0.98) and the presence of an ACS service (OR 13.6; 95% CI 7.5–24.8) were statistically significant.

A total of 342 patients received definitive surgical management for GSP. The re-admission rate and the number of ER visits for GSP were significantly reduced with the addition of an ACS service, Table 3 and Fig. 1. When considering index, elective, and non-surgery groups, the rates of re-admission were 3, 30, and 29%, respectively ($p < 0.001$). OR duration, postoperative stay, and total length of stay were no different between time periods, Table 3. There was significant cost savings realized when both sites had an ACS service compared to when neither did, Table 3. When comparing influence on patient quality of life, all periods with an ACS service resulted in improved QALY over the fully non-ACS period. During period 2, the average per patient improved by 0.032 QALY ($p < 0.001$) vs period 1 and period 3 the average patient improved by 0.039 QALY ($p = 0.013$), Fig. 2. Regarding costs, implementation of ACS at site A during period 2 resulted in a non-significant average cost increase of \$52 ($p = 0.954$). During period 3, when both sites had established ACS, there was a cost savings of \$1162 ($p = 0.05$) per case compared to period 1. The primary outcome of ICER for period 2 compared to that for period 1 was \$1626/QALY. The ICER for period 3 compared to that for period 1 was negative, and thus, the magnitude is not meaningful and therefore not reported (dominant strategy). Figure 2 displays a cost by QALY chart where the bottom right quadrant represents the ideal scenario of simultaneous cost saving with improved QALY outcomes. ACS at both sites (period 3) suggests both a significant cost saving and improved quality of life for patients.

There was an increase in Monday to Friday, daytime (7 a.m.–5 p.m.) operating room use, 46 to 62% when IC was performed, although this was not significant ($p = 0.32$). There were more ultrasounds performed on patients undergoing an elective operation compared to IC; >25% of patients undergoing an elective operation required more than one ultrasound compared to <10% of patients undergoing an IC ($p < 0.001$). ERCP rates were not statistically different between periods although less ERCPs were performed when both sites had ACS. Patients who did not undergo operative management were more likely to undergo ERCP compared to those undergoing operative management of GSP, 53% compared to 34% ($p < 0.001$).

Table 2 Patient demographics of the three periods, based on the presence of an ACS service

	Period 1	Period 2	Period 3	p value
Number, n	139	241	55	–
Site A, n (%)	73 (53)	127 (53)	32 (58)	0.74
Age, year, mean (SD)	55 (21)	58 (20)	57 (21)	0.45
Male, n (%)	50 (36)	97 (40)	23 (40)	0.65

Period 1: 2008–2010 (no ACS at either site)
Period 2: 2010–2014 (ACS at site A)
Period 3: 2014–2015 (ACS at both sites)

Discussion

The standard of care for uncomplicated GSP is IC, and our results confirm that the presence of ACS services can enable high rates of IC which are robust over time and replicable. Further, our results suggest that IC is exceptionally cost effective, resulting in both fiscal cost savings and improved patient quality of life outcomes. The most favorable ICER was the final period of study, where both sites had an ACS service, suggesting that ACS services deliver high quality and cost-effective care for GSP.

GSP management has shifted over the past decade from the previous preference for a "cooling off" period prior to outpatient cholecystectomy to the modern approach of performing early IC [23, 31–34]. The PONCHO trial, a randomized trial comparing IC to outpatient cholecystectomy confirms the safety and efficacy of definitive management for non-severe GSP on the index admission. Even with the short delay (25–30 days) for elective operation, 18% of patients in this study

Table 3 Comparison of clinical outcomes and total cost between three time periods, based on the presence of an ACS service

	Period 1	Period 2	Period 3	*p* value
Number, *n*	139	241	55	–
Index OR, *n* (%)	22 (16)	120 (50)	42 (76)	<0.001
Elective OR, *n* (%)	85 (61)	67 (28)	6 (11)	<0.001
Inpatient ERCP, *n* (%)	61 (44)	87 (36)	16 (29)	0.11
ER to OR, d, mean (SD)	95 (194)	32 (66)	23 (107)	<0.001
OR duration, minutes	65 (32)	68 (29)	63 (34)	0.44
Open, *n* (%)	6 (4)	9 (4)	0 (0)	–
Postoperative stay, d, mean (SD)	1.5 (1.8)	1.4 (5.7)	1.1 (1.9)	0.87
Total LOS on index admission, days, mean (SD)	5 (3)	6 (9)	5 (3)	0.10
More than one admission for GSP, *n* (%)	47 (34)	30 (12)	4 (7)	<0.001
More than one ER visit for GSP, *n* (%)	58 (42)	32 (13)	9 (16)	<0.001
Time of index OR				
Mon–Fri (7 a.m.–5 p.m.)	10 (46)	73 (61)	26 (62)	0.675
Mon–Fri (5 p.m.–Midnight)	2 (9)	9 (8)	2 (5)	
Mon–Fri (Midnight–7 a.m.)	0 (0)	0 (0)	0 (0)	
Weekend	10 (46)	38 (32)	14 (33)	
Total cost (2011 dollars), mean (SD)	\$9255 (324)	\$9307 (648)	\$8093 (505)	<0.001

Period 1: 2008–2010 (no ACS at either site)
Period 2: 2010–2014 (ACS at site A)
Period 3: 2014–2015 (ACS at both sites)
LOS Length of stay, *ERCP* endoscopic retrograde cholangiopancreatography, *ER* emergency room, *OR* operating room

required re-admission for gallstone-related problems. Our re-admission rate for patients undergoing planned elective surgery was significantly higher, likely due to an even longer delay (194 days) to definitive management in this group. This was similar to the re-admission rate of ~30% seen in the group of patients who did not undergo surgical management. Our findings are consistent with other reports on mild non-severe gallstone pancreatitis [14, 15, 35]. Our previous work demonstrated that our institution had very low IC rates historically, and that the passage of time following the publication of mounting evidence and guidelines encouraging IC only marginally improved our IC rates [4]. It was clear, that at our institution, barriers to IC performance included a lack of operative resources accessible to emergency patients and competition with busy elective practices. Encountering intraoperative surgical difficulty with the "hot gallbladder" has been suggested as another potential additional barrier but has not been confirmed as a valid reason for delaying surgery. Numerous reports suggest cholecystectomy may be easier in the setting of GSP [36, 37]. Indeed, the PONCHO trial included a rating scale of intraoperative surgical difficulty and found no difference [4]. We also did not see an increase in operative time, length of stay, or rate of conversion associated with the increased rate of IC. Implementation of an ACS service with dedicated daytime emergency operative time allowed surgeons to suspend elective practice and facilitated IC achievement.

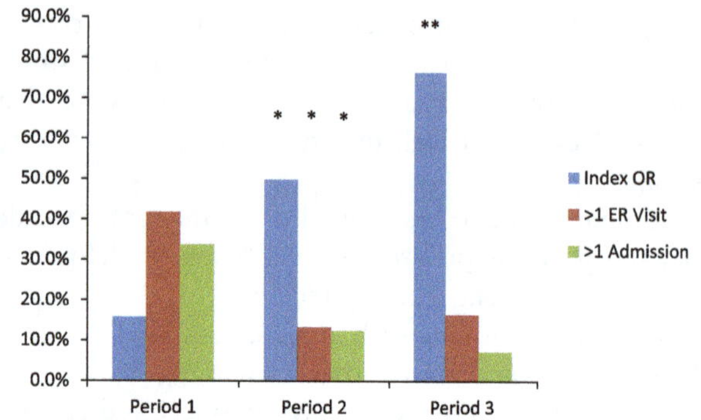

Fig. 1 Rate of index cholecystectomy, emergency room visits, and admissions across the three time periods. (*<0.05 compared to period 1, **<0.05 compared to period 2

De Mestral et al. clearly demonstrate the variation in management of acute biliary disease. In this study, the authors found a fourfold difference in the likelihood of IC at various centers within the province of Ontario, Canada, even for young, healthy male patients with acute cholecystitis [25]. While our study represents some of the first work to demonstrate the increase of IC for uncomplicated GSP resulting from ACS adoption, others have demonstrated similar findings in acute cholecystitis. Pepingco et al. found an increase from 55 to 90% in the rate of IC for acute cholecystitis after the

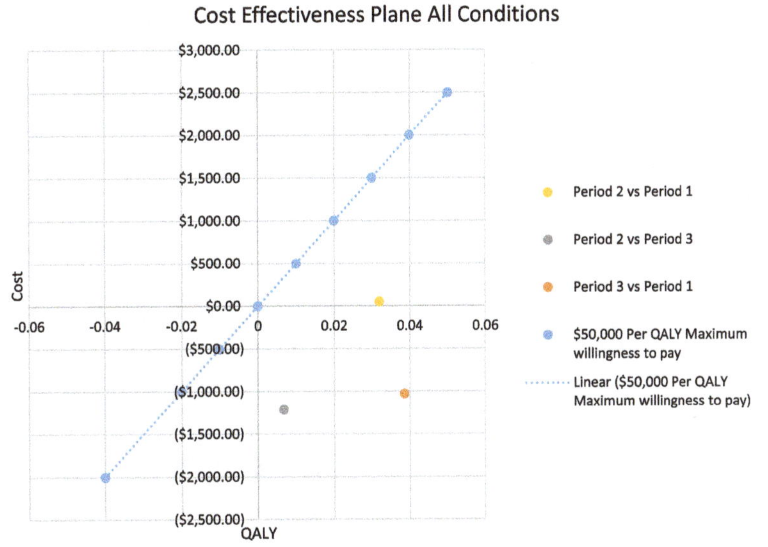

Fig. 2 Cost effectiveness plane for each time period; period 3 (ACS at both sites favored)

addition of an ACS service [5]. Our ACS service has dedicated daytime operating time at one site which we believe facilitates our improved IC rate. We obtained a rate of 76% without a subsequent increase in after-hours or weekend operations. Reports of operative timing for acute cholecystitis vary with some centers reporting an increase in after-hours/weekend operations [38], and others reporting a decrease [5, 9, 11]. Unfortunately, the role of a dedicated operating room is challenging to discern as the reporting on the design of the ACS services in the collective literature is generally poor.

Waiting for an elective operation, including cholecystectomy, significantly impacts quality of life from both potential physical and emotional aspects [39]. Further, quality of life can be impacted by the financial implications of missing work due to emergency room visits, outpatient clinic visits, and hospital re-admissions [40, 41]. For example, the number of patients reporting pain while waiting for surgery in the interval cholecystectomy group in the PONCHO trial was >50%. While other studies have demonstrated the cost savings associated with an ACS service for acute cholecystitis, none have done so for gallstone pancreatitis. We demonstrate significant cost savings of over $1000 per patient when both sites had an ACS service (period 3). This has significant health care resource utilization implications on a national scale given: (1) the number of cholecystectomies are performed on an annual basis and (2) gallstone-related disease is the leading cause of gastrointestinal admission to hospital [42]. Coupled with improved quality of life following cholecystectomy, the resulting negative incremental cost effectiveness ratio suggests both improvement of quality of life and a net cost benefit. Using the results of a Cochrane review on the management of GSP, Morris et al. demonstrated divergent results. In the analysis performed by Morris et al., early laparoscopic cholecystectomy (<72 h) demonstrated a cost reduction which was attributed to decreased length of stay [26]. In contrast, our cost savings results were largely driven by decreased re-admission rates, imaging utilization, and ER visits (while length of stay remained largely unchanged).

Our study is retrospective and is limited by the inherent biases associated with this study design, including identification of GSP patients. Further, we cannot be completely certain that the care of the study patients was contained to our institution and that they did not present elsewhere. Our electronic record does include most neighboring community hospitals and as such, we believe that the potential to miss re-presentations to nearby hospitals is very low but not impossible. Therefore, our results represent a minimum re-admission rate for GSP. In addition, we cannot adequately discern the reason for not undergoing IC and certainly mitigating factors such as patient preference may influence the timing of an operation. Finally, there are numerous other patient and societal factors that we cannot measure directly such as missed work and social welfare costs.

Conclusions

A dedicated ACS service significantly improves rates of IC for GSP in a cost-effective manner that improves quality of life for patients. The increased rate of IC is associated with a similar magnitude in decreased re-admissions, ER visits, and ancillary testing. We believe that our results provide an important quality benchmark (rate of IC) and moreover, suggests that financial costs may no longer be (or at least less of) a barrier to the creation of ACS services than some may have previously thought. In fact, ACS adoption may allow surgical hospitals to achieve the "ultimate outcome", generation of cost savings while providing better quality of care. General surgeons seeking to improve their care of emergency surgery patients via the adoption of an ACS service should consider our results when advocating and negotiating for resources with hospital administration and other stakeholders.

Abbreviations

ACS: Acute care surgery; EGS: Emergency general surgery; ER: Emergency room; ERCP: Endoscopic retrograde cholangiopancreatography; GSP: Gallstone pancreatitis; IC: Index cholecystectomy; ICER: Incremental cost effectiveness ratio; LOS: Length of stay; OR: Operating room; QALY: Quality-adjusted life years

Acknowledgements

Not applicable.

Funding

There was no funding source.

Authors' contributions

All authors contributed to the study design. PM and JK performed data collection and data analysis. RH performed the cost analysis. All authors critically interpreted all data analysis. PM and JK composed the manuscript, and all the remaining authors provided critical edits to the final draft. All authors read and approved the final manuscript.

Competing interests

The authors declare that they have no competing interests.

Author details

[1]Division of General Surgery, Department of Surgery, Schulich School of Medicine and Dentistry, Western University, London, Canada. [2]Divisions of General Surgery Trauma & Critical Care Medicine, University of Toronto, Toronto, Canada. [3]Divisions of Critical Care, Department of Surgery, Schulich School of Medicine and Dentistry, Western University, London, Canada.

References

1. Dinan KA, Davis JW, Wolfe MM, Sue LP, Cagle KM. An acute care surgery fellowship benefits a general surgical residency. J Trauma Acute Care Surg. 2014;77:209–12.
2. Earley AS, Pryor JP, Kim PK, et al. An acute care surgery model improves outcomes in patients with appendicitis. Ann Surg. 2006;244:498–504.
3. Murphy PB, Vogt KN, Mele TS, Hameed SM, Ball CG, Parry NG. Timely Surgical Care for Acute Biliary Disease: An Indication of Quality. Ann Surg. 2016;264(6):913–4.
4. Murphy PB, Paskar D, Parry NG, et al. Implementation of an acute care surgery service facilitates modern clinical practice guidelines for gallstone pancreatitis. J Am Coll Surg. 2015;222:975–81.
5. Pepingco L, Eslick GD, Cox MR. The acute surgical unit as a novel model of care for patients presenting with acute cholecystitis. Med J Aust. 2012;196:509–10.
6. Chana P, Burns EM, Arora S, Darzi AW, Faiz OD. A systematic review of the impact of dedicated emergency surgical services on patient outcomes. Ann Surg. 2015;261:1.
7. Britt RC, Bouchard C, Weireter LJ, Britt LD. Impact of acute care surgery on biliary disease. J Am Coll Surg. 2010;210:595–9. 599–601.
8. Kulvatunyou N, Joseph B, Gries L, et al. A prospective cohort study of 200 acute care gallbladder surgeries: the same disease but a different approach. J Trauma Acute Care Surg. 2012;73:1039–45.
9. Lau B, Difronzo LA. An acute care surgery model improves timeliness of care and reduces hospital stay for patients with acute cholecystitis. Am Surg. 2011;77:1318–21.
10. Lehane CW, Jootun RN, Bennett M, Wong S, Truskett P. Does an acute care surgical model improve the management and outcome of acute cholecystitis? ANZ J Surg. 2010;80:438–42.
11. Lim DW, Ozegovic D, Khadaroo RG, Widder S. Impact of an acute care surgery model with a dedicated daytime operating room on outcomes and timeliness of care in patients with biliary tract disease. World J Surg. 2013; 37:2266–72.
12. Burch JM, Feliciano DV, Mattox KL, Jordan GL. Gallstone pancreatitis. The question of time. Arch Surg. 1990;125:853–9. discussion 859–60.
13. Yadav D, Lowenfels AB. Trends in the epidemiology of the first attack of acute pancreatitis: a systematic review. Pancreas. 2006;33:323–30.
14. Mustafa A, Begaj I, Deakin M, et al. Long-term effectiveness of cholecystectomy and endoscopic sphincterotomy in the management of gallstone pancreatitis. Surg Endosc. 2014;28:127–33.
15. van Baal MC, Besselink MG, Bakker OJ, et al. Timing of cholecystectomy after mild biliary pancreatitis: a systematic review. Ann Surg. 2012;255:860–6.
16. Ito K, Ito H, Whang E. Timing of cholecystectomy for biliary pancreatitis: do the data support current guidelines? J Gastrointest Surg. 2008;12:2164–70.
17. Sanjay P, Yeeting S, Whigham C, et al. Management guidelines for gallstone pancreatitis. Are the targets achievable? JOP. 2009;10:43–7.
18. Sakowska M, McKay J, Lake S, Deacon A. Index cholecystectomy: a continuing challenge for a provincial hospital. N Z Med J. 2013;126:53–9.
19. Creedon L, Neophytou C, PC L, Awan A. Are we meeting the British Society of Gastroenterology guidelines for cholecystectomy post-gallstone pancreatitis? ANZ J Surg. 2016;86(12):1024–7.
20. Tucker JJ, Grim R, Bell T, Martin J, Mueller M, Ahuja V. Changing demographics in laparoscopic cholecystectomy performed in the United States hospitalizations from 1998–2010. J Surg Res. 2014;186:611–2.
21. de Mestral C, Rotstein OD, Laupacis A, Hoch JS, Zagorski B, Nathens AB. A population-based analysis of the clinical course of 10,304 patients with acute cholecystitis, discharged without cholecystectomy. J Trauma Acute Care Surg. 2013;74:26–30. discussion 30–1.
22. da Costa DW, Bouwense S a, Schepers NJ, et al. Same-admission versus interval cholecystectomy for mild gallstone pancreatitis (PONCHO): a multicentre randomised controlled trial. Lancet. 2015;386:1261–8.
23. Gurusamy KS, Nagendran M, Davidson BR. Early versus delayed laparoscopic cholecystectomy for acute gallstone pancreatitis. Cochrane Database Syst Rev. 2013;9:CD010326.
24. Lankisch PG, Weber-Dany B, Lerch MM. Clinical perspectives in pancreatology: compliance with acute pancreatitis guidelines in Germany. Pancreatology. 2005;5:591–3.
25. de Mestral C, Laupacis A, Rotstein OD, et al. Early cholecystectomy for acute cholecystitis: a population-based retrospective cohort study of variation in practice. CMAJ. 2013;1:E62–7.
26. Morris S, Gurusamy KS, Patel N, Davidson BR. Cost-effectiveness of early laparoscopic cholecystectomy for mild acute gallstone pancreatitis. Br J Surg. 2014;101:828–35.
27. National Institute for Health and Clinical Excellence. Methods for the development of NICE public health guidance. London: National Institute for Health and Clinical Excellence; 2012.

28. Ministry of Health and Long Term Care. Ontario Case Costing Program. Available at: https://hsimi.on.ca/hdbportal/. Accessed 15 Oct 2015.
29. Cook J, Richardson JRJ, National Centre for Health Program Evaluation. Quality of life measurement of patients receiving treatments for gallstone disease: options, issues and results. Fairfield: National Centre for Health Program Evaluation; 1993.
30. Bass EB, Pitt HA, Lillemoe KD. Cost-effectiveness of laparoscopic cholecystectomy versus open cholecystectomy. Am J Surg. 1993;165:466–71.
31. Tenner S, Baillie J, DeWitt J, Vege S. American College of Gastroenterology guideline: management of acute pancreatitis. Am J Gastroenterol. 2013;108:1400–15.
32. Forsmark CE, Baillie J. AGA Institute technical review on acute pancreatitis. Gastroenterology. 2007;132:2022–44.
33. UK Working Party on Acute Pancreatitis. UK guidelines for the management of acute pancreatitis. Gut. 2005;54:iii1–9.
34. Uhl W, Warshaw A, Imrie C, et al. IAP guidelines for the surgical management of acute pancreatitis. Pancreatology. 2002;2:585–73.
35. Hwang S, Bonnie H, Philip I. Gallstone pancreatitis without cholecystectomy. JAMA Surg. 2013;148:867–72.
36. Sinha R. Early laparoscopic cholecystectomy in acute biliary pancreatitis: the optimal choice? HPB (Oxford). 2008;10:332–5.
37. Monkhouse SJW, Court EL, Dash I, Coombs NJ. Two-week target for laparoscopic cholecystectomy following gallstone pancreatitis is achievable and cost neutral. Br J Surg. 2009;96:751–5.
38. Michailidou M, Kulvatunyou N, Friese RS, et al. Time and cost analysis of gallbladder surgery under the acute care surgery model. J Trauma Acute Care Surg. 2014;76:710–4.
39. Gurusamy KS, Koti R, Fusai G, Davidson BR. Early versus delayed laparoscopic cholecystectomy for uncomplicated biliary colic. Cochrane Database Syst Rev. 2013;6:CD007196.
40. Garner JP, Sood SK, Robinson J, Barber W, Ravi K. The cost of ignoring acute cholecystectomy. Ann R Coll Surg Engl. 2009;91:39–42.
41. Oudhoff JP, Timmermans DRM, Knol DL, Bijnen AB, van der Wal G. Waiting for elective general surgery: impact on health related quality of life and psychosocial consequences. BMC Public Health. 2007;7:164.
42. Shaheen NJ, Hansen RA, Morgan DR, et al. The burden of gastrointestinal and liver diseases, 2006. Am J Gastroenterol. 2006;101:2128–38.

Introduction of a mass burn casualty triage system in a hospital during a powder explosion disaster

Chip-Jin Ng[1], Shih-Hao You[1], I-Lin Wu[2], Yi-Ming Weng[1,3,4*], Chung-Hsien Chaou[1], Cheng-Yu Chien[5] and Chen-June Seak[1]

Abstract

Background: The triage system used during an actual mass burn casualty (MBC) incident is a major focus of concern. This study introduces a MBC triage system that was used by a burn center during an actual MBC incident following a powder explosion in New Taipei City, Taiwan.

Methods: This study retrospectively analyzed data from patients who were sent to the study hospital during a MBC incident. The patient list was retrieved from a national online management system. A MBC triage system was developed at the study hospital using the following modifiers: consciousness, breathing, and burn size. Medical records were retrieved from electronic records for analysis. Patient outcomes consisted of emergency department (ED) disposition and intervention.

Results: The patient population was predominantly female (56.3%), with an average age of 24.9 years. Mean burn sizes relative to the TBSA of triage level I, II, and III patients were 57.9%, 40.5%, and 8.7%, respectively. ICU length of stay differed markedly according to triage level (mean days for levels I vs II vs III: 57.9 vs 39.9 vs 2.5 days; $p < 0.001$). Triage system levels I and II indicate ICU admission with a sensitivity of 93.9% (95%CI 80.4–98.3%) and a specificity of 86.7% (62.1–96.3%).

Overall, 3 (6.3%) patients were under-triaged. Two (4.2%) patients were over-triaged. Sixteen (48.5%) and 21 (63.6%) patients of triage levels I and II received endotracheal intubation and central venous catheterization, respectively. Sorting of the study population with simple triage and rapid treatment (START) showed great sensitivity (100.0%) but poor specificity (53.3%). The Taiwan Triage and Acuity Scale (TTAS) presented 87.9% sensitivity and 93.9% specificity.

Conclusions: The current MBC triage algorithm served as a good indicator of ED disposition but might have raised excessive immediate attention and had the potential to exhaust the available resources. These findings add to our knowledge of the MBC triage system and should help future researchers in adjusting the triage criteria to fit actual disasters.

Keywords: Triage, Mass casualty incidents, Burns, Explosions, Outcome assessment

* Correspondence: wengym33@gmail.com; yiming33@adm.cgmh.org.tw
[1]Department of Emergency Medicine, Chang Gung Memorial Hospital and Chang Gung University, Linko, Taiwan
[3]Department of Emergency Medicine, Prehospital Care Division, Taoyuan General Hospital, Ministry of Health and Welfare, No. 1492 Zhongshan Rd., Taoyuan Dist, Taoyuan City 330, Taiwan
Full list of author information is available at the end of the article

Background

Mass casualty triage helps first responders to sort victims during a mass casualty incident [1, 2]. The priority of care according to the triage scale indicates response time, transportation, resource allocation, and patient treatment [3, 4]. "Simple triage and rapid treatment" (START), which was developed in the 1980s, is a widely used method [1, 5]. A responder first identifies walking wounded patients (green), followed by sorting patients into immediate (red) and delay (yellow) based on respiratory rate, perfusion, and mental status. A previous study, which evaluated the performance of START via a retrospective review, showed poor agreement between triage levels and outcomes [6–8]. There were concerns about the insufficiency of using START triage in mass burn casualty (MBC) incidents [2]. A universal triage system used in a mass burn casualty (MBC) incident during a gas leak or powder explosion has not been validated [9]. In addition to inhalation injuries, the burn matrix uses age and burn size to classify patients in such circumstances [4, 10, 11]. However, it might not be feasible to rapidly determine a precise burn size when confronted with numerous patients [12]. Nevertheless, the burn matrix might be appropriate for use by a specialist to determine the tier of care 48 h following injury [10]. In short, the optimum approach to MBC triage remains unclear [5]. The development of a MBC triage system based on an actual event should be validated.

Importance

The triage system used during an actual MBC incident is a major focus of concern. Examination of the relationship between triage level and patient outcome can improve the triage system to promote future disaster preparedness.

Goals of this investigation

This study introduces and validates the MBC triage system that was used by a burn center during an actual MBC incident following a powder explosion in New Taipei City, Taiwan.

Methods

Study design and setting

This study retrospectively analyzed data from patients who were sent to the study hospital during a MBC incident on June 27, 2015. The study was approved by the Chang Gung Memorial Hospital (CGMH) Institutional Review Board and was exempted from requiring informed consent and full committee review.

At 20:32 on June 27, 2015, a colored cornstarch powder explosion occurred during a party at the Formosa Fun Water Park in New Taipei City and injured 499 people. Of the injured, 75% suffered from second- to third-degree burns. The Ministry of Health and Welfare activated the regional Emergency Medical Operation Center and informed designated hospitals to prepare for the MBC incident. In total, 48 patients were sent to the study hospital. The first injured patient was registered at the emergency department (ED) at 21:21. Others were admitted over the following 4 h. The hospital activated its mass casualty incident response at 22:00 and ended the incident command system at 01:04 on June 28, 2015.

All triage nurses were trained in a departmental teaching program using the "Taiwan Triage and Acuity Scale" (TTAS). This included reading a manual and participating in workshops twice per year. All triage nurses had completed the program. Patients suffering from burn injuries were classified under the chief complaint category of burn injury (TTAS T1301) with the primary modifiers of respiratory distress (oxygen saturation), level of consciousness (Glasgow Coma Scale, GCS), hemodynamic status (blood pressure), and pain (a numeric pain rating scale). The secondary modifiers included the size of second- to third-degree burns relative to the total body surface area (TBSA). The detailed criteria of different TTAS levels for burn injury are as follows:

TTAS level 1 for burn injury: severe respiratory distress (oxygen saturation < 90%), hemodynamic collapse, or coma (GCS 3–8)
TTAS level 2 for burn injury: moderate respiratory distress (oxygen saturation < 92%), hemodynamic instability, unclear consciousness (GCS 9–13), 2nd- and 3rd-degree burns with a size of > 25%, burn over face/genital area/hand/foot, or suspected inhalation injury.
TTAS level 3 for burn injury: mild respiratory distress (oxygen saturation 92–94%), abnormal blood pressure measurement without signs of shock, pain scale 9–10, or 2nd- and 3rd-degree burns with a size of 5–25%.
TTAS level 4 for burn injury: pain scale 4–7, or 2nd- and 3rd-degree burns with a size of < 5%.
TTAS level 5 for burn injury: pain scale < 4.

However, there was no specific triage system for a MBC incident at the study hospital. Therefore, a MBC triage system, based on the consensus of triage nurses, was developed at the study hospital during this incident (Fig. 1). The triage nurses immediately sorted the patients after a primary survey during the mass casualty incident response. Patients were triaged as level I (emergency), II (urgent), or III (less urgent). Patients who presented with an altered level of consciousness or with any breathing difficulty were considered level I. Patients were then classified according to the individual burn size and body part involved. A burn size of TBSA > 50% or a burn injury over the head and neck area was classified as level I. Instead of a cutoff value of a burn size of > 25%, a TBSA > 50% was considered easier to identify and would garner higher levels of agreement

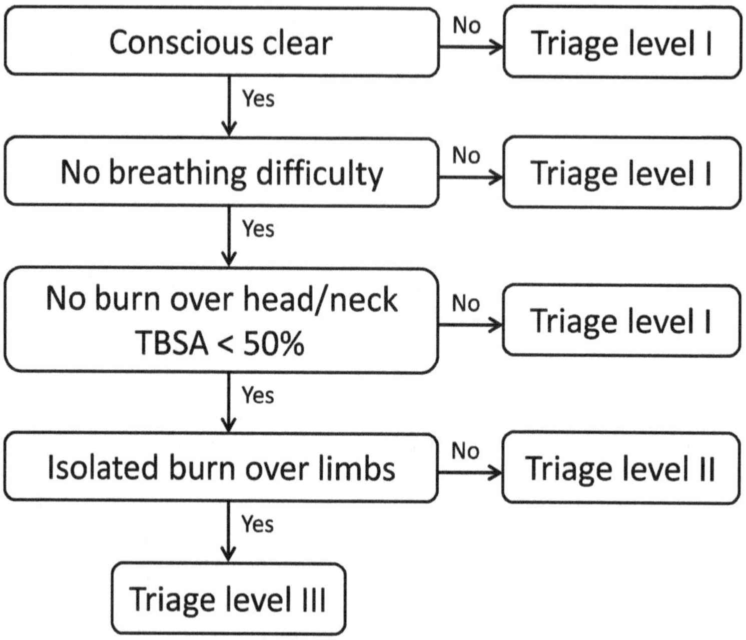

Fig. 1 A mass burn casualty triage system was developed at the study hospital during this incident

among staff. Patients suffering from a burn injury that involved the torso area with TBSA < 50% were classified as level II. Those who presented with isolated limb burn injuries were classified as level III. In contrast to those with isolated limb burn injuries, patients with torso burn injuries might need a bed for further treatment and wound dressing changes.

Patients were then sent to red, yellow, and green zones for treatment according to triage levels I, II, and III, respectively. Patients received endotracheal intubation, central venous line access, and wound care from ED personnel according to their individual conditions. Patients were then either admitted to the intensive care unit (ICU)/ ward or discharged, according to physicians' assessments.

Data collection and processing

Data were collected using several methods. First, on-duty emergency medical technicians registered patients who were affected by the MBC incident. The patient list, designated hospital, and time of registration were abstracted via an online emergency medical management system. Second, the patient list was then confirmed with the ED boarding system of the study hospital. All patients sent to CGMH from the MBC incident at the Formosa Fun Water Park explosion on June 27, 2015, were enrolled. Those who were transferred from other hospitals were excluded. Third, we reviewed the medical records and collected data using a standardized reporting template with clear definitions and codes. Data were retrieved from electronic records.

Background demographic characteristics of the enrolled patients, including age, gender, triage level, 2nd- or 3rd-degree burn size relative to the TBSA, escharotomy or tangential excision of necrotic tissue, number of procedures, abbreviated burn severity index (ABSI), and injury severity score (ISS), were abstracted. Data on ED interventions with endotracheal intubation and/or central venous catheterization (CVC) were recorded. Patient outcomes, including ED disposition (admitted to ICU/ ward, discharged), ICU/ward length of stay (LOS), and mortality, were collected.

To compare the performance of START, TTAS, and the MBC triage used in the study hospital, the study population was assigned to different START/TTAS levels according to the records. The sensitivity and specificity of START and TTAS triage to predict ICU admission were calculated. The TTAS criteria for burn injury are listed above. The study population was retrospectively assigned into different START triage categories based on certain assumptions and the collected data as follows: START triage category immediate (red): unclear consciousness (GCS < 14), respiratory rate > 30, radial pulse absent or mean arterial pressure less than 65 mmHg and START triage category minor (green): patients allocated to the treatment area without beds.

All others patients were assigned to "delay (yellow) category".

Outcome measures

The primary outcome measure was ED disposition, including the proportion of ICU/ward admissions. Secondary outcome measures included ED interventions (i.e., endotracheal intubation, CVC, ICU/hospital LOS, and mortality).

Primary data analysis

Data were analyzed using SPSS software (ver. 13.0 for Windows; SPSS Inc., Chicago, IL, USA). In the descriptive analysis, normality tests for continuous variables were performed. Means and standard deviations were used to describe the central tendency and spread of continuous variables. Categorical variables are presented as counts and percentages and were compared using the chi-squared test or Fisher's exact test. Comparisons between groups in terms of the continuous variables were performed using analysis of variance (ANOVA) as appropriate. A trend test was also used to examine the sequential effect of the triage levels. A Kaplan–Meier survival curve was used to describe relationships between the length-of-stay curves of patients at different triage levels. A log-rank test was used to confirm differences in survival curves. A p value < 0.05 was considered to indicate statistical significance.

Results

Data from 48 patients were analyzed, and the patients' demographic characteristics are presented in Table 1. The study population was predominantly female (56.3%), with an average age of 24.9 years. The mean of 2nd- and 3rd-degree burn sizes relative to the TBSA of triage level I, II, and III patients were 57.9%, 40.5%, and 8.7%, respectively. The outcomes of different triage levels were compared. There was a trend toward a difference between groups at different triage levels with regard to ICU admission (level I vs II vs III, 100.0 vs 89.5 vs 20.0%; $p < 0.001$). There was a significant difference in ED intervention between the groups (level I vs II vs III: endotracheal intubation, 92.9 vs 15.8 vs 6.7%, $p < 0.001$; CVC, 71.4 vs 57.9 vs 6.7%, $p < 0.001$). Overall, 3 (9.1%) patients, who were admitted to the ICU with initial triage level III, were under-triaged. Two patients were admitted to the ICU at the ED, and one was admitted to the ICU via a ward. The first patient, who experienced a

Table 1 Patient characteristics and outcomes comparison between triage levels

	Overall		Triage level I		Triage level II		Triage level III		p value for
	$N = 48$		$N = 14$		$N = 19$		$N = 15$		Difference
Gender, N (%)									0.623
Female	27	(56.3)	9	(64.3)	11	(57.9)	7	(46.7)	
Male	21	(43.7)	5	(35.7)	8	(72.7)	8	(53.3)	
Age in years, mean (SD)	24.9	(8.8)	26.6	(11.6)	25	(9.0)	23.1	(3.5)	0.588
TBSA of 2nd to 3rd-degree of burn (%), mean (SD)	35.6	(23.8)	57.9	(15.4)	40.5	(15.9)	8.7	(7.8)	< 0.001
ED intervention, N (%)									
Endotracheal intubation	17	(35.4)	13	(92.9)	3	(15.8)	1	(6.7)	< 0.001
CVC	22	(45.8)	10	(71.4)	11	(57.9)	1	(6.7)	< 0.001
Surgery, N (%)									< 0.001
Escharotomy	22	(45.8)	12	(85.7)	9	(47.4)	1	(6.7)	
Tangential excision of necrotic skin	17	(35.4)	2	(14.3)	10	(52.6)	5	(33.3)	
No surgery	9	(18.8)	0	(0)	0	(0)	9	(60.0)	
Overall procedures, N (%)	4.3	(3.6)	6.2	(2.3)	5.3	(3.9)	1.0	(1.4)	< 0.001
ED disposition, N (%)									< 0.001
ICU	34	(70.8)	14	(100)	17	(89.5)	3	(20.0)	
Ward	5	(10.4)	0	(0)	2	(10.5)	3	(20.0)	
Discharge	8	(16.7)	0	(0)	0	(0)	8	(53.3)	
Transfer	1	(2.1)	0	(0)	0	(0)	1	(6.7)	
ABSI, mean (SD)	7.3	(2.9)	10.3	(1.6)	7.6	(1.7)	4.1	(1.1)	< 0.001
ISS, mean (SD)	16.5	(13.2)	27.3	(14.1)	19.4	(6.8)	2.7	(2.8)	< 0.001
LOS in days, mean (SD)									
ICU	32.2	(30.9)	57.9	(16.6)	39.9	(30.9)	2.5	(6.6)	< 0.001
Hospital	48.6	(37.0)	73.9	(15.3)	62.2	(36.4)	12.0	(17.1)	< 0.001
Mortality, N (%)	2	(4.2)	2	(14.3)	0	(0)	0	(0)	0.081

Abbreviations: SD standard deviation, *TBSA* total body surface area, *ICU* intensive care unit, *ED* emergency department, *CVC* central venous catheterization, *ABSI* abbreviated burn severity index, *ISS* injury severity score, *LOS* length of stay

20% TBSA burn injury, had full consciousness and normal breathing and was without head or neck burn injury. This patient was triaged as level III at the ED and suffered from shortness of breath during ED boarding 6 h after the accident. The patient received nasal intubation and was then admitted to the ICU. The second and third patients, who experienced 24 and 18% TBSA burn injuries, respectively, were admitted to the ICU. These two patients were admitted due to difficult wound care according to a plastic surgeon's judgment.

In contrast, 2 (6.1%) patients were over-triaged and were classified as levels I and II without mortality or ICU admission. Only one of 15 (6.7%) patients at triage level III received endotracheal intubation and CVC in the ED, whereas 16 (48.5%) and 21 (63.6%) patients at triage levels I and II received endotracheal intubation and CVC, respectively. A total of 22 (45.8%) patients received escharotomy. Table 2 demonstrates the performance of the triage system regarding the prediction of ICU admission, endotracheal intubation, and CVC at the ED. The overall MBC triage system, which indicated levels I and II vs level III, predicted ICU admission with a sensitivity of 93.9% (95%CI 80.4–98.3%) and a specificity of 86.7% (62.1–96.3%).

Both ICU and total hospital LOSs significantly differed between groups. Patients at triage level I had the longest ICU and hospital LOSs, with mean LOSs of 32.2 and 48.6 days, respectively. There was no mortality in the triage level II and III groups, and two deaths occurred in the level I patients. The percentage of time in the ICU according to the total number of hospitalization days in the different groups is plotted in Fig. 2 using a Kaplan–Meier estimate. The survival curves (probability of remaining in the ICU) differed markedly among the triage levels ($p < 0.001$, log-rank test).

Table 3 demonstrates the sensitivity and the specificity of START, TTAS, and the MBC triage categories in predicting ICU admission. While START had 100.0% sensitivity but poor specificity (53.3%), the MBC triage category showed comparable performance with TTAS. The predictability of ED intervention and escharotomy among different triage systems revealed similar findings (TTAS: endotracheal intubation sensitivity/specificity: 94.1%/54.8%; CVC: 90.9%/61.5%; escharotomy: 95.5%/65.4%; START: endotracheal intubation: 100.0%/28.6%; CVC: 100.0%/34.8%; escharotomy: 100.0%/33.3%).

Discussion

Mass casualty incidents have the potential to overwhelm the medical resources of even highly developed nations; thus, a feasible triage strategy is important to ensure that resources are used effectively [1, 13]. Focusing on patient outcomes, this retrospective study examined a triage method used by a medical center during a colored cornstarch powder explosion MBC incident. Several aspects should be discussed in relation to the MBC triage system addressed in this study. During a MBC incident, it might not be practical to determine the triage level by inputting all the modifiers using a computer system or coding book according to the TTAS criteria. TTAS was developed and modified based on the Canada Triage and Acuity Scale (CTAS), which is widely used in Taiwan [14–16]. There was no specific triage method for such a MBC incident. Thus, a modified triage system based on the current method was developed. A MBC triage system developed in such a short period should be simple and easy to use without developing new measurement tools [6, 7]. Additionally, the criteria for different triage levels should be easy to identify and recall and result in as little inter-rater variation as possible. Testing for

Table 2 The performance of the MBC triage system in the study

	ICU admission (%), 95%CI	ET Intubation (%), 95%CI	CVC (%), 95%CI	Escharotomy (%), 95%CI
Triage category I				
Sensitivity	42.4 (27.2–59.2)	76.5 (52.7–90.4)	45.5 (26.9–65.3)	54.6 (34.7–73.1)
Specificity	100.0 (79.6–100.0)	96.8 (83.8–99.4)	84.6 (66.5–93.3)	92.3 (75.9–97.9)
Triage category II				
Sensitivity	51.5 (35.2–67.5)	17.7 (6.2–41.0)	50.0 (30.7–69.3)	40.9 (23.3–61.3)
Specificity	86.7 (62.1–96.3)	48.4 (32.0–65.2)	69.2 (50.0–83.5)	61.5 (42.5–77.6)
Triage category III				
Sensitivity	6.1 (1.7–19.6)	5.9 (1.1–27.0)	4.6 (8.0–21.8)	4.6 (8–21.8)
Specificity	13.3 (3.7–37.9)	54.8 (37.8–70.8)	46.2 (28.8–64.5)	46.2 (28.8–64.5)
Triage category MBC*				
Sensitivity	93.9 (80.4–98.3)	94.1 (73.0–99.0)	95.5 (78.2–99.2)	95.5 (78.2–99.2)
Specificity	86.7 (62.1–96.3)	45.2 (29.2–62.2)	53.9 (35.5–71.2)	53.9 (35.5–71.2)

Abbreviations: MBC mass burn casualty, *ICU* intensive care unit, *CI* confidence interval, *ET* endotracheal tube, *CVC* central venous catheterization

*Triage category MBC indicates the triage categories I and II vs III in predicting ICU admission and interventions

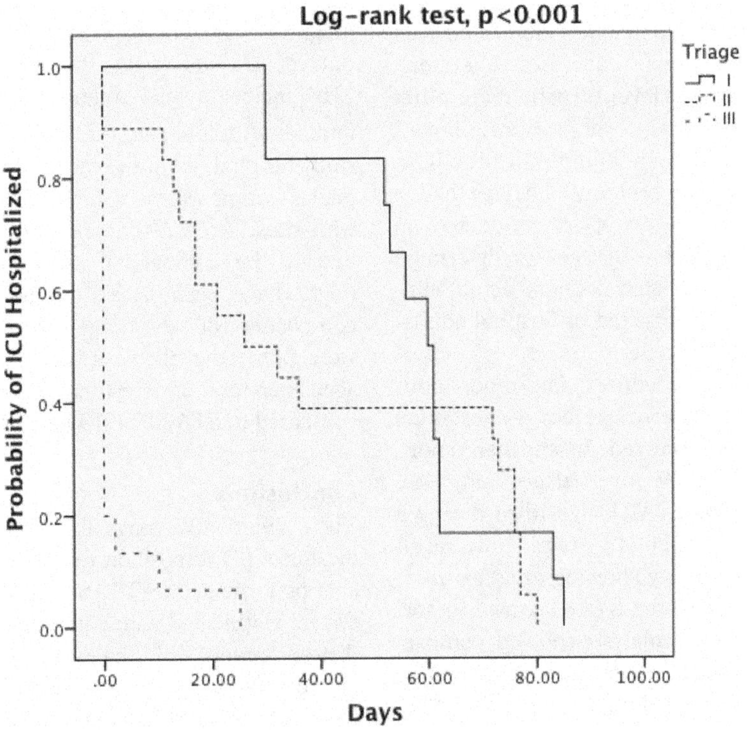

Fig. 2 A Kaplan–Meier survival curve was used to describe relationships between the length-of-stay curves of patients at different triage levels

responsiveness is the universal first step when a first responder approaches a victim [17]. Patients with altered level of consciousness were triaged as level I (red); these patients may require immediate intervention. Second, breathing is assessed. A patient suffering from an inhalation injury might initially present with a normal breathing pattern. Thus, inhalation injuries should be evaluated in terms of any suspicious signs, such as facial burns, nose hair burns, and hoarseness. Once respiratory distress progresses, laryngeal edema might result in a difficult airway, possibly requiring surgical airway establishment [18]. As a result, the study triage protocol stipulated emergency evaluation and management for those who presented with any difficulty in breathing. Third, patients with full consciousness and normal breathing were further classified according to second- and third-degree burn size and body part. TTAS, a five-level triage scale [14], considers a TBSA of > 25% as a secondary modifier to classify patients as level II without age adjustment. More than 40% TBSA affected by second- and third-degree burns in patients aged 20–29.9 years was considered to present a medium-to-low survival rate according the American Burn Association benefit-to-resources grid, which indicates a severe form of injury [9, 10]. This study used a cut-off criterion of 50% TBSA to sort the study population in such a young age group. The current triage algorithm appeared to be a robust screening tool for ED implementation while facing a MBC incident.

Outcome assessment was performed for the enrolled patients. For the primary outcome of ICU admission, the results revealed an acceptable sensitivity (93.9%) but insufficient specificity (86.7%). There was an obvious trend toward a different length of hospital stay between triage levels. The ABSI and ISS also revealed a significant difference between triage levels, which indicated the survival and prognosis. One patient (2.1%) was intubated, and 3 (6.3%) were admitted to the ICU with an initial triage level of III. Approximately half of patients

Table 3 The comparison between different triage systems to predict the ICU admission

	Triage category MBC*	TTAS#	START$
Sensitivity (%), 95% CI	93.9 (80.4–98.3)	87.9 (72.7–95.2)	100.0 (87.1–100.0)
Specificity (%), 95% CI	86.7 (62.1–96.3)	93.3 (70.2–98.8)	53.3 (30.1–75.2)

Abbreviations: ICU intensive care unit, *MBC* mass burn casualty, *CI* confidence interval, *TTAS* Taiwan Triage Acuity Scale, *START* simple triage and rapid treatment
*Triage category MBC indicates the triage categories I and II vs III in predicting ICU admission
#TTAS levels 1 and 2 vs levels 3–5 in predicting ICU admission
$START triage red (immediate) and yellow (delayed) vs green (minor) in predicting ICU admission

in triage level III were admitted for further care. Under-triage may endanger patient safety due to delayed treatment, promoting unfavorable outcomes. Therefore, it is not feasible to divert triage level III patients to other resources. Regarding over-triage, all patients but 2 (4.2%) of triage levels I and II were admitted to the ICU. Previous studies showed that prehospital triage had a high over-triage rate [6–8]. Kahn et al. conducted an outcome assessment after a true disaster to determine whether START triage levels match patients' actual clinical status [6]. The outcome consisted of hospital admission and modified Baxt criteria, such as chest decompression and airway procedures. The report concluded that an acceptable under-triage but a substantial amount of over-triage had occurred. In another report, Hoff et al. also noted 23.3% over-triage and 5.8% under-triage by applying the START algorithm during a state triage tag exercise in 2011 [19]. Our study result echoes that of the previous study showing great sensitivity but very poor specificity of the START triage to sort the study population. Further analysis showed comparable performance of the MBC triage used in this study to that of TTAS but much better specificity than START. However, TTAS and START were applied retrospectively with 100% compliance using all available measurements at ED, which might not be available at the triage area. Therefore, overestimation of the performance of TTAS and START might have occurred. The current MBC triage system performed comparably to TTAS but better than START.

Regarding endotracheal intubation, triage level I identified that 76.4% (13/17) of patients required endotracheal intubation. In contrast, only 45.5% (10/22) of patients who received CVC had been classified as triage level I. Overall triage levels I and II identified approximately 95% patients who required emergent endotracheal intubation and CVC. A validated triage system should be consistent with patient outcomes, and the MBC triage tool used in this study might not precisely identify the immediate intervention needed at ED [20, 21]. Although the current MBC triage algorithm may contribute to ED disposition, resources may be exhausted due to over-triage for immediate needs.

Limitations

This study should be interpreted in the context of the following limitations. First, due to its retrospective nature, small sample size, and specific age group of patients from a single medical center, selection bias may have affected the results. Second, there may have been unmeasured confounders, such as triage nurse experience, the triage criteria used for each patient, the influential factor of physician judgment, and ED disposition. Third, this study was conducted at a university-affiliated teaching hospital after a MBC incident, which might limit the generalizability of the findings. Additionally, the number of patients sent to the study hospital did not exceed the surge capacity of the hospital. A comparison of the validity of these study results with those from a different setting would be of interest. Fourth, the comparison among different triage systems might have been based on assumptions, including full compliance with the triage criteria. In addition, some data were gathered at the treatment area rather than during triage. Therefore, underestimation of the MBC triage system compared to START or TTAS might have occurred.

Conclusions

The current MBC triage algorithm served as a superior indicator of ED disposition relative to START with a comparable performance to TTAS in a MBC incident. This triage system is validated with patient outcomes instead of immediate attention with the potential for resource depletion. The outcomes analysis of the triage system should extend beyond ED disposition and prognosis and encompass emergent intervention. These findings add to our knowledge of the MBC triage system and should help future research to adjust the triage criteria to fit actual disasters.

Abbreviations

ABSI: Abbreviated burn severity index; CGMH: Chang Gung Memorial Hospital; CVC: Central venous catheterization; ED: Emergency department; ICU: Intensive care unit; LOS: length of stay; MBC: Mass burn casualty; START: Simple triage and rapid treatment; TBSA: Total body surface area; TTAS: Taiwan Triage and Acuity Scale

Acknowledgements

We thank the Ministry of Health and Welfare for helping with data collection.

Authors' contributions

YSH, WIL, NCJ, and WYM conceived the study. NCJ supervised the data collection. CCY, CCH, and WIL recruited the participating patients and managed the data, including quality control. NCJ, CCH, and CCY provided statistical advice and analyzed the data. NCJ and SCJ chaired the data oversight committee. NCJ, YSH, and WYM drafted the manuscript, and all authors contributed substantially to its revision. NCJ take responsibility for the paper as a whole. All authors read and approved the final manuscript.

Competing interests

The authors declare that they have no competing interests.

Author details

[1]Department of Emergency Medicine, Chang Gung Memorial Hospital and Chang Gung University, Linko, Taiwan. [2]Department of Emergency, Taoyuan

Armed Forces General Hospital, Taoyuan, Taiwan. [3]Department of Emergency Medicine, Prehospital Care Division, Taoyuan General Hospital, Ministry of Health and Welfare, No. 1492 Zhongshan Rd., Taoyuan Dist, Taoyuan City 330, Taiwan. [4]Faculty of Medicine, National Yang-Ming University School of Medicine, Taipei, Taiwan. [5]Department of Emergency Medicine, Ton-Yen General Hospital, Zhubei, Hsinchu County, Taiwan.

References

1. Schultz CH, Koenig KL, Noji EK. A medical disaster response to reduce immediate mortality after an earthquake. N Engl J Med. 1996;334(7): 438–44.
2. Atiyeh B, Gunn SW, Dibo S. Primary triage of mass burn casualties with associated severe traumatic injuries. Ann Burns Fire Disasters. 2013;26(1): 48–52.
3. Kearns RD, Hubble MW, Holmes JH, Cairns BA. Disaster planning: transportation resources and considerations for managing a burn disaster. J Burn Care Res. 2014;35(1):e21–32.
4. Cairns BA, Stiffler A, Price F, Peck MD, Meyer AA. Managing a combined burn trauma disaster in the post-9/11 world: lessons learned from the 2003 West Pharmaceutical plant explosion. J Burn Care Rehabil. 2005; 26(2):144–50.
5. Benson M, Koenig KL, Schultz CH. Disaster triage: START, then SAVE––a new method of dynamic triage for victims of a catastrophic earthquake. Prehosp Disaster Med. 1996;11(2):117–24.
6. Kahn CA, Schultz CH, Miller KT, Anderson CL. Does START triage work? An outcomes assessment after a disaster. Ann Emerg Med. 2009;54(3):424–30. 30 e1
7. Bhalla MC, Frey J, Rider C, Nord M, Hegerhorst M. Simple triage algorithm and rapid treatment and sort, assess, lifesaving, interventions, treatment, and transportation mass casualty triage methods for sensitivity, specificity, and predictive values. Am J Emerg Med. 2015;33(11):1687–91.
8. Hong R, Sexton R, Sweet B, Carroll G, Tambussi C, Baumann BM. Comparison of START triage categories to emergency department triage levels to determine need for urgent care and to predict hospitalization. Am J Disaster Med. 2015;10(1):13–21.
9. McGregor JC. Major burn disasters: lessons to be learned from previous incidents and a need for a national plan. Surg J R Coll Surg Edinb Irel. 2004; 2(5):249–311.
10. Conlon KM, Ruhren C, Johansen S, Dimler M, Frischman B, Gehringer E, et al. Developing and implementing a plan for large-scale burn disaster response in New Jersey. J Burn Care Res. 2014;35(1):14–20.
11. Taylor S, Jeng J, Saffle JR, Sen S, Greenhalgh DG, Palmieri TL. Redefining the outcomes to resources ratio for burn patient triage in a mass casualty. J Burn Care Res. 2014;35(1):41–5.
12. Cairns BA, Stiffler A, Price F, et al. Managing a combined burn trauma disaster in the post-9/11 world: lessons learned from the 2003 West Pharmaceutical plant explosion. J Burn Care Rehabil. 2005;26(2):144–50.
13. Garner A, Lee A, Harrison K, Schultz CH. Comparative analysis of multiple-casualty incident triage algorithms. Ann Emerg Med. 2001;38(5):541–8.
14. Ng CJ, Yen ZS, Tsai JC, Chen LC, Lin SJ, Sang YY, et al. Validation of the Taiwan triage and acuity scale: a new computerised five-level triage system. Emerg Med J. 2011;28(12):1026–31.
15. Jimenez JG, Murray MJ, Beveridge R, Pons JP, Cortes EA, Garrigos JB, et al. Implementation of the Canadian Emergency Department Triage and Acuity Scale (CTAS) in the Principality of Andorra: can triage parameters serve as emergency department quality indicators? CJEM. 2003;5(5):315–22.
16. Bullard MJ, Unger B, Spence J, Grafstein E, Group CNW. Revisions to the Canadian Emergency Department Triage and Acuity Scale (CTAS) adult guidelines. CJEM. 2008;10(2):136–51.
17. Kleinman ME, Brennan EE, Goldberger ZD, Swor RA, Terry M, Bobrow BJ, et al. Part 5: adult basic life support and cardiopulmonary resuscitation quality: 2015 American Heart Association Guidelines Update for Cardiopulmonary Resuscitation and Emergency Cardiovascular Care. Circulation. 2015;132(18): 414–35.
18. Cancio LC. Airway management and smoke inhalation injury in the burn patient. Clin Plast Surg. 2009;36(4):555–67.
19. Hoff JJ, Carroll G, Hong R. Presence of undertriage and overtriage in simple triage and rapid treatment. Am J Disaster Med. 2017;12(3):147–54.
20. Dong SL, Bullard MJ, Meurer DP, et al. Predictive validity of a computerized emergency triage tool. Acad Emerg Med. 2007;14:16–21.
21. Wuerz RC, Milne LW, Eitel DR, et al. Reliability and validity of a new five-level triage instrument. Acad Emerg Med. 2000;7:236–42.

Focus on the prophylaxis, epidemiology and therapy of methicillin-resistant *Staphylococcus aureus* surgical site infections and a position paper on associated risk factors: the perspective of an Italian group of surgeons

G. Sganga[1*], C. Tascini[2], E. Sozio[3], M. Carlini[4], P. Chirletti[5], F. Cortese[6], R. Gattuso[7], P. Granone[8], C. Pempinello[9], M. Sartelli[10] and S. Colizza[11]

Abstract

Background: The aim of this research was to study the epidemiology, microbiology, prophylaxis, and antibiotic therapy of surgical site infections (SSIs), especially those caused by methicillin-resistant *Staphylococcus aureus* (MRSA), and identify the risk factors for these infections. In Italy SSIs occur in about 5 % of all surgical procedures. They are predominantly caused by staphylococci, and 30 % of them are diagnosed after discharge. In every surgical specialty there are specific procedures more associated with SSIs.

Methods: The authors conducted a systematic review of the literature on SSIs, especially MRSA infections, and used the Delphi method to identify risk factors for these resistant infections.

Results: Risk factors associated with MRSA SSIs identified by the Delphi method were: patients from long-term care facilities, recent hospitalization (within the preceding 30 days), Charlson score > 5 points, chronic obstructive pulmonary disease and thoracic surgery, antibiotic therapy with beta-lactams (especially cephalosporins and carbapenem) and/or quinolones in the preceding 30 days, age 75 years or older, current duration of hospitalization >16 days, and surgery with prothesis implantation. Protective factors were adequate antibiotic prophylaxis, laparoscopic surgery and the presence of an active, in-hospital surveillance program for the control of infections. MRSA therapy, especially with agents that enable the patient's rapid discharge from hospital is described.

Conclusion: The prevention, identification and treatment of SSIs, especially those caused by MRSA, should be implemented in surgical units in order to improve clinical and economic outcomes.

Keywords: Surgical site infection, MRSA, Dalbavancin

* Correspondence: gsganga@sepsi.org
[1]Istituto Clinica Chirurgica, Divisione Chirurgia Generale e Trapianti d'Organo, Università Cattolica del Sacro Cuore, Fondazione Policlinico Universitario Agostino Gemelli, Rome, Italy
Full list of author information is available at the end of the article

Background

Surgical site infections (SSIs) remain a major clinical problem in terms of morbidity, mortality, time spent in hospital and overall direct and indirect costs [1–3]. Despite progress in their prevention, SSIs remain one of the most common adverse events in hospitals, accounting for 11 % to 26 % of all healthcare-associated infections [4]. Surgical patients can develop several post-operative infections; wound infections, are common causes of post-operative morbidity and prolonged hospitalization. SSIs increase the total hospital bill by an additional 10–20 % [5], lead to 80,000 deaths and are associated with an annual treatment cost of two billion US dollars [6]. *S. aureus* SSIs can be life-threatening, being associated with a mortality rate of 5 %, more than 2 extra weeks of time spent in hospital and around an extra cost of 50,000 US dollars [7].

Nearly 60 % of SSIs are diagnosed after discharge from the hospital. This percentage is rising as the post-operative stay in hospital is getting shorter and the number of 1-day surgical procedures is increasing over time [8]. The Diagnosis Related-Group (DRG) system underestimates the rate of SSIs because of the very early discharge of surgical patients. The exact incidence of SSIs is, therefore, difficult to determine. According to current literature, active SSI surveillance is useful in reducing the incidence of SSIs by surveillance-induced infection control efforts [9]. When any prosthesis is implanted into the body during general surgery, cardiac surgery, orthopaedics, etc., beside *S. aureus*, Coagulase-negative Staphylococci, especially *S. epidermidis*, may be the cause of severe infections that can necessitate removal of the prosthesis.

Classification of surgical site infections

The identification of SSIs involves interpretation of clinical and laboratory findings. The Centers for Disease Control and Prevention's (CDC) National Nosocomial Infections Surveillance system has developed standardized surveillance criteria for defining SSIs [10]. According to these criteria, SSIs are classified as being either incisional or organ/space. Incisional SSIs are further divided into those involving only skin and subcutaneous tissue (superficial incisional SSIs) and those involving deeper soft tissues of the incision (deep incisional SSIs).

Superficial incisional surgical site infections

The infection occurs within 30 days after the operation and involves only the skin or subcutaneous tissue at the incision and at least one of the following:

1. purulent drainage, with or without laboratory confirmation, from the superficial incision;
2. organisms isolated from an aseptically obtained culture of fluid or tissue from the superficial incision;
3. at least one of the following signs or symptoms of infection: pain or tenderness, localized swelling, redness, or heat; the site is deliberately opened by the surgeon, unless ithe incision is culture-negative.

Deep incisional surgical site infections

The infection occurs within 30 days after the operation if no implant is left in place or within 1 year if an implant is left in the body and the infection appears to be related to the operation and involves deep soft tissues (e.g., fascial and muscle layers) at the incision site and at least one of the following:

1. purulent drainage from the deep incision but not from the organ/space component of the surgical site;
2. a deep incision spontaneously dehisces or is deliberately opened by a surgeon when the patient has at least one of the following signs or symptoms: fever (>38 °C), localized pain, or tenderness, unless the site is culture-negative.
3. an abscess or other evidence of infection involving the deep incision is found on direct examination, during reoperation, or by histopathological or radiological examination.

Organ/space surgical site infections

The infection occurs within 30 days after the operation if no implant is left in place or within 1 year if an implant is left in the body and the infection appears to be related to the operation and involves any part of the anatomy (e.g., organs or spaces), other than the incision, which was opened or manipulated during an operation and at least one of the following:

1. purulent drainage from a drain that is placed through a stab wound into the organ/space.
2. organisms isolated from an aseptically obtained culture of fluid or tissue in the organ/space.
3. an abscess or other evidence of infection involving the organ/space that is found on direct examination, during reoperation, or by histopathological or radiological examination.

Recently, the Food and Drug Administration (FDA) proposed a new classification of skin and soft tissue infections, namely acute bacterial skin and skin structure infections (ABSSSIs), incorporating erysipelas, cellulitis, major subcutaneous abscesses and wound infections including SSIs. An ABSSSI is a bacterial infection of the skin with a lesion area of at least 75 cm^2, measured by redness, edema, or induration [11]. ABSSSIs represent a significant burden for the health-care system, with increasing incidence and severity in recent years, and they have become a challenging medical problem associated with high direct and indirect costs to both the medical system and society. Among the various ABSSSIs, SSIs caused by MRSA may have an important impact on hospital budgets and on patients' health. The rationale for introducing this terminology was to provide a consistent means of identifying infections for which a reliable drug treatment effect can be estimated and of correctly stratifying patients with this kind of infection included in clinical trials.

Microbiological epidemiology

According to the National Nosocomial Infection Surveillance system reports, Gram-positive cocci (particularly *S. aureus*, coagulase-negative staphylococci and *Enterococcus* spp.), followed by *Escherichia coli, Pseudomonas aeruginosa* and *Enterobacter* spp., are the most commonly encountered pathogens in SSIs [12]. In most cases, the source of pathogens is the endogenous flora of the patient's skin, mucous membranes, or hollow viscera [13]. When mucous membranes or the skin are incised, the exposed tissues are at risk of contamination by endogenous flora [14]. These micro-organisms are usually aerobic Gram-positive cocci (e.g., staphylococci), but may include fecal flora (e.g., anaerobic bacteria and Gram-negative aerobes) when incisions are made near the perineum or groin. Exogenous sources of SSI pathogens include surgical personnel (especially members of the surgical team), the operating room environment (including air), and all equipment, instruments, and materials brought to the sterile field during an operation. Exogenous flora consists primarily of aerobes, especially Gram-positive organisms (e.g., staphylococci and streptococci) [15].

Table 1 presents the more frequent pathogens according to the surgical procedure.

Methicillin-resistant *Staphylococcus aureus*

Methicillin-resistant *Staphylococcus aureus (*MRSA) is a versatile and dangerous bacterial pathogen, combining virulence, antibiotic resistance, and survival fitness [16]. Its spread is facilitated by cross-transmission through health-care workers' hands and selection pressure exercised by broad-spectrum antibiotic treatment. MRSA infections represent a substantial burden, because they increase treatment costs and can cause excess morbidity and mortality. Since MRSA carriers without symptomatic infection are an important reservoir and source of spread of infections, risk profiles to identify patients at high risk of carrying MRSA might improve prevention of MRSA infections [17].

The control of SSIs within the hospital is important, as is identifying patients at risk of being colonized and subsequently infected by multi-drug resistant microorganisms such as MRSA; surveillance itself, even without any specific intervention, has been associated with a

Table 1 More frequent pathogens according to the surgical procedure

Type of surgery	Likely Pathogens
Placement of all grafts, prostheses, or implants	*S. aureus*, coagulase negative staphylococci
Cardiac	*S. aureus*, coagulase negative staphylococci
Neurosurgery	*S. aureus*, coagulase negative staphylococci
Breast	*S. aureus*, coagulase negative staphylococci
Ophthalmic (limited data, however, commonly used in procedures such as anterior segment resection, vitrectomy, and scleral buckles)	*S. aureus*, coagulase negative staphylococci, streptococci, gram-negative bacilli
Orthopedic (Total joint replacement, closed fractured/use of nails, bone plates, other internal fixation device, functional repair without implant/device trauma)	*S. aureus*, coagulase negative staphylococci, gram-negative bacilli
Non-cardiac thoracic (lobectomy, pneumonectomy, wedge resection, other non-cardiac mediastinal procedures) Closed tube thoracotomy	*S. aureus*, coagulase negative staphylococci, *S. pneumoniae*, gram-negative bacilli
Vascular	*S. aureus*, coagulase negative staphylococci
Appendectomy	Gram-negative bacilli, anaerobes
Biliary tract	Gram-negative bacilli, anaerobes
Colorectal	Gram-negative bacilli, anaerobes
Gastroduodenal	Gram-negative bacilli, streptococci, oropharyngeal anaerobes (e.g. peptostreptococci)
Head and neck (majorly procedures with incision through oropharyngeal mucosa)	*S. aureus*, streptococci, oropharyngeal anaerobes (e.g. peptostreptococci)
Obstetric and gynecologic	Gram-negative bacilli, enterococci, group B streptococci, anaerobes
Urologic	Gram-negative bacilli

reduction in the incidence of SSIs, which is another reason to recommend implementation of surveillance systems [18].

According to the new ABSSSI classification, erysipelas and cellulitis are mostly due to Gram-positive organisms whereas SSIs and subcutaneous abscesses are due to mixed flora including Gram-positive microbes.

The epidemiology of surgical site infections in Italy

In Italy the incidence rate of SSIs might be around 5 % (Table 2). Hospitals without a surveillance system that report rates less than 5 % probably underestimate the problem. In fact many SSIs are diagnosed more than 30 days after surgery, when the patient has already been discharged from hospital. The overall incidence rate of SSIs in Italy in the past was higher, ranging from 5.4 % up to 12.8 % [19, 20]. In Europe, considering only general, gynecological (including Cesarean sections), and vascular surgery, SSIs rates are higher and range from 6.34 % to 14.8 % [21].

Petrosillo et al. reported that SSIs occurred in 5.2 % of 4,665 patients. Of these SSIs, 148 (61.4 %) developed during the patients' stay in hospital, and 93 (38.6 %) within 30 days after discharge. Of the 148 in-hospital SSIs, 87, 37, and 24 were classified as superficial, deep, and organ/space, respectively. Post-discharge SSIs observed at medical follow-up were all superficial [21].

This study also produced information on post-discharge SSIs; the authors found that 38.6 % of SSIs were diagnosed after the patients' discharge from hospital; this rate is comparable to the 34.8 % reported by Fiorio et al. [22] in Italian general surgery in-patients, although other similar surveillance studies [23] found considerably higher post-discharge SSIs rates, ranging from 34.8 % to 60 %.

Marchi et al. reported data on non-prosthetic surgery from the Italian SSI surveillance program for the period 2009 to 2011. In the 355 surgical wards included in the study, 60,460 operations were recorded. SSIs were observed in 1,628 cases (2.6 %) and 60 % of the infections were diagnosed through 30-day post-discharge surveillance. Operations performed in hospitals with at least 2 years of surveillance showed a 29 % lower risk of SSIs, confirming that surveillance is a protective factor for preventing SSIs [24].

Table 3 reports the probability of developing a post-discharge SSI according to type of surgery performed. Used vascular surgery as the benchmark (0 % of infections after discharge) each number represents the probability of a post-discharge diagnosis of a SSI.

Specific types of surgical procedures and surgical site infections

Hernia and abdominal wall surgery

Although this type of surgery is "clean and easy" to perform, the usual application of meshes might expose patients to a higher risk of SSIs.

According to the Italian Society of Hernia and Abdominal Wall Surgery, 210,000 surgical procedures per year are performed on the abdominal wall in Italy; this kind of procedure is, therefore, the most common type in Italy. These procedures comprise 170,000 inguinal hernia repairs per year, and 40,000 parietal hernia repairs, with this latter group including 20,000 incisional hernias. Almost all of these procedures are performed using meshes in order to reduce the incidence of recurrence and to achieve closure of the abdominal wall defect avoiding abdominal hypertension and respiratory complications. The use of meshes may increase the risk of SSIs caused by difficult-to-treat microorganisms such as *S. aureus*, coagulase-negative staphylococci and multidrug-resistant nosocomial Gram-negative organism [25], leading to infection of the mesh itself.

Despite hernia repairs being classified as "clean" operations, the use of synthetic material has been associated with a theoretical increase in infectious risk. Although routine use of prophylactic antibiotics is not recommended for open, non-implant herniorrhaphy, there is little direct clinical evidence on which to base recommendations when an implantable mesh is used. No SSIs occurred following 120 mesh herniorrhaphies performed without routine antibiotic administration [26]; however, the incidence of SSIs varies, depending on the different case series, ranging from 1–2 % to 3–4 %.

Mesh infection, although infrequent, is a devastating complication of mesh hernioplasties. The crude mesh infection rate was 5 % in a recent meta-analysis. Statistically significant risk factors were smoking, American Society of Anesthesiologists (ASA) score C3 and emergency operation; mesh infections were also significantly correlated with the patients' age and the duration of the

Table 2 SSI epidemiology in Italy

Authors	Country	Period	Number of surgeries	SSIs
Petrosillo et al.	Italy, multicenter	2002, Prospectively for one month in 48 hospitals	4.665	241 (5,2 %)
Marchi et al.	Italy, multicenter	2009–2001, retrospective, 355 surgical departments	60.460	1.628 (2,6 %)
Fiorio et al.	Italy, multicenter	2002, Prospectively for one month in 48 hospitals, 32 surgical departments	2.972	158 (5,2 %)

Table 3 Probability to have a post-discharge SSIs according to type of surgery performed

Surgery	Ratio between post-discharge SSIs and in-hospital SSIs
Vascular surgery	0
Breast surgery	3,4
Cesarean section	2,5
Cholecistectomy	1,2
Gastric surgery	0,4
Appendectomy	0,2
Colon surgery	0,1
Hernia repair	1,4
Abdominal hysterectomy	0,6
Vaginal hysterectomy	1

hernioplasty. A trend toward higher mesh infection rates was observed in obese patients. The usual causative organisms associated with cases of mesh infection are *Staphylococcus* spp., especially *S. aureus*, *Streptococcus* spp. (including group B streptococci), Gram-negative bacteria (mainly Enterobacteriaceae), and anaerobic bacteria (including *Peptostreptococcus* spp.) [25]. In a study of mesh-related infections following incisional herniorrhaphy, 63 % of the microorganisms isolated were MRSA [27].

Table 4 shows the microbiology of prosthetic infection after hernia or ventral mesh repair.

Theoretically, surgical treatment of infected mesh hernioplasties requires removal of the implant and then implantation of a new mesh; conservative treatments, such as drainage or sinus resection, are usually unsuccessful. Tolino et al. reported on 51 operations to treat 32 patients with mesh infections: removal of the mesh, recurrence and bowel fistulas were described [28].

Every year in Italy there are probably about 1,700 infections of inguinal hernioplasties and 4,000 infections of ventral hernioplasties (for %1 and 10 % rates of infective complications, respectively). The role of *S. aureus* and MRSA in the etiology of these complications is very strong [28, 29].

Table 4 Microbiology of prosthetic infection (1 day- > 1 year) after haernia or ventral mesh repair

Microbiology of prosthetic infection (1 day- > 1 year) after haernia or ventral mesh repair	
Staphylococcus aureus	50–60 %
Staphylococcus spp	10–20 %
Enterococcus spp	10–20 %
Gram-neg	5–10 %
Pseudomonas, *Streptococcus spp*, *Mycobacteria spp*, mixed flora	rare

Vascular surgery

The incidence of SSIs at the groin after vascular procedures ranges from 3 % to 44 % [30]. Factors contributing to the increased incidence of SSIs in this subset of patients include disruption of the lymphatic system, proximity of the surgical site to the perineum and external urinary organs, and prosthetic graft placement. It must be emphasized that the groin area contains a substantial number of lymph nodes which have a priority role in draining the entire lower limb and an incorrect surgical technique often leads to lymphorrhea with a subsequent SSI. A SSI following vascular surgery is a complication that may lead not only to healing problems, but also to limb loss and the risk of death. Furthermore, it is assumed to be a risk factor for deeper infections extending to the graft, which are associated with catastrophic consequences: a death rate between 15 % and 75 % and a major amputation rate of up to 70 %. Even when treatment is successful, the morbidity associated with vascular graft infection is considerable, the outcomes often being worse than the natural history of the vascular condition that led to implantation of the graft.

A SSI always implies prolongation of the time spent in hospital, higher hospital costs and greater morbidity for the patient. Groin incisions play a central role in various vascular operations. In addition to their traditional use in bypass procedures, endarterectomies and thromboembolectomies, more than 95 % of all percutaneous interventions are performed via the femoral access. The increasing prevalence of infections by multiresistant bacteria has been associated with worsened outcomes. Although the management of groin SSIs is well documented, there is little published information about the incidence and classification of these infections. Many authors consider that diabetes, as well as obesity, has a relatively minor role in initiating groin wound infections. Besides general aseptic measures, the only strategy that significantly reduces the incidence of SSIs is prophylactic systemic antibiotics, administered only preoperatively. There is no "gold standard" treatment of these infections. The initial treatment generally includes surgical debridement and antibiotics. Pharmacological therapy is very often prolonged for several weeks but with uncertain results. Secondary interventions have been attempted with limited success; such interventions include rotational flaps, wound vacuum-assisted closure, alginate dressing, graft excision and extra-anatomic or in situ bypass or patch replacement using autologous, rifampin-soaked or silver-impregnated materials.

Thoracic surgery

Thoracic surgery includes a wide variety of operations involving the lungs and pleural cavities, mediastinum, oesophagus and neck.

The most common surgical incisions in thoracic surgery are thoracotomies, cervicotomies, and thoraco-abdominal incisions; sternotomies are less common.

The overall incidence of SSIs in thoracic surgery has been estimated to be around 2–4 %.

Esophageal surgery, especially when the indication is cancer, is the operation most frequently complicated by SSIs, accounting for up to 15 % of cases due to radical dissection, difficult reconstruction, frequent concomitant colonization, and patients being at higher risk because of concomitant conditions (age, smoking, alcoholism, malnutrition, etc.).

The most common procedure, thoracotomy for lung cancer, has been estimated to be complicated by SSIs in only 2 % to 5 % of cases. However, this type of SSI can produce serious discomfort for the patient, due to the need for ongoing medication, pain, difficulty with breathing with the risk of developing more serious infections such as pneumonia, pleural empyema and mediastinitis.

Most recently mini-invasive thoracic approaches and video-assisted thoracoscopic surgery have reduced the overall wound infection rate to a mean of 1.7 % [31].

Deep sternal infections in cardiothoracic surgery, despite accounting only for 1–4 % cases, can be associated with ten-fold higher mortality rate.

An American study from 2002 showed that risk factors for deep and superficial chest SSIs after coronary artery bypass surgery differ, suggesting different etiopathogenesis. However, some of the risk factors for thoracic SSIs are well known, such as age, smoking, diabetes, obesity and, in particular, chronic obstructive pulmonary disease requiring pre-operative treatment with systemic antibiotics and nebulisers [32]. The need for neoadjuvant chemoradiotherapy in advanced cancer is another independent risk factor.

It seems obvious that all the risk factors for postoperative infections in such fragile patients become even more critical because the infections are caused by multi-resistant organisms. The main sources of multi-resistant infections are Gram-positive bacteria, particularly MRSA, but other sources, such as fungi, are becoming increasingly common.

Orthopedic surgery

Because orthopedic procedures are performed in a variety of inpatient and outpatient settings, increased vigilance, strict adherence to aseptic technique, attention to adequacy of reprocessing and management of intraoperative breaches of sterile technique are vitally important to ensure a safe and consistent standard of care.

According to the National Healthcare Safety Network report, which includes data from 2006 to 2008 in the USA, the total number of patients who develop SSIs following any type of orthopedic surgery is somewhere between 31,000 and 35,000 [33]. SSIs in orthopedic surgery prolong total hospital stay by a median of 2 weeks per patient, approximately double readmission rates, and increase health care costs by more than 300 %. Moreover, patients with SSIs have substantially greater physical limitations and significant reductions in their quality of life [33].

The rates of SSIs following orthopedic procedures appear to be increased when certain risk factors are present. Risk factors can be either patient modifiable or not modifiable and/or procedure-specific, in which case they may again be modifiable or not modifiable.

Hair removal, perioperative normothermia, preoperative skin preparation, nasal decolonization, health problems and situations predisposing the patient to infection, skin antisepsis, surgical hand antisepsis, antibiotic prophylaxis, air quality, double gloves, traffic pattern gowns and drapes, bone cement, and sterility assurance are key factors for controlling the risk of infections.

Although the use of antimicrobial sutures is not routine practice, the benefits of this strategy are becoming increasingly apparent [34]. Likewise, advances in antimicrobial coatings for implants, instruments, equipment and the environment may provide additional support to reach the goal of no SSIs. The practice of prescreening patients prior to surgery is recommended, as part of a comprehensive program to eliminate SSIs in orthopedic surgery, especially in cases involving an implantable device.

Type of surgery and risk of surgical site infections

Attempts have been made to quantify the risk of SSIs following types of surgery other than operations to the abdominal wall..

De Lissovoy et al. performed a study with the aim of analyzing the surgical procedures associated with the highest rate of SSIs; they studied 723,490 discharges from surgery units in 2005, identifying SSIs from the presence of The International Classification of Diseases, Ninth Revision, Clinical Modification (ICD-9-CM) code 998.59. They divided surgical procedures into seven categories: neurological; cardiovascular, colorectal, skin, subcutaneous and breast; gastrointestinal, orthopedic and obstetric-gynecological. This made it possible to quantify the risk of SSIs according to the type of surgical procedure used.

Table 5 lists the five most frequent surgical procedures by category with respect to the incidence of SSIs.

Antimicrobial prophylaxis

The prevention of SSIs is an important issue in surgery. Besides general strategies aimed at reducing the rate of SSIs (hair removal, asepsis of the operating room,

Table 5 The 5 most frequent surgical procedures for categories with respect to the incidence of SSIs

Surgery category	Procedure	Percent of discharge	Percent with SSI
Neurologic	03.59 Spinal structure repair not elsewhere classified	1,34	2.53
	81.05 Other dorsolum fusion	0,27	2,29
	02.12 Brain meninges repair not elsewhere classified	0,75	2,25
	01.25 Other craniectomy	0,22	2,1
	01.53 Brain lobectomy	0,29	2,09
Cardiovascular	35.14: Open heart valvuloplasty of tricuspid valve without replacement	0,3	4,32
	35.84: Total correction of transposition of great vessels	0,35	4,09
	35.91: Interatrial venous return transposition	0,08	3,85
	37.22: Left heart cardiac catherization	0,17	3,74
	35.28: Replace tricuspid valve not elsewhere classified	0,09	3,7
Colorectal	46.74: Closure small bowel fistula not elsewhere classified	0,28	10,0
	45.93: Small-to-large bowel not elsewhere classified	0,55	9,24
	45.61: Multiple segmental small bowel excision	0,55	8,73
	46.20: Ileostomy not otherwise specified	0,19	8,59
	46.01: Small bowel exteriorization	0,84	6,34
Breast Skin and subcutaneous tissue	54.11: Exploratory laparotomy	0,5	2,5
	84.15: Below knee amputation not elsewhere classified	0,32	1,96
	40.11: Lymphatic structure biopsy	0,35	1,79
	85.45: Unilateral radical mastectomy	0,6	1,57
	54.30: Destruction abdominal wall lesion	0,42	1,49
Gastrointestinal	52.70: Radical pancreaticoduodenectomy	0,78	7,74
	43.70: Partial gastrectomy with jejunum anastomosis	0,89	5,63
	42.41: Partial esophagectomy	0,25	5,03
	43.99: Total gastrectomy not elsewhere classified	0,49	4,99
	86.22: Wound debridement	0,44	4,97
Orthopedic	80.05: Arthrotomy/prosthesis removal-hip	0,22	1,74
	79.85: Open reduction-hip dislocatation	0,64	1,19
	77.85: Partial ostectomy-femur	0,5	0,76
	77.25: Femoral wedge osteotomy	0,55	0,69
	80.15: Other arthrotomy-hip	0,88	0,66
Obstetric/ gynecologic	68.80: Pelvic evisceration	0,04	10,48
	68.40: Total abdominal hysterectomy	0,03	4,3
	40.54: Radical groin dissection	0,01	4,17
	71.50: Radical vulvectomy	0,2	3,42
	40.52: Radical dissection periaortic lymph node	0,08	2,3

glucose control, blood transfusions, and smoking cessation) antibiotic prophylaxis plays a pivotal role in reducing SSIs.

The degree of bacterial contamination during surgery, together with the ASA score and duration of surgery, define the appropriateness of antibiotic prophylaxis: surgical procedures are classified, as well-known, into clean, clean-contaminated, contaminated and dirty.

Dirty surgery should be treated as therapy of the infection involved (no prophylaxis).

Clean surgery usually does not need prophylaxis, unless comorbidities are present and/or prostheses are used.

The main indication for prophylaxis is, therefore, clean-contaminated or contaminated surgery. The purpose of antibiotic prophylaxis is only to avoid SSIs, not to prevent any other post-operative infectious complications (pneumonia, urinary tract infections, etc.).

The choice of antibiotic for prophylaxis should be directed towards the more probable pathogens for the particular type of surgery. Furthermore, antibiotics with a broad spectrum of action should not be used, because such these are the drugs of choice to treat an infection empirically.

Prophylaxis should be administered intravenously, half an hour before the start of surgery and should not be continued for more than 24 h.

Table 6 lists the recommended antibiotics for antimicrobial prophylaxis [35] according to the type of surgery, and the alternative drugs in case of allergy to penicillin and/or cephalosporins. It is clear that the most frequently used antibiotic is cefazolin alone, combined with metronidazole when anti-anaerobe coverage is required and with vancomycin in selected cases of cardiovascular, orthopedic or neurosurgery when devices and/or prostheses are used.

According to the guidelines, if the surgical procedure lasts more than 3–4 h, there is an indication to administer another dose of prophylactic antibiotic, during surgery. In the case of renal impairment, this interval should be modified according to the creatinine clearance.

Therapy for methicillin-resistant *Staphylococcus aureus* infections

The guidelines of the Infectious Diseases Society of America recommend treatment with a beta-lactam or clindamycin for mild/moderate, non-purulent ABSSSIs and vancomycin plus piperacillin/tazobactam for severe, non-purulent ABSSSIs [36]. Treatment of purulent ABSSSIs should cover MRSA empirically with doxycycline or trimethoprim/sulfamethoxazole in moderate cases and vancomycin, daptomycin, linezolid, or ceftaroline in severe cases. With the increase of clinical MRSA isolates with decreased susceptibility or resistance to these drugs, treatment of ABSSSIs, especially SSIs, is now challenged by antibiotic resistance, toxicity, few oral options, and greater need for hospitalization and its associated costs [37]. Dalbavancin, a recent addition to the antimicrobial armamentarium that could meet these challenges, is a novel lipoglycopeptide approved by the FDA in May 2014 and by the European Medicines Agency (EMA) in February 2015 for ABSSSIs caused by susceptible Gram-positive organisms [38].

Antimicrobials available in Italy for treating ABSSSIs with activity against MRSA and other resistant Gram-positive pathogens include vancomycin, teicoplanin, daptomycin, linezolid, and ceftaroline. Of the antimicrobials listed, only linezolid has an oral formulation, and some have significant potential for toxicity, including renal impairment from vancomycin, bone marrow suppression, and drug interactions (e.g., selective serotonin re-uptake inhibitors) from linezolid, and myopathy from daptomycin. While doxycycline and trimethoprim/sulfamethoxazole have MRSA activity, their activity against beta-hemolytic streptococci is poorly, limiting their use as monotherapy for ABSSSIs. Dalbavancin is a recently approved, novel lipoglycopeptide which could be an important addition to the antimicrobial armamentarium. It has well-established activity against the Gram-positive organisms commonly involved in superficial and deep SSIs, including MRSA and other multidrug-resistant pathogens, and the MIC_{90} values for these organisms have remained stable over the past decade. Dalbavancin's

Table 6 The recommendations for antimicrobial prophylaxis [30]

Surgical category	Routine antibiotic prophylaxis	Penicillin or cephalosporin allergy
Cardiac	Cefazolin plus vancomycin (device only)	Vancomycin or Clindamycin plus gentamicin
Thoracic	Cefazolin	Vancomycin or Clindamycin
Colorectal	Cefazolin plus metronidazole	Clindamycin plus gentamicin
Otorlaryngology	Cefazolin alone or plus metronidazole	Clindamycin alone or plus ciprofloxacin
General surgery	Cefazolin	Clindamycin alone or plus gentamicin
Hepatobiliary (complicated)	Cefazolin	Vancomycin plus tobramycin
Neurosurgery	Cefazolin plus vancomycin (device only)	Vancomycin
Orthopedic	Cefazolin plus vancomycin (artroplasties only)	Vancomycin or Clindamycin
Obstetric/gynecologic	Cefazolin	Clindamycin
Vascular	Cefazolin plus vancomycin (syntetic graft only)	Vancomycin
Plastics, Reconstructive & Hand Surgery	Cefazolin	Clindamycin
Urology	Cefazolin	Ciprofloxacin alone or plus vancomycin

high protein binding and prolonged half-life allow for easily and consistently attainable therapeutic levels. Several clinical trials have demonstrated its tolerability, efficacy, and non-inferiority compared to standard therapy for ABSSSIs. The DISCOVER 1 and DISCOVER 2 studies showed that once-weekly intravenous dalbavancin was not inferior to twice-daily intravenous vancomycin followed by oral linezolid for the treatment of ABSSSIs. Adverse events were reported less frequently in patients treated with dalbavancin than in those treated with vancomycin–linezolid [39]. Indeed, dalbavancin's most unique feature is its once weekly dosing; thus far it had been approved as a 1000 mg dose followed by 500 mg 1 week later.

Dalbavancin is also approved by the EMA for a 1500 mg, one-shot, single dose [40, 41].

Factors promoting its use as an anti-MRSA treatment are its bactericidal activity, partial activity on biofilm increased by combination with rifampin, no interactions and adverse events and the possibility of an early discharge.

The main characteristics of anti-MRSA drugs used for SSIs are reported in Table 7.

Methods

Three of us (GS, CT and SC) analyzed the literature on the field of SSIs (randomized clinical trials, case–control studies, recommendations and clinical cases) and proposed some major and minor risk factors for SSIs to a board of general and specialist surgeons. We used the Delphi method [42–44] to make operative decisions through different steps of convergence, depending on the consensus reached in each round of consultation of the board.

The board was composed of one vascular surgeon, one orthopedic surgeon, one thoracic surgeon, six general and emergency surgeons and one infectious diseases specialist.

Results

We identified the major and minor risk factors for MRSA SSIs using the Delphi method. The level of consensus acceptable for approval by the group was more than 80 %. Beside the risk factors we also identified protective factors for these kind of infections.

Table 8 reports the risk factors with rates of agreement in the Delphi consultation.

These factors should be validated in prospective studies, in order to refine the identification of patients at higher risk of developing MRSA SSIs or to identify patients with a SSI due to MRSA earlier so that effective antibiotic therapy can be administered promptly.

Discussion

S. aureus is consistently the leading cause of nosocomial infections, including SSIs, and the incidence of MRSA strains is rising dramatically. Admissions to hospital because of MRSA infections have more than doubled in the past decade, and MRSA is the leading cause of SSIs in many academic and community hospitals [45].

Table 7 The main characteristics of anti MRSA drugs used for SSIs

Antibiotic	Battericidal activity/Pharmacodynamic/ anti-biofilm activity	Route of administration	Doses	Adverse events	Interaction	Cost (70 kg)
Teicoplanin	Bactericidal with low MIC/time dependent/none	iv im	7-10 mg/Kg die, loading dose	Renal toxicicty	None	50–70 E/die
Vancomycin	Bactericidal with low MIC/time dependent/none	Iv	1 g x 2 die 500 mg x 4 die	Renal toxicicty	Other nephrotoxic drugs	5 E/die
Daptomycin	Bactericidal/concentration dependent/yes	Iv	4-6 mg/kg	Tossicità muscolare	Statine	80–120 E/die
Linezolid	Bacteriostatic/time dependent/none	Iv/oral	1200 mg die	Bome marrow toxicity, neuropathy, serotoninergic syndrome	SSRI	120 E/die
Tigecycline	Bacteriostatic/time dependent/partial	Iv	50 mg x 2 die; 100 mg loading dose	Nausea, vomit, pancreatitis	None	120 E/die
Ceftaroline	Bactericidal/time dependent/none	Iv	600 mg x 2 die	rash	None	96 E/die
Dalbavancin	Bactericidal/concentration dependent/ partial (in association with rifampin)	Iv	1000 mg giorno 1, 500 mg giorno 7	No	None	NA
Cotrimoxazole	Bactericidal/time dependent/none	Iv, oral	800/160 mg 3 times a dai	anemia	None	15 E/die
Rifampin	Bactericidal/time dependent/yes	Iv/oral	600 mg once a day	Liver toxicity	Several	6 E/die

Table 8 Risk factors and protective factors according to italian literature

Risk factors	Marchi et al. OR	Petrosillo et al. OR	Fiorio et al. OR
Duration of surgery > 75 percentile (minor criteria)	1,52	–	–
Hospitalization before major surgery	>48 h 1,22	>24 h 1,45	>48 h statistically significant
Urgent surgical intervention	1,29	1,73	–
ASA ≥ 3 (minor criteria)	1,71	–	–
Age > 70 years (major criteria)	–	1,5	–
Drainage > 3 days	–	2,17	–
NNIS score 2-3	–	3,34	–
diabetes (minor criteria)	–	–	statistically significant
Obesity (minor criteria)	–	–	statistically significant
Protective factors			
Laparoscopy	0,49	–	–
SSIs hospital with active surveillance for at least 2 years	0,71	–	–
Adequate prophylaxis	–	0,68	–

MRSA as a cause of a SSI was also shown to be a significant independent risk factor for adverse economic outcomes. The risk-adjusted attributable increase in duration of hospitalization was approximately 1 day and the increase in hospitalization costs was over $1,000. Other studies support the finding that patients with MRSA infections require more health care resources than patients with methicillin-sensitive *S. aureus* (MSSA) infections [46]. Kirkland et al. estimated that the excess hospital costs associated with MRSA SSIs ranged from $3,089 to $35,367 [2]. Engemann et al. found that, among surgical patients, those with MRSA infections were hospitalized 5 days longer than those with MSSA [47]. Hospital charges for patients with MRSA infections were also $62,908 greater than those for patients without an infection and $40,000 greater than for patients with MSSA infections.

Weigelt et al. found that significant independent risk factors increasing cost and duration of hospitalization SSIs due to MRSA included illness severity, transfer from another health care facility, previous admissions (within the preceding 30 days), and other polymicrobial infections ($p < 0.05$) [48].

Because universal, rapid MRSA screening is not recommended by all authors, identifying patients at risk of colonization by MRSA and subsequently of SSIs could be very useful.

Harbarth et al. found that emergency surgery, presence of comorbid condition, immunosuppressive therapy, contaminated surgery, and a surgical duration longer than the 75th percentile were the strongest risk factors for MRSA colonization in surgical patients and these factors were confirmed in a validation cohort. [49] We also tried to identify risk factors for colonization and/or infection by MRSA. We analyzed the literature in order to list and quantify the risks of colonization and/or infection by MRSA in surgical patients. The risk factors and protective factors that emerged from Italian literature are presented in Table 9.

An algorithmic method may be useful for identifying patients without risk factors (high negative predictive model) but could be less useful for identifying true positive cases (low positive predictive value). We, therefore, tried to assign a different importance to specific risk factors dividing them into major and minor risk factors for MRSA infection in surgical patients in general and in Italy in particular.

After a review of the specific literature, using the Delphi method we attempted to quantify the importance of risk factors and protective factors for MRSA SSIs. This information could be useful for a surgeon in the daily evaluation of patients who have to undergo surgery or patients who are suspected of having a SSI. This instrument is not an alternative to the current, recommended hygiene measures or to adequate, correctly timed antibiotic prophylaxis. In the case of a SSI, after debridement of the wound and culture of the material obtained from the wound, empirical antibiotic therapy should be started, especially if there is a high risk that the pathogenic agent is MRSA. Dalbavancin, with its long half-life (186 h), should also be administered in the case of programmed discharge of the patient. According to the current summary of product characteristics, a second dose is indicated after 7 days. This second administration might also be a useful occasion for the second surgical evaluation of the wound. Because early discharge is almost always recommended for surgical patients, dalbavancin could be a further

Table 9 Risk factors with the rate of agreement at the Delphy method

Major risk factors	Rate of agreement
Surgery with elevate risk of MRSA infection	100 %
SSIs with signs of systemic infections	100 %
Patients from long term care facilities	100 %
Previous hospitalization (less than 30 days)	89 %
Charlson score > 5 points	100 %
COPD and thoracic surgery	100 %
Antibiotic therapy with beta-lactams (especially cefalosporins and carbapenem) and/or quinolones in the previous 30 days	89 %
Current lengt of stay > 16 days	100 %
Age 75 years or older	100 %
Surgery with prothesis implantation	100 %
Minor risk factors	
Not compensated diabetes or complicated diabetes	100 %
Body mass index > 30	100 %
Previous hospitalization (>30 days, < 12 months)	100 %
Steroids (prednisone 15 mg/die or equivalent dose for at least 15 days)	100 %
Other immunosoppressive therapy	100 %
Renal insufficiency	100 %
COPD not in thoracic surgery	100 %
Antibiotic therapy not with beta-lactams and/or quinolones in the previous 30 days	89 %
Lenght of surgery > 75 percentile (for surgical procedures that last more than 4 h)	100 %
External biliary drainage	100 %
Protective factors	
Hospital with surveillance system of SSIs	100 %
Correct antibiotic prophylaxis	100 %
Laparoscopic surgery	100 %

beneficial tool to treat SSIs correctly, without increasing the duration of hospitalization, especially for those patients who require continued hospitalization only to complete intravenous antibiotic therapy.

Conclusion

SSIs are still important diseases in the context of ABSSSIs. These infections have a strong impact from both clinical and economic points of view. Therefore, in the pre-operative and post-operative evaluation of patients suspected of developing a SSI, recognizing whether the patient has risk factors for a SSI and especially one caused by MRSA, the most important pathogen in this field, might be very important in the management of surgical patients.

In the case of a SSI, after debridement of the wound and culture of the material obtained from the wound, empirical antibiotic therapy should be started especially if there is a high probability of the pathogenic agent being MRSA. Dalbavancin, with its long half-life (186 h), should also be administered in the case of programmed discharge of the patient. A second dose is indicated after 7 days according to the drug's summary of product characteristics.

Abbreviations

SSIs, surgical site infections; MRSA, methicillin-resistant Staphylococcus aureus; S. aureus, staphylococcus aureus; US dollars, United States dollars; DRG, diagnosis related-group; S. epidermidis, staphylococcus epidermidis; CDC, centers for disease control and prevention's; FDA, food and drug administration; ABSSSIs, acute bacterial skin and skin structure infections; ASA, American Society of anesthesiologists; ICD-9-CM, International classification of diseases, ninth revision, clinical modification; EMA, European medicines agency; MIC_{90},-minimum inhibitory $concentration_{90}$; MSSA, methicillin-sensitive S. aureus

Acknowledgements

Not applicable.

Funding

No fundings to declare.

Authors' contributions

GS and CT wrote the manuscript. All authors read and approved the final manuscript.

Competing interests

The authors declare that they have no competing interests.

Author details

[1]Istituto Clinica Chirurgica, Divisione Chirurgia Generale e Trapianti d'Organo, Università Cattolica del Sacro Cuore, Fondazione Policlinico Universitario Agostino Gemelli, Rome, Italy. [2]U.O. Malattie Infettive, Azienda Ospedaliera Universitaria Pisana, Pisa, Italy. [3]U.O. Medicina d'Urgenza Universitaria, Azienda Ospedaliera Universitaria Pisana, Pisa, Italy. [4]Chirurgia generale Ospedale Sant'Eugenio di Roma, Rome, Italy. [5]Dipartimento di Chirurgia Università La Sapienza, Policlinico Umberto I, Rome, Italy. [6]UOC Chirurgia di Urgenza Ospedale San Filippo Neri, Rome, Italy. [7]Dipartimento di Chirurgia Generale e Trapianti d'Organo, UOC Chirurgia Vascolare, Università La Sapienza, Policlinico Umberto I, Rome, Italy. [8]Istituto Patologia Chirurgia, Unità Operativa Complessa Chirurgia Toracica, Università Cattolica del Sacro Cuore, Fondazione Policlinico Universitario Agostino Gemelli, Rome, Italy. [9]Ortopedia e Traumatologia dell'Ospedale S. Gennaro ASL Napoli 1 Centro, Naples, Italy. [10]U.O Chirurgia Generale Ospedale di Macerata, Macerata, Italy. [11]Master Sepsi in Chirurgia, Università Cattolica, Rome, Italy.

References

1. Astagneau P, Rioux C, Golliot F, Brucker G. for the INCISO Network Study Group: Morbidity and mortality associated with surgical site infections: results from the 1997–1999 INCISO surveillance. J Hosp Infect. 2001;48:267–74.
2. Kirkland KB, Briggs JP, Trivette SL, Wilkinson WE, Sexton DJ. The impact of surgical-site infections in the 1990s: attributable mortality,

excess length of hospitalization, and extra costs. Infect Control Hosp Epidemiol. 1999;20:725–30.

3. Leaper DJ, van Goor H, Reilly J, Petrosillo N, Geiss HK, Torres AJ, Berger A. Surgical site infection-a European perspective of incidence and economic burden. Int Wound J. 2004;1:247–73.
4. Emmerson AM, Enstone JE, Griffin M, Kelsey MC, Smyth ET. The Second National Prevalence Survey of infection in hospitals – overview of the results. J Hosp Infect. 1996;32:175–90.
5. Sganga G, Brisinda G, Castagneto M. Practical aspects of antibiotic prophylaxis in high-risk surgical patients. In: van Saene HK, Sganga G, Silvestri L, editors. Infection in the Critically Ill: An Ongoing Challenge. Berlin: Springer Verlag; 2001. p. 47–58.
6. Howard RJ, Simmons RL. Surgical Infectious Diseases. Norwalk, NJ: Appleton and Lange; 1988.
7. Sganga G. New perspectives in antibiotic prophylaxis for intra-abdominal surgery. J Hosp Infect. 2002;50(Suppl A):S17–21.
8. Delgado-Rodriguez M, Gomez-Ortega A, Sillero-Arenas M, Llorca J. Epidemiology of surgical-site infections diagnosed after hospital discharge: a prospective cohort study. Infect Control Hosp Epidemiol. 2001;22:24–30.
9. Brandt C, Sohr D, Behnke M, Daschner F, Ruden H, Gastmeier P. Reduction of surgical site infection rates associated with active surveillance. Infect Control Hosp Epidemiol. 2006;27:1347–51.
10. Horan TC, Gaynes RP, Martone WJ, et al. CDC definitions of nosocomial surgical site infections, 1992: a modification of CDC definitions of surgical wound infections. Infect Control Hosp Epidemiol. 1992;13:606–8.
11. Food and Drug Administration. Guidance for industry acute bacterial skin and skin structure infections: developing drugs for treatment. 2013. Available from: http://www.fda.gov/downloads/Drugs/Guidances/ucm071185.pdf. October 2013.
12. National Nosocomial Infections Surveillance (NNIS). system report, data summary from January 1992 through June 2004. Am J Infect Control. 2004; 32:470–85.
13. Altemeier WA, Culbertson WR, Hummel RP. Surgical considerations of endogenous infections sources, types, and methods of control. Surg Clin North Am. 1968;48:227–40.
14. Wiley AM, Ha'eri GB. Routes of infection: a study of using "tracer particles" in the orthopedic operating room. Clin Orthop. 1979;139:150–5.
15. Guideline for prevention of surgical site infection, Mangram AJ, Horan TC, Pearson ML, Silver LC, Jarvis WR. Hospital Infection Control Practices Advisory Committee. Infect Control Hosp Epidemiol. 1999;20:250–78.
16. Albrich W, Harbarth S. Health-care workers: source, vector, or victim of MRSA? Lancet Infect Dis. 2008;8:289–301.
17. Cosgrove SE, Qi Y, Kaye KS, et al. The impact of methicillin resistance in Staphylococcus aureus bacteremia on patient outcomes: mortality, length of stay, and hospital charges. Infect Control Hosp Epidemiol. 2005;26:166–74.
18. Gastmeier P, Schwab F, Sohr D, Behnke M, Geffers C. Reproducibility of the surveillance effect to decrease nosocomial infection rates. Infect Control Hosp Epidemiol. 2009;30:993–9.
19. Greco D, Moro ML, Tozzi AE, De Giacomi GV. Effectiveness of an intervention program in reducing postoperative infections. Infection. 2003; 31 Suppl 2:164–9.
20. Nicastri E, Petrosillo N, Martini L, Larosa M, Gesu GP, Ippolito G, the INF-NOS Study Group. Prevalence of nosocomial infections in 15 Italian hospitals: first point prevalence study for the INF-NOS Project. Infection. 2003;31 Suppl 2:16–22.
21. Petrosillo N, Drapeau CM, Nicastri E, et al. Surgical site infections in Italian hospitals: a prospective multicenter study. BMC Infect Dis. 2008;8:34.
22. Fiorio M, Marvaso A, Viganò F, Marchetti F. Incidence of surgical site infections in general surgery in Italy. Infection. 2006;34:310–4.
23. Prospero E, Cavicchi A, Bacelli S, Barbadoro P, Tantucci L, D'Errico MM. Surveillance for surgical site infection after hospital discharge: a surgical procedure-specific perspective. Infect Control Hosp Epidemiol. 2006;27: 1313–7.
24. Marchi M, Pan A, Gagliotti C, Morsillo F, Parenti M, Resi D, Moro ML. Sorveglianza Nazionale Infezioni in Chirurgia (SNICh) Study Group]: The Italian national surgical site infection surveillance programme and its positive impact, 2009 to 2011. Euro Surveill. 2014;29:19.
25. Mavros MN, Athanasiou S, Alexiou VG, Mitsikostas PK, Peppas G, Falagas ME. Risk factors for mesh-related infections after hernia repair surgery: a meta-analysis of cohort studies. World J Surg. 2011;35:2389–98.
26. Limson AA, Relos RP, Balo SA, Fojas MC. Tension-free herniorrhaphy for primary and recurrent inguinal hernias: a prospective study of 120 patients. Philipp J Surg Spec. 1996;51:93–6.
27. Cobb WS, Harris JB, Lokey JS, McGill ES, Klove KL. Incisional herniorrhaphy with intraperitoneal composite mesh: a report of 95 cases. Am Surg. 2003; 69:784–7.
28. Tolino MJ, Tripoloni DE, Ratto R, Garcia MI. Infections associated with prosthetic repairs of abdominal wall hernias: pathology, management and results. Hernia. 2009;13:631–7.
29. Lovecchio F, Farmer R, Souza J, Khavanin N, Dumanian GA, Kim JY. Risk factors for 30-day readmission in patients undergoing ventral hernia repair. Surgery. 2014;155:702–10.
30. van der Slegt J, Kluytmans JA, Mulder PG, Veen EJ, Ho GH, van der Laan L. Surgical site infection after multiple groin incisions in peripheral vascular surgery. Surg Infect. 2014;15:752–6.
31. Rovera F, Imperatori A, Militello P, Morri A, Antonini C, Dionigi G, Dominioni L. Infections in 346 consecutive video-assisted thoracoscopic procedures. Surg Infect. 2003;4:45–51.
32. Olsen MA, Lock-Buckley P, Hopkins D, et al. The risk factors for deep and superficial chest surgical-site infections after coronary artery bypass graft surgery are different. J Thorac Cardiovasc Surg. 2002;124:136–45.
33. L R Greene, R Mills, R Moss, K Sposato, M Vignari. Guide to the Elimination of the Orthopedic Surgical Site Infections *APIC Guide* 2010
34. Edminston Jr CE, Seabrook GR, Goheen M, Krepel C, Johnson CP, Lewis B, et al. Bacterial adherence to surgical sutures: can antibacterial coated sutures reduce the risk of microbial contamination. J Am Coll Surg. 2006;203:481–9.
35. Solomkin JS, Mazuski JE, Bradley JS, Rodvold KA, Goldstein EJC, Baron E, O'Neill PG, et al. Diagnosis and management of complicated intra-abdominal infection in adults and children: guidelines by the Surgical Infection Society and the Infectious Diseases Society of America. Clin Infect Dis. 2010;50:133–64.
36. Stevens DL, Bisno AL, Chambers HF, et al. Practice guidelines for the diagnosis and management of skin and soft tissue infections: 2014 update by the Infectious Diseases Society of America. Clin Infect Dis. 2014;59:e10–52.
37. Long SW, Olsen RJ, Mehta SC, et al. PBP2a mutations causing high-level ceftaroline resistance in clinical methicillin-resistant Staphylococcus aureus isolates. Antimicrob Agents Chemother. 2014;58:6668–74.
38. Food and Drug Administration. FDA approves dalvance to treat skin infections. 2014. European Medicines Agency. Available from: http://www.ema.europa.eu/ema/index.jsp?curl=pages/medicines/human/medicines/002840/human_med_001848.jsp&mid=WC0b01ac058001d124. 25 May 2016.
39. Boucher HW, Wilcox M, Talbot GH, et al. Once-weekly dalbavancin versus daily conventional therapy for skin infection. N Engl J Med. 2014;370:2169–79.
40. Dunne MW, Puttagunta S, Giordano P, Krievins D, Zelasky M, Baldassarre J. A Randomized Clinical Trial of Single-Dose Versus Weekly Dalbavancin for Treatment of Acute Bacterial Skin and Skin Structure Infection. Clin Infect Dis. 2016;62(1 March):545–51.
41. EMA Community register of medicinal products for human use. Auth. number: EU/1/14/986. Active substance: Dalbavancin. Available at: http://ec.europa.eu/health/documents/community-register/html/h986.htm. 11 May 2016.
42. Fink A, Kosecoff J, Chassin M, et al. Consensus Methods: characteristics and guideline for use. Am J Public Health. 1984;74:979–83.
43. Dixon E, Armstrong C, Maddern G, et al. Development of quality indicators of care for patients undergoing hepatic resection for metastatic colorectal cancer using a Delphi process. J Surg Res. 2009;156:32–8.
44. Helmer O, Rescher N. On the epistemology of the inexact science. Management Science. 1959;6:25–53.
45. Klein E, Smith DL, Laxminarayan R. Hospitalizations and deaths caused by methicillin-resistant *Staphylococcus aureus*, United States, 1999–2005. Emerg Infect Dis. 2007;13:1840–6.
46. Rubin RJ, Harrington CA, Poon A, Dietrich K, Greene JA, Moiduddin A. The economic impact of *Staphylococcus aureus* infection in New York City hospitals. Emerg Infect Dis. 1999;5:9–17.
47. Engemann JJ, Carmeli Y, Cosgrove SE, Fowler VG, Bronstein MZ, Trivette SL, et al. Adverse clinical and economic outcomes attribut- able to methicillin resistance among patients with *Staphylococcus aureus* surgical site infection. Clin Infect Dis. 2003;36:592–8.

27

Defining our destiny: trainee working group consensus statement on the future of emergency surgery training in the United Kingdom

A. E. Sharrock[1,2*], V. J. Gokani[1], R. L. Harries[1], L. Pearce[1], S. R. Smith[1], O. Ali[1], H. Chu[1], A. Dubois[1], H. Ferguson[1], G. Humm[1], M. Marsden[1], D. Nepogodiev[1], M. Venn[1], S. Singh[1], C. Swain[1] and J. Kirkby-Bott[2]

Abstract

The United Kingdom National Health Service treats both elective and emergency patients and seeks to provide high quality care, free at the point of delivery. Equal numbers of emergency and elective general surgical procedures are performed, yet surgical training prioritisation and organisation of NHS institutions is predicated upon elective care. The increasing ratio of emergency general surgery consultant posts compared to traditional sub-specialities has yet to be addressed. How should the capability gap be bridged to equip motivated, skilled surgeons of the future to deliver a high standard of emergency surgical care? The aim was to address both training requirements for the acquisition of necessary emergency general surgery skills, and the formation of job plans for trainee and consultant posts to meet the current and future requirements of the NHS.

Twenty nine trainees and a consultant emergency general surgeon convened as a Working Group at The Association of Surgeons in Training Conference, 2015, to generate a united consensus statement to the training requirement and delivery of emergency general surgery provision by future general surgeons. Unscheduled general surgical care provision, emergency general surgery, trauma competence, training to meet NHS requirements, consultant job planning and future training challenges arose as key themes. Recommendations have been made from these themes in light of published evidence. Careful workforce planning, education, training and fellowship opportunities will provide well-trained enthusiastic individuals to meet public and societal need.

Keywords: Emergency general surgery, Surgical training, Surgical education, NHS National Health Service, Management and job planning

Introduction

In the United Kingdom (UK), the National Health Service (NHS) seeks to provide high quality healthcare, funded by the taxpayer. Trainees are 'invaluable eyes and ears in the hospital setting' [1] and are well placed to evaluate day to day practice and areas for improvement. However, they remain an under-utilised resource in planning services. This Emergency General Surgery consensus document has utilised trainee perspectives of Emergency General Surgeons and the current provision of care for NHS acute surgical patients. Obstacles to a dedicated, high-quality future workforce, equipped to manage acutely unwell patients requiring surgical care have been identified, and strategies to overcome them have been recommended. The key overarching considerations at the Working Group meeting were; how can competency be reached and enthusiasm retained, and who is responsible for ensuring that each clinician maintains the high standard of skills expected by the UK population?

The working group

A Working Group of 29 trainees ranging from Foundation Year (recently qualified) to the point of obtaining a certificate of completion of training (CCT), alongside a Consultant Emergency General Surgeon convened on 01 March 2015 during the Association of Surgeons in Training (ASiT) International Conference in Glasgow,

* Correspondence: sharrock@doctors.org.uk
[1]Association of Surgeons in Training (ASiT), Royal College of Surgeons England, 35 – 43 Lincoln's Inn Fields, London WC2A 3P3, UK
[2]Department of Emergency Surgery, Southampton General Hospital, Tremona Road, Southampton, Hampshire SO16 6YD, UK

UK. The aims of the Group were to address the training requirements for attaining the necessary emergency general surgery skills, and the formation of job plans for trainee and consultant posts. To achieve this, the Group was divided into four and all considered the following prompt questions:

- Will all newly appointed consultant general surgeons be emergency general surgeons?
- Can emergency surgical training be delivered through elective surgery?
- How should surgeons demonstrate emergency competence for completion of training?
- What should a job plan in emergency general surgery look like?
- What experience is necessary in trauma surgery, how should trainee surgeons obtain it, and how should this training be separate to emergency general surgery training?

The discussion was distilled with the full Working Group. Themes arising from the prompt questions are reported with concerns raised and relevant recommendations as bullet points.

To put these recommendations into context a thorough literature review of the clinical, service and training aspects of emergency surgical care provision was undertaken. The National Institute for Health and Care Excellence (NICE), Ovid (Medline and EMBASE) and PubMed libraries were searched to provide a clinical background. NHS England and the National Audit Office in conjunction with National Confidential and Public enquires were used to provide an insight of service provision. The Academy of Medical Royal Colleges, the four UK Royal Surgical Colleges, the Association of Surgeons of Great Britain and Ireland and the Intercollegiate Surgical Curriculum Project publications were reviewed for manning and training requirements. Searches were expanded through publication reference lists and related documents. This consensus statement seeks to identify the perceived ideal training and educational requirements of general surgical trainees to meet the current and future requirements of the NHS.

Unscheduled general surgical care provision

In the UK the estimated population density is 413 people per square kilometre, compared to 35 and 3 people per square kilometre in the USA and some African nations respectively [2]. The relative density of the UK population means patients are often within a short distance of medical care, and that there is little requirement for the pan-specialty general surgeon. Instead, emergency orthopaedic, neurosurgical, cardiothoracic, ear nose and throat (ENT), maxillofacial, urological, vascular, and burns and plastics procedures are usually referred directly to the relevant speciality, and it is the remaining surgical conditions which are the responsibility of the general surgeon. This configuration is reflected by many European countries, who similarly have recognised the importance of providing training for emergency general surgeons, in an increasingly subspecialised environment [3]. Whilst the specifics of surgical provision vary between nations, the core need is to provide an emergency service with a well-defined range of skills.

Patients attending NHS hospitals with such emergency general surgical conditions make up half of all general surgery admissions in the UK [4]. Despite this, current models of UK healthcare tariffs and commissioning prioritise elective care over the care of emergency patients, through preferential financial agreements. A patient admitted as an emergency may not be physiologically prepared for a procedure, and particular consideration should be given to the growing demographic of the elderly patient, who may have multiple co-morbidities, cognitive impairment and frailty and whose mortality rate from emergency laparotomy currently sits at 24 % [5]. Equally concerning, is the wide variation in mortality for all-cause emergency laparotomy across UK trusts ranging from 3.6 – 41.7 %. This reflects the diverse range of models and standards used to deliver emergency surgical care [4, 5].

Some forward thinking institutions are developing and evolving their acute surgical care provision with dedicated specialist emergency general surgical clinical teams improving patient flow, treatments and outcomes. A recent single institution analysis of the hospital length of stay outcome of a new 'acute surgical unit' showed a 10 % reduction in bed days and cost saving of £475,848 per annum [6]. Whilst the NHS should evolve with evidence of best medical practice, it is a public institution, and therefore targets and restructuring are sensitive to manipulation by political agendas. It will take time to optimise the system. Going forward, consensus groups are a powerful tool to reflect on current systems and advise on the future direction of travel to improve patient care.

- Outcomes from emergency general surgery operations vary considerably across the UK
- The current system requires modification to improve outcomes and cost

Emergency general surgery competency

Emergency surgery forms up to half of the general surgical workload in some specialities [4]. By its very nature it embodies an array of cross-specialty pathology, often in patients with multiple co-morbidities. Most of these admissions result from infective complications of disease processes. This is an area of pathology that has recently faded in significance, as political targets focus upon cancer care. We have now reached a point where a thorough re-evaluation of the management of surgical infection is required, as novel antibiotics developed in the second half of the twentieth century and new techniques gained through cancer surgery can be applied with a fresh approach to surgical infection in the twenty first century. Operations for such infective complications include laparoscopic cholecystectomies, laparoscopic or open appendicectomies and abscess drainages; they form the majority of procedures undertaken and are predictable in terms of training requirements. It is possible for transferrable skills in laparoscopic and open surgery and endoscopy to be instigated and developed in the elective setting, with other skills to be acquired during on-call shifts, providing staffing levels do not preclude training activities. Aside from these procedures and less complex intra-abdominal surgery, for example a perforated duodenal ulcer, there lacks a definition of what an emergency general surgeon should be capable of. Should the management of sepsis and surgical infection, as well as a more specialist gastrointestinal or trauma surgery skillset be an integral part of every emergency general surgeons' abilities?

The minority of emergency cases include complex intra-abdominal pathology and trauma. Within this group it has been shown that most procedures (70 %) are performed for colorectal or small bowel pathology, whilst subspecialist oesphagogastric surgery, for example, comprises only 5 % of emergency laparotomies [7]. The emergency general surgeon is therefore required to know how to surgically intervene and perform a damage limitation procedure, with the ability to perform more sub-specialist surgery such as complex colonic or gastric resections if competent. It is entirely appropriate, and arguably expected, that a sub-specialist be contacted in complex cases, and that they may take the lead in the emergency context.

Every doctor who practises emergency surgery should be able to make timely, appropriate plans, and the surgical training pathway should provide the challenges and encouragement to equip each individual trainee with this skill. Consultant-delivered care is the accepted standard for high-quality expedient emergency surgery [8, 9], but this must be tempered with the opportunity for surgical trainees to safely accumulate the experience and skill necessary for future independent consultant practice.

- The exact competencies of the Emergency General Surgeon are yet to be defined
- Many emergency general surgery skills can be learnt in the elective setting.
- Management of sepsis and infective complications is an important aspect of care
- Consultant delivered care must be balanced with the need to train the next generation

Trauma competence

The success of the British military trauma services in recent years [10], and a review of trauma services in 2007 [9, 11] sparked political interest in UK trauma management. The UK Major Trauma Centre (MTC) network was implemented in April 2012, and despite a significant proportion of injured patients now being treated in MTCs, a study of four large UK centres has shown that mortality, critical care requirements and length of stay are yet to significantly improve [12]. It is unknown what the role of limited UK trauma training will be on outcomes but it is clear that training in this area could be improved.

The technical skills required for competency in trauma surgery are far ranging and include surgical airway insertion, control of non-compressible haemorrhage through thoracotomy (left lateral and clam-shell), laparotomy and retroperitoneal access (pre-peritoneal packing and medial visceral rotation manoeuvres as examples), and control of contamination. The development of a list of trauma competencies was not within the remit of the Working Group, but questions were raised regarding the depth of training required to deliver a trauma service in the UK and how these skills are to be maintained. A focused trauma training curriculum should be developed and delivered in selected MTCs, and overseen with assessment criteria by the Intercollegiate Surgical Curriculum Project (ISCP) [13]. Future workforce planning can predict the number of trauma surgeons required at the MTCs; as only 22 of the 190 trusts providing an emergency surgery service also provide an adult major trauma service, only a proportion of emergency trained surgeons will need significant trauma training. It is not possible or necessary to train all emergency surgeons as trauma surgeons. Conversely, it may be possible that a flourishing trauma interest is developed in surgeons from other specialties, such as vascular surgery. Fellowships within high intensity trauma centres, or deployments to areas of operational theatres (in the case of military trainees), may be provided to bridge perceived knowledge gaps. Additionally, advanced trauma courses, simulation training and workshops need to be developed to augment the training available in the UK. All emergency general surgeons should be trained in the principles of surgical trauma care, and this could be delivered as a rotation to an MTC in higher surgical training.

- Trauma surgery and emergency surgery are distinct, and the definition of competence requires further work.
- Although many technical emergency surgical skills can be taught in the elective setting, this is not the case for trauma surgery proficiencies. Focused trauma surgical training curricula, to be delivered in highly selected units, should be developed.

- All emergency general surgeons should be aware of the principle of surgical trauma care, but not necessarily trained as trauma surgeons.

Training to meet NHS requirements

The ratio of new to replacement consultant posts has increased [14], as have the number of 'emergency general surgery' consultant posts advertised since 2009 [15]. In response, there have been calls from some clinicians [16] for emergency general surgery to be a specialty in its own right. Following the implementation of the European Working Time Directive [17] it has been estimated that the exposure to surgical emergencies by the time of completion of higher surgical training is approximately 50 % less than those training 20 years ago [18]. There is currently no recognised higher surgical training programme for emergency general surgery, and consequently the emergency surgery and trauma competencies of those applying for emergency general surgery posts is largely unregulated.

Cognisant of the lack of consensus over the future of training for emergency general surgeons, the working group considered models in other countries. In Europe, there are a number of different models and the issues relating to operative exposure, training time and super-specialisation remain prevalent [3]. In the last few years the USA have trained Acute Care Surgeons who are competent in trauma surgery, surgical critical care and emergency general surgery. This has been partly driven by the profound decline in General Surgical Residency Applications and a shift in the desires of junior surgeons to have an acceptable work-life balance throughout their career. There was also recognition of the wide geographical variation in the provision of surgical trauma services and the need to address shortages [19, 20]. Consequently, the Acute Care Surgery training models are varied to suit local healthcare requirements whilst maintaining a minimum standard within the curriculum [21]. Geographical population density is less varied in the UK, so this flexible model of training less relevant.

Until now, the majority of emergency surgery training in the UK has been delivered yhrough time 'on-call'. This model is no longer tenable in the reduced working hours models that have been instigated since the advent of the European Working Time Directive. Poorer patient outcomes for those admitted outside traditional working hours has created the current impetus for a seven day-working week for consultants and trainees [22]. Whilst it is difficult to separate service provision from training, the Working Group considered most on-call experience as service provision rather than an opportunity to obtain training proficiencies. This is beneficial to the organisation, and in some part to the individual, but must be balanced with the acquisition of clinical competency through training. Formal six-month rotations in emergency surgery with a targeted curriculum have provided some trainees with an immersion in the discipline. It is important that these placements are organised to complement the training of other trainees at the institution. This allows a sequential progression of skill acquisition rather than 'ad hoc' tuition. As Emergency units are set up and new knowledge is acquired, significant training opportunities for emergency surgery training in general surgery will present themselves. The decision-making and practical skills learnt in this context are transferable and add value to the trainees' elective sub-specialty progression.

Prompted by a growing trend towards consultant-delivered care, trainees have found themselves supervised in the operating theatre more often than ever before. Undoubtedly, this is of patient benefit in the short term. Consultants need to pass on their knowledge to the next generation such that on completion of training, new consultants are not only capable of performing potentially complex procedures under pressure, but can also make informed, reproducible decisions throughout the operative process. This type of knowledge and processing is developed through repeated exposure to clinical challenges, and may not be refined in newly appointed consultants who have been sheltered from independent clinical practice. Surgeons in training need to be able to take the lead as well as being part of the team. The trainer-trainee relationship is key in providing the appropriate level of training for the individual. This raises the question as to whether all consultants are capable of training trainees to such a standard [23]. Uncoupling of the traditional 'firm' structure means that trainers may not be familiar with the competency of the trainee they are working with for a set day. This adds to the challenge of providing the appropriate level of training as trainers and trainees are increasingly unfamiliar with others experiences and expertise. Six month modular training in Emergency General Surgery may go some way to improving the working relationship between trainee and trainer and allow a structured progression of skills and experiences.

- The training pathway must be modified and monitored to meet the requirement to fill 'Emergency General Surgery' posts
- Formal placements in emergency general surgery may be suitable in structured surgical training programs.
- Training in non-technical skills, especially in the emergency setting, is essential.

Emergency surgery consultant job planning

Emergency general surgeons may wish to have another sub-specialty interest that augments their emergency capability. This offers increased value to the population the surgeon serves and their employer. Importantly, some may experience a relative rest period from the intensity of continual emergency practice. Whilst possible, it is unlikely that sub-specialty interests such as Breast surgery and Vascular surgery (achieved via the new curriculum) will lend themselves to emergency general surgery due to their nature of elective practice, and specialty specific emergency workload in the case of vascular surgery. Some academic surgeons whose interests lie outside of the emergency field may also be unable to align themselves with emergency general surgery, equally others may pursue an academic interest in emergency surgery. Currently, as emergency general surgery posts are being established, there are almost as many different consultant job plans as posts [15]. Additionally, sub-specialty interest need not be limited to clinical sub-specialties: it may include academic, medical leadership, training and education fields. A survey of general surgical consultants and trainees showed that pure emergency general surgery job plans are not attractive to the current or future workforce [15]. There is a need for flexibility. Concerns have also been raised over the ability and desire to continue a high intensity high pressure work pattern in the later years of a surgeon's career [24, 25]. To remain sustainable and attractive jobs, emergency general surgery roles will need to be flexible in terms of working hours (full-time or less than full-time), the combination of emergency and elective practice with variability over the course of a career, and welcome non-clinical sub-speciality interests.

- Job plans involving solely emergency general surgery are likely to be unattractive to the majority of surgeons and a sub-speciality interest (clinical or non-clinical) will need to be incorporated into job plans and the skillset maintained.
- Job plans will need to be flexible in terms of their component parts over the course of a career.
- It may be inappropriate to include emergency surgery in all consultants' job plans: such as those undertaking significant academic or leadership roles.

Future training challenges

The 'Shape of Training' review ('ShoT') [26] seeks to outline how doctors' training pathways might be altered to meet a perceived change in patient needs. However, it is imperative that during this process, which risks shortening the length of training time further, quality and competence are not eroded. ShoT has recommended restructuring UK training in all specialties to form a broader base of practice, and has entertained the concept of credentialing to provide specialist qualification and capability later on. Whilst this remains contentious amongst some trainee groups, including ASiT, partly due to a lack of clarity over its implementation, it may represent an opportunity to redefine training in emergency surgery to meet an increasing service demand. However, no benefit can be gained from a training system producing unprepared sub-consultants requiring mandatory extra training before independent practise is truly possible. Whilst the Working Group does not agree that training should be shortened, if implemented it would mandate that focused, active, consultant-delivered training and reflective practice would be required alongside formal assessment through the Annual Review of Competence Progression (ARCP) process. Despite the difficulties it poses, this would most likely need to occur outside of prescribed service duties. The changes taking place in emergency general surgery provision may lend themselves to ShoT restructuring, but down-grading the quality assurance of a consultant by cutting corners and delivering a premature end product while maintaining the title does not benefit patients [27]. At best it would result in less competent consultants; at worst, accepted mediocrity and poorer quality healthcare. Patents rightly expect high standards from both consultants and trainees, and both require support to provide this level of care.

- The Working Group opposes the creation of a sub-consultant grade, but advocates quality training for independent consultant practice.

Summary

This Working Group set out to address the training requirements for attaining the necessary emergency general surgery skills, and the formation of job plans for trainee and consultant posts. Through discussion and consensus, unscheduled general surgical care provision, emergency general surgery, trauma competence, training to meet NHS requirements, consultant job planning and future training challenges have been key themes. Recommendations have been based on evidence where possible and inferences drawn by group discussion. Trainees are well placed to consider how to bridge the training gap between their current state of competence and the 'ideal' breadth and depth of ability for an emergency surgeon. The training process for emergency general surgery and trauma should be tailored to service needs, but must be an attractive career option for ambitious and successful surgeons in training. Through combination of an interest in a related surgical discipline, workable job plan, and integration of training courses and a fellowship, well equipped highly capable emergency general surgeons will be available for work-force planning.

Conclusions

The consultant workforce of the future must meet the patient demands for the NHS to work. Surgical trainees should be consulted regarding changes to surgical training; they are willing to engage in the process of optimising the training pathway. Careful workforce planning and design of education, training and fellowship opportunities, and flexible consultant job plans will enable the supply of well-trained individuals to meet demand, and retain enthusiasm. Above all, doctors who work within the NHS should not be overlooked to provide information on the functionality of a service, and forecast the direction of travel for future service improvement.

As a major stakeholder, ASiT is committed to pursuing high quality curricula, including that of emergency general surgery. ASiT opposes a sub-consultant grade or equivalent by another name, and does not agree that training should be shortened. Instead emergency general surgeons should be on the same contract and pay scale with the same opportunities for progression as their consultant colleagues in other sub-speciality areas.

Competing interests
Some co-authors have an affiliation to ASiT, whilst others do not. This Working Group was hosted by ASiT but represents the views of the Working Group and not necessarily the views of ASiT, whose position is summarised in the paragraph above. The authors declare that they have no financial competing interests.

Authors' contributions
AES co-chaired the working group and wrote the manuscript. JKB was the facilitating consultant emergency surgeon, conceived the project, and was involved in the project's organisation, commissioning, and structuring. Likewise VG and RH were involved in the project organisation and redrafting of the manuscript. HF co-chaired and redrafted the manuscript. LP and SS were members of the working group who contributed to the acquisition of reference material and restructuring of the manuscript. All other authors were members of the working group who made substantial contributions to redrafting of the manuscript. All authors read and approved the final version of the manuscript.

References

1. Francis R. Report of the Mid Staffordshire NHS Foundation Trust Public Inquiry. http://webarchive.nationalarchives.gov.uk/20150407084003/http://www.midstaffspublicinquiry.com/report: 2013.
2. Food and Agrigculture organisation and World Bank population estimates 2015, 1818 H Street, NW Washington, DC 20433 USA. http://data.worldbank.org/indicator/EN.POP.DNST
3. Soreide K. Trauma and the acute care surgery model–should it embrace or replace general surgery? Scand J Trauma Resusc Emerg Med. 17. England 2009. p. 4. doi:10.1186/1757-7241-17-4. PubMed PMID: 19193218; PubMed Central PMCID: PMC2646681
4. Royal College of Surgeons England Separating Emergency and Elective Surgical Care Working Party. Separating Emergency and Elective Surgical Care: Recommendations for Practice. England, London: Royal College of Surgeon; 2007.
5. Saunders DI, Murray D, Pichel AC, Varley S, Peden CJ. Variations in mortality after emergency laparotomy: the first report of the UK Emergency Laparotomy Network. Br J Anaesth. 2012;109:368–75.
6. Pearson KCG, Trompetas V, Bailey I, Kirkby Bott J. Cost benefit of setting up a dedicated acute surgery unit. Short Papers Br J Surg. 2015;102:9–118. doi:10.1002/bjs9729.
7. Barrow E, Anderson ID, Varley S, Pichel AC, Peden CJ, Saunders DI, et al. Current UK practice in emergency laparotomy. Ann R Coll Surg Engl. 2013;95(8):599–603.
8. Academy of Medical Royal Colleges. The benefits of consultant delivered care. http://www.aomrc.org.uk/doc_view/9450-the-benefits-of-consultant-delivered-care: 2012.
9. National Confidential Enquiry into Patient Outcomes and Deaths. Trauma: Who cares? 2007.
10. National Audit Office, Ministry of Defence. Treating Injury and Illness arising on Military Operations. London: The Stationay Office; 2010. Contract No.: HC 294.
11. Darzi A. High Quality Care For All: Next Stage Review Final Report. http://webarchive.nationalarchives.gov.uk/20130107105354/http:/www.dh.gov.uk/prod_consum_dh/groups/dh_digitalassets/@dh/@en/documents/digitalasset/dh_085826.pdf. 2008
12. Metcalfe D, Bouamra O, Parsons NR, Aletrari MO, Lecky FE, Costa ML. Effect of regional trauma centralization on volume, injury severity and outcomes of injured patients admitted to trauma centres. Br J Surg. 2014;101(8):959–64.
13. The Intercollegiate Surgical Curriculum Project, Educating the surgeons of the future. https://www.iscp.ac.uk/static/syllabus2013/gs_curric_2013.pdf.
14. Kirkby-Bott J, Nelson M. Trends in consultant posts advertised and SPRs completing training in general surgery. Bull Royal College Surgeons. 2010;92(6):1–4.
15. Pearce L, Smith SR, Parkin E, Kennedy J, MacDonald A. Emergency General Surgery: emergence of a speciality by stealth (ASGBI abstract in print 2015). Association of Surgeons of Great Britain and Ireland conference abstract (ahead of print)
16. Behar N, King D. Proposal for a new specialty: emergency general surgery. http://careers.bmj.com/careers/advice/view-article.html?id=20007882. 2012.
17. Directive 2003/88/EC of the European Parliament and of the Council of 4 November 2003 concerning certain aspects of the organisation of working time. Official Journal of the European Union L 299, 18/11/2003. p. 0009–0019
18. Association of Surgeons of Great Britain and Ireland. Issues in Professional Practice: Emergency General Surgery. Association of Surgeons of Great Britain and Northern Ireland. http://www.asgbi.org.uk/download.cfm?docid=A76F042A-0F5D-4D06-82BE71360E973708.
19. Napolitano LM, Fulda GJ, Davis KA, Ashley DW, Friese R, Van Way 3rd CW, et al. Challenging issues in surgical critical care, trauma, and acute care surgery: a report from the critical care committee of the american association for the surgery of trauma. J Trauma. 2010;69(6):1619–33.
20. Green SM. Trauma surgery: discipline in crisis. Ann Emerg Med. 2009;53(2):198–207.
21. TraumaSource. The American Association for the Surgery of Trauma. Acute Care Surgery. http://www.aast.org/AcuteCareSurgery.aspx
22. NHS England. NHS Services, Seven Days a Week Forum. Evidence base and clinical standards for the care and onward transfer of acute inpatients. http://www.england.nhs.uk/wp-content/uploads/2013/12/forum-summary-report.pdf.
23. McIlhenny C, Pitts D. Standards for Surgical Trainers. Faculty of surgical trainers, Royal College of Surgeons of Edinburgh. http://fst.rcsed.ac.uk/media/9403/surgical-trainers-lr.pdf.
24. Harkin D, Beard J, Wyatt M, Shearman C. Vascular Society UK Workforce Report. In: Society V, editor. http://www.vascularsociety.org.uk/wp-content/uploads/2014/07/VS-UK-Workforce-Report.pdf. p. p.25.
25. Garrett K, Kaups KL. The aging surgeon: when is it time to leave active practice? Bull Am Coll Surg. 2014;99(4):32–5.
26. Greenaway D. Securing the future of excellent patient care. The Shape of Training. http://www.shapeoftraining.co.uk/static/documents/content/Shape_of_training_FINAL_Report.pdf_53977887.pdf.
27. Ferguson H, Fitzgerald E, Shalhoub J, Gokani V, Beamish A. The Shape of Training Review 2013: A Response on behalf of the Council of the Association of Surgeons in Training. http://www.asit.org/assets/documents/ShoT20Response20Final20Draft.pdf. 2013

28

First clinical experiences of concurrent bleeding control and intracranial pressure monitoring using a hybrid emergency room system in patients with multiple injuries

Takahiro Kinoshita[1*], Kazuma Yamakawa[1], Jumpei Yoshimura[1], Atsushi Watanabe[1], Yosuke Matsumura[2], Kaori Ito[3], Hiroyuki Ohbe[4], Kei Hayashida[5], Shigeki Kushimoto[4], Junichi Matsumoto[6], Satoshi Fujimi[1] and on behalf of the Japanese Association for Hybrid Emergency Room System (JA-HERS) Scientific Promotion Committee

Abstract

Background: The outcomes of multiple injury patients with concomitant torso hemorrhage and traumatic brain injury (TBI) are very poor. The hybrid emergency room system (HERS) is a trauma management system designed to complete resuscitation, computed tomography (CT), surgery, angioembolization, and intracranial pressure (ICP) monitoring all in one trauma resuscitation room without patient transfer. We aimed to review the outcomes of polytrauma patients who underwent concurrent bleeding control and ICP monitoring using the HERS.

Methods: In this retrospective observational study, we enrolled patients who underwent concurrent bleeding control and ICP monitoring using the HERS between August 2011 and June 2018. Initial data on vital signs, Injury Severity Score (ISS), probability of survival (Ps) calculated by the Trauma and Injury Severity Score (TRISS), intervention type, 28-day mortality, and Extended Glasgow Outcome Scale at 6 months after injury were collected. Continuous variables were expressed as the median (25th and 75th percentiles) and categorical variables as numbers (%).

Results: Ten patients were included in the analysis. The injury severity of the patients was as high as an ISS of 58 (50–64) and TRISS Ps of 0.15 (0.02–0.36). Seven of the 10 (70%) patients had hemodynamic instability within 30 min from arrival. The recorded durations from arrival to events were CT examination 9 (6–16) min, bleeding control procedure 29 (22–42) min, and neurosurgical intervention 39 (31–53) min. Four of the 10 patients (40%) survived to discharge, and two of them (20%) were able to live independently at 6 months after injury.

Conclusions: The concurrent performance of bleeding control procedure and ICP monitoring would be feasible in HERS settings among polytrauma patients with exsanguinating hemorrhage and TBI.

Keywords: Concurrent treatment, Functional outcome, HERS, Mortality, Polytrauma

Background

Advanced Trauma Life Support guidelines have long been used in the initial management of patients with suspicions of severe injury [1]. These guidelines emphasize limiting the use of computed tomography (CT) as a detailed secondary survey examination only in hemodynamically stable patients without an apparent indication for emergency surgery. Thus, CT scanning for hemodynamically unstable patients is not practical until the completion of emergency bleeding control surgery even in cases with a decreased level of consciousness; traumatic brain injury (TBI) in conjunction with torso hemorrhage is often left untreated or even unidentified. This notion is based on the concern that CT is a time-consuming procedure that involves the considerable risk of deterioration during CT scanning itself and/or patient transfer to CT suites. Although the emergence of multidetector-row CT has dramatically reduced the

* Correspondence: ogmc.dmat.t.kinoshita@gmail.com
[1]Division of Trauma and Surgical Critical Care, Osaka General Medical Center, 3-1-56 Bandai-Higashi, Sumiyoshi-ku, Osaka 558-8558, Japan
Full list of author information is available at the end of the article

time required for CT scanning [2], the time delay to definitive surgery associated with the transfer of patients to a room with CT equipment remains unacceptable in those with hemodynamic instability.

The hybrid emergency room system (HERS) is a novel trauma management system that is potentially suitable for the evaluation and care of severe multiple injury patients [3–5]. The key component of this system is the trauma resuscitation room that is designed for the completion of all the examinations and treatments in a single place and which includes angio-CT equipment, a ventilator, a vital sign monitor, ultrasonography equipment, and surgical, neurosurgical, and interventional radiology (IR) instruments. Our novel trauma workflow using the HERS enables the performance of whole-body CT even in hemodynamically unstable patients with hemodynamic resuscitation under monitoring [4]. Furthermore, it is possible to concurrently perform bleeding control procedures including thoracotomy, laparotomy, preperitoneal pelvic packing, and endovascular intervention and surgical intracranial pressure (ICP) monitoring without patient transfer, based on CT findings. This progress allows for the advancement of titrating neuroprotective therapies formulated according to the CT findings, ICP, and cerebral perfusion pressure (CPP) in the bleeding control intervention phases.

Previously, we reported that a novel trauma workflow using the HERS was significantly associated with reduced mortality in severe blunt trauma patients [4] and improved functional outcomes in patients with severe TBI [5]. In the present study, we aimed to review a series of patients with hemorrhagic torso injury in conjunction with TBI, who underwent concurrent bleeding control and ICP monitoring.

Methods

Study population

In this retrospective observational study, we enrolled consecutive blunt polytrauma patients who underwent concurrent bleeding control and ICP monitoring using the HERS in the Osaka General Medical Center from August 2011 to June 2018. We defined concurrent treatment as a combination of interventions in which the recorded durations of bleeding control (through direct surgery or endovascular embolization) and ICP monitoring and/or ventriculostomy overlapped, whichever started first. Patients with cardiopulmonary arrest on arrival, who underwent bleeding control and ICP monitoring separately and who were transferred from other hospitals, were excluded from the analysis. The study was approved by the Institutional Review Board of the Osaka General Medical Center (#30-S07-001). The board waived the need for informed consent, as this was a retrospective study.

Treatment strategy for polytrauma patients

In the Osaka General Medical Center, an original approach was formulated for polytrauma patients with concomitant exsanguinating hemorrhage and TBI. First, airway and breathing abnormalities were evaluated and fixed at the earliest after patients' arrival. We fundamentally performed whole-body CT to detect all life-threatening injuries including torso hemorrhages and TBIs even in patients with shock since CT could be conducted within approximately 10 min from arrival through the use of angio-CT equipment, with hemodynamic resuscitation under continuous monitoring [4]. If patients' vital signs were too unstable for 10-min CT scanning, we proceeded to more aggressive resuscitation including blood transfusion, resuscitative thoracotomy, and resuscitative endovascular balloon occlusion of the aorta (REBOA). When REBOA was used prior to CT examination, a self-propelled C-arm was manipulated to the patient table for the insertion of the REBOA catheter with a fluoroscopic guide. The aorta was occluded partially rather than fully, targeting a systolic blood pressure (BP) of 90–100 mmHg for the preservation of cerebral blood flow and also the prevention of possible intracranial hemorrhage expansion.

When life-threatening torso hemorrhage and TBI were observed on CT, we embarked upon the simultaneous treatment of both injuries. An attending trauma surgeon decided on the performance of direct surgery (thoracotomy, laparotomy, and preperitoneal pelvic packing), angioembolization, or both based on CT findings. At the same time, an attending neurosurgeon initiated intracranial surgery for ICP monitoring and/or ventriculostomy without waiting for the completion of the bleeding control procedure (Fig. 1). If a space-occupying lesion with a midline shift was identified in the CT images, the neurosurgeons created two burr holes in the frontal bone and attempted to evacuate epidural or subdural hematomas to the greatest extent possible. Discussions were held with trauma surgeons for the provision of the best available neurocritical care for each patient guided by early ICP monitoring. More specifically, neuroprotective treatments to maintain a CPP ≥ 60 mmHg were selected from among 30° head elevation, sedation, analgesia, hyperosmolar treatment, and the administration of fluid, blood, and inotropes, with attention to hemodynamic status and the anatomical sites of injuries. After the completion of concurrent treatment, we routinely re-evaluated the brain CT and determined if craniotomy was to be added in an operating room or if continued critical/neurocritical care was to be provided in an intensive care unit.

Data collection

Initial data on vital signs (Glasgow Coma Scale total score, BP, and heart rate [HR]) were collected for the first

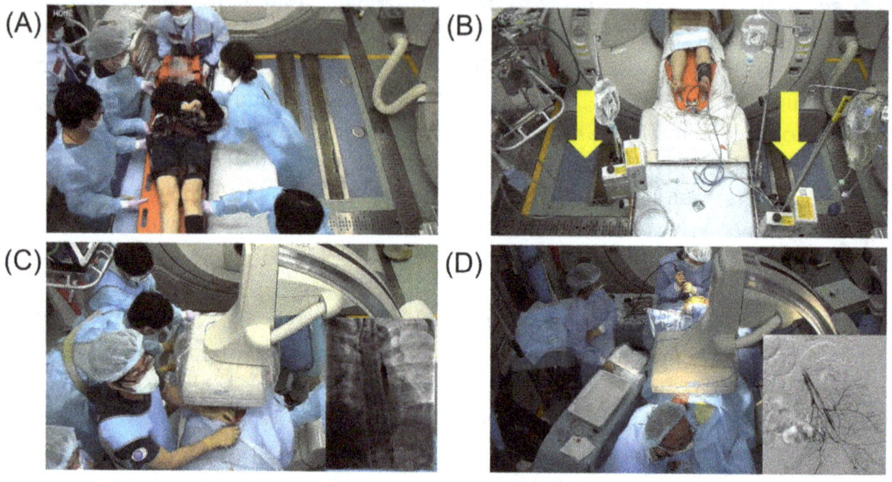

Fig. 1 Photographs of the concurrent treatments performed using the HERS. **a** All doctors and nurses wear radiation protection products before patients' arrival. Patients are directly accommodated in the hybrid emergency room on arrival. Chest X-ray, pelvic X-ray, and FAST are not performed routinely preceding CT scanning. **b** After intravenous access is achieved, whole-body CT examination is performed as soon as possible. Head and neck CT are routinely performed without contrast and chest, abdominal, and pelvic CT with contrast. The gantry of the CT scanner moves instead of the patients' table during CT scanning. **c** A REBOA catheter is inserted with fluoroscopic guidance to avoid complications. The balloon inflation volume is controlled to maintain a systolic BP of 90–100 mmHg before ICP measurement and to preserve a CPP ≥ 60 mmHg after ICP monitoring. **d** Bleeding control procedures and ICP monitoring and/or ventriculostomy are performed simultaneously if active torso bleeding and significant intracranial lesion are detected by CT. Neurosurgeons make sure not to interfere with surgical procedures and IR since priority is always given to hemostasis. BP, blood pressure; CPP, cerebral perfusion pressure; CT, computed tomography; FAST, focused assessment with sonography for trauma; HERS, hybrid emergency room system; ICP, intracranial pressure; IR, interventional radiology; REBOA, resuscitative endovascular balloon occlusion of the aorta

measurement. The lowest BP within 30 min from arrival was also extracted from patients' records. Unstable vital signs were defined as hypotension (systolic BP ≤ 90 mmHg), tachycardia (HR ≥ 120 beats per minutes), or deterioration of BP (systolic BP ≤ 90 mmHg) within 30 min after arrival, indicating the high risk associated with transferring patients to a CT room in the conventional trauma workflow. The results of laboratory tests including platelet counts, prothrombin time-international normalized ratio, and activated partial thromboplastin time were collected. The Abbreviated Injury Scale of each body region was recorded to measure the Injury Severity Score (ISS). Findings from the initial CT examination were categorized based on Marshall CT classification: diffuse injury I, II, III, IV, and non-evacuated mass lesion [6]. The probability of survival (Ps) was calculated using the Trauma and Injury Severity Score (TRISS) (coefficients were b0 − 1.2470, b1 0.9544, b2 − 0.0768, and b3 − 1.9052) [7]. Data on the type of surgery, IR, and neurosurgical intervention conducted in the hybrid emergency room were recorded. The intervals from patient arrival to CT examination, the bleeding control procedure, and ICP measurement were described. Data on 24-h mortality were extracted from patient records, and the Extended Glasgow Outcome Scale at 6 months post injury was evaluated from records, referral documents, or telephone interviews.

Descriptive statistics

Continuous variables were expressed as the median (25th and 75th percentiles) as the data were not normally distributed. Categorical variables were described as numbers (%). Descriptive statistics were performed with R software packages (version 3.1.0; R Foundation for Statistical Computing, Vienna, Austria).

Results

Of 2686 eligible patients admitted for trauma in the Osaka General Medical Center during the 8-year study period, 10 were identified for the reception of concurrent bleeding control and ICP monitoring (Fig. 2). Table 1 shows the patients' baseline characteristics. The age of the patients was 43 (30–60) years. The injury severity of the patients was extremely high, as indicated by the ISS 58 (50–64) and TRISS Ps 0.15 (0.02–0.36). Most of the included patients had high risks for the performance of whole-body CT in conventional trauma settings, since all but three had hemorrhagic shock status on arrival or their condition deteriorated within 30 min of arrival.

Table 2 shows the contents and timelines of interventions and patients' outcome. The recorded durations from patient arrival to events were CT examination, 9 (6–16) min; bleeding control procedure, 29 (22–42) min; and neurosurgical intervention, 39 (31–53) min. ICP monitoring was used not only to guide patients'

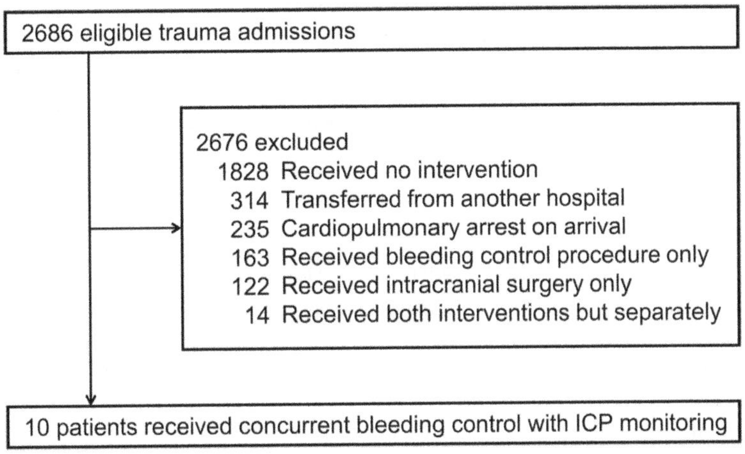

Fig. 2 Patient enrollment flow diagram. ICP, intracranial pressure

neurocritical care but also to prepare for further neurosurgical interventions, with concerns of expanded intracranial hemorrhage during the bleeding control procedure in one patient (No. 5), in whom the ICP was elevated to 40 mmHg in the midst of an endovascular intervention, suggesting the indication for emergency craniotomy. Two of the patients (Nos. 7 and 9) underwent REBOA for hemodynamic stabilization before CT scanning. In these patients, partial REBOA was applied to avoid an excessive increase in the ICP and intracranial hemorrhage exacerbations. Specifically, we attempted to control the balloon inflation volume to maintain a systolic BP of 90–100 mmHg before ICP measurement and to preserve a CPP ≥ 60 mmHg after ICP monitoring (see video, Additional file 1: Digital Content 1, which demonstrates the trauma workflow in one patient with concomitant torso exsanguinating hemorrhage and severe TBI [No. 7]).

Four of the 10 patients (40%) survived to discharge and two of them (Nos. 7, 8) were able to live independently at 6 months after injury. None of the patients was considered to have perished from exsanguination since the CPP decreased to less than 20 mmHg before hemodynamic collapse in all patients who did not survive.

Discussions

In this study, we reported the clinical courses of multiple injury patients who underwent the simultaneous performance of a bleeding control procedure and rigorous ICP/CPP-oriented neuroprotective management. We confirmed that concurrent treatment for the exsanguination of torso hemorrhage and TBI was feasible in HERS settings. Furthermore, four of our patients had survival to discharge and two had favorable functional outcomes at 6 months post injury. Notably, we were able to successfully treat two patients with the most severe injuries,

Table 1 Baseline characteristics of the multiple injury patients who underwent concurrent treatment

Case	Age (years)	Sex	GCS total score	Initial BP (mmHg)	HR (bpm)	Lowest BP within 30 min (mmHg)	Platelet count (× 10^4/L)	PT-INR	aPTT (s)	Marshall CT classification	ISS	Ps
1	52	Female	6	183/137	140	66/52	13.9	1.5	65	Diffuse injury IV	59	0.37
2	62	Female	3	154/88	56	74/40	12.3	1.7	> 200	Non-evacuated mass lesion	66	0.01
3	72	Female	10	155/116	113	112/45	17.4	1.3	56	Non-evacuated mass lesion	59	0.15
4	36	Male	3	142/59	133	88/42	12.8	1.7	63	Diffuse injury III	66	0.07
5	49	Male	8	126/78	97	107/65	16.0	1.2	35	Non-evacuated mass lesion	45	0.65
6	34	Male	4	194/147	116	52/20	21.2	1.4	54	Non-evacuated mass lesion	50	0.36
7	29	Female	3	46/25	151	30/20	18.3	1.7	74	Non-evacuated mass lesion	57	0.02
8	18	Female	8	110/80	155	105/79	17.0	1.5	52	Diffuse injury II	50	0.49
9	29	Female	3	60/30	117	58/37	15.2	1.4	44	Non-evacuated mass lesion	66	0.02
10	74	Male	6	175/111	102	97/70	17.2	1.1	50	Non-evacuated mass lesion	45	0.25

Ps was calculated using the Trauma and Injury Severity score

aPTT activated partial thromboplastin time, *BP* blood pressure, *CT* computed tomography, *GCS* Glasgow Coma Scale, *HR* heart rate, *ISS* Injury Severity Score, *Ps* probability of survival, *PT-INR* prothrombin time-international normalized ratio

Table 2 Contents and timelines of interventions and patients' outcomes

Case	Time to CT scan (min)	Bleeding control procedure	Time to bleeding control procedure (min)	Intracranial surgery	Time to intracranial surgery (min)	24-h mortality	GOS-E at 6 months
1	5	Angioembolization (IIA)	54	ICP measurement, burr hole drainage	53	Dead	D
2	7	Angioembolization (ICA, IIA)	28	ICP measurement, craniotomy	28	Dead	D
3	10	Angioembolization (IIA)	43	ICP measurement	51	Dead	D
4	6	PPP, angioembolization (IIA)	21	ICP measurement, ventricular drainage	29	Alive	VS
5	9	Angioembolization (ICA)	30	ICP measurement, craniotomy	35	Alive	Upper SD
6	18	Angioembolization (ICA, SA, IIA)	25	ICP measurement, burr hole drainage	26	Alive	D
7	24	REBOA, angioembolization (HA, IIA), PPP	18	ICP measurement, burr hole drainage	56	Alive	Lower MD
8	5	Angioembolization (ITA)	47	ICP measurement	43	Alive	Lower MD
9	18	REBOA, PPP, angioembolization (IIA)	13	ICP measurement, burr hole drainage	35	Dead	D
10	9	PPP, angioembolization (IIA)	40	ICP measurement, craniotomy	59	Alive	D

CT computed tomography, *D* death, *GOS-E* Extended Glasgow Outcome Scale, *HA* hepatic artery, *ICA* intercostal artery, *ICP* intracranial pressure, *IIA* internal iliac artery, *ITA* internal thoracic artery, *MD* moderate disability, *PPP* preperitoneal pelvic packing, *REBOA* resuscitative endovascular balloon occlusion of the aorta, *SA* splenic artery, *SD* severe disability, *VS* vegetative state

who had TRISS Ps as low as 0.02 and 0.07. To the best of our knowledge, this is the first study to report on the outcomes of patients who received concurrent surgery/angioembolization with neurocritical care following ICP monitoring in HERS settings.

Exsanguination and TBI are reciprocally harmful, creating a vicious circle; hemorrhage causes hypotensive secondary brain injury that increases the mortality associated with TBI [8–13] while TBI leads to coagulopathy that precludes hemorrhagic injuries from hemostasis [14–17]. These relations lead to extremely poor outcomes in polytrauma patients with active thoracic, abdominal, and retroperitoneal hemorrhage and severe TBI. For example, a recent post hoc study of a randomized control trial reported that patients with concomitant TBI and hemorrhagic shock had significantly higher mortality, received higher amounts of transfusion, and developed a higher proportion of respiratory complications than patients without TBI and hemorrhagic shock [18]. Nevertheless, there is no consensus regarding an effective method that can be used to reduce the associated mortality and improve the functional outcomes of these patients. Concurrent treatment is potentially beneficial in the provision of appropriate neurocritical care based on ICP/CPP without the need to wait for the completion of bleeding control procedures. However, the performance of this treatment is basically impractical in hemorrhagic shock patients because the evaluation of TBI by CT is considered a prerequisite for neurosurgical intervention even though patients with an unstable condition require bleeding control before CT.

The HERS was designed to overcome this problem. The installation of a CT scanner in a trauma resuscitation room enabled the performance of CT, which is indispensable for TBI management even in hemodynamically unstable patients. Furthermore, the introduction of surgical and neurosurgical instruments as well as a C-arm in this room allowed for the simultaneous provision of damage control surgery, endovascular intervention including REBOA and angioembolization, and invasive ICP measurement and/or ventriculostomy. That is to say, we were able to perform concurrent treatment for multiple injury patients by combining the functions of a CT scan room with the recently reported-upon hybrid operating room [19]. We believe the HERS, which was invented with high aspiration to provide resuscitation, CT examination, damage control surgery, IR, and ICP monitoring "all in one room", is an ideal trauma suite setting for the realization of this innovative intervention.

The present study has several limitations. First, we could not find a well-matched comparative group due to the retrospective nature of the study design. It was impossible to demonstrate an existence of TBI in patients in whom we suspected multiple injuries within the conventional period, because these patients frequently died during or soon after bleeding control procedure without CT scanning. Therefore, the effectiveness of concurrent treatment, using the HERS, on patient outcomes should be investigated in a prospective study. Second, we did not determine the indication for concurrent treatment. We provided it when an attending surgeon and neurosurgeon who participated in trauma resuscitation decided that both a bleeding control procedure and ICP monitoring were required and feasible based on CT findings. The objective indication for concurrent treatment should be investigated in a future study. Third, the management strategy other than concurrent treatment may have changed during the study period since the 8-year observational period was relatively long. Finally, we did not provide this treatment to penetrating trauma patients. As the efficacy of whole-body CT scanning in penetrating trauma is still not well-explored, we could not discuss the effect of the present treatment in this population.

Conclusions

We described the first clinical case series of patients who underwent concurrent bleeding control and ICP monitoring using the HERS. The HERS could be a breakthrough in the treatment of the most severe polytrauma cases requiring both bleeding control and neurosurgical procedures. The effect of the concurrent treatment on patients' clinical outcomes should be investigated in a prospective interventional study.

Abbreviations

BP: Blood pressure; CPP: Cerebral perfusion pressure; CT: Computed tomography; HERS: Hybrid emergency room system; HR: Heart rate; ICP: Intracranial pressure; IR: Interventional radiology; ISS: Injury severity score; Ps: Probability of survival; REBOA: Resuscitative endovascular balloon occlusion of the aorta; TBI: Traumatic brain injury; TRISS: Trauma and Injury Severity Score

Acknowledgements

We would like to thank all of the members in the Japanese Association for Hybrid Emergency Room System.

Funding

The authors have no funding to report.

Authors' contributions

TK and KY conceived, designed, and coordinated the study. TK wrote the initial draft of the manuscript. AW, JY, YM, KI, and HO contributed to the interpretation of data and assisted in the preparation of the manuscript. KH, SK, and JM critically reviewed the manuscript. SF provided critical appraisal of the manuscript. All authors have read and approved the final manuscript.

Competing interests

TK has received lecture fees and travel expenses from Canon Medical Systems for lectures given at national and international conferences. YM was a Clinical Advisory Board Member of Tokai Medical Products (2015–2017). The remaining authors declare that they have no competing interests.

Author details

[1]Division of Trauma and Surgical Critical Care, Osaka General Medical Center, 3-1-56 Bandai-Higashi, Sumiyoshi-ku, Osaka 558-8558, Japan. [2]Department of Emergency and Critical Care Medicine, Chiba University Graduate School of Medicine, 1-8-1 Inohana, Chuo-ku, Chiba 260-0856, Japan. [3]Department of Emergency Medicine, Division of Acute Care Surgery, Teikyo University School of Medicine, 2-11-1 Kaga, Itabashi-ku, Tokyo 173-8606, Japan. [4]Division of Emergency and Critical Care Medicine, Tohoku University Graduate School of Medicine, 1-1 Seiryo-cho, Aoba-ku, Sendai 980-8574, Japan. [5]Department of Emergency and Critical Care Medicine, School of Medicine, Keio University, 35 Shinanomachi, Shinjuku-ku, Tokyo 160-8582, Japan. [6]Department of Emergency and Critical Care Medicine, St. Marianna University School of Medicine, 2-16-1 Sugao, Miyamae-ku, Kawasaki 216-8511, Japan.

References

1. American College of Surgeons Committee on Trauma. ATLS Advanced Trauma Life Support program for doctors. Student course manual. 10th ed. Chicago, IL: American College of Surgeons; 2018.
2. Rieger M, Czermak B, El Attal R, Sumann G, Jaschke W, Freund M. Initial clinical experience with a 64-MDCT whole-body scanner in an emergency department: better time management and diagnostic quality? J Trauma. 2009;66:648–57.
3. Wada D, Nakamori Y, Yamakawa K, Fujimi S. First clinical experience with IVR-CT system in the emergency room: positive impact on trauma workflow. Scand J Trauma Resusc Emerg Med. 2012;20:52.
4. Kinoshita T, Yamakawa K, Matsuda H, Yoshikawa Y, Wada D, Hamasaki T, et al. The survival benefit of a novel trauma workflow that includes immediate whole-body computed tomography, surgery, and interventional radiology, all in one trauma resuscitation room: a retrospective historical control study. Ann Surg. 2017. https://doi.org/10.1097/SLA.0000000000002527.
5. Kinoshita T, Hayashi M, Yamakawa K, Watanabe A, Yoshimura J, Hamasaki T, et al. Effect of the hybrid emergency room system on functional outcome in patients with severe traumatic brain injury. World Neurosurg. 2018;118: e792–9.
6. Marshall LF, Marshall SB, Klauber MR, Van Berkum Clark M, Eisenberg H, Jane JA, et al. The diagnosis of head injury requires a classification based on computed axial tomography. J Neurotrauma. 1992;9:S287–92.
7. Champion HR, Copes WS, Sacco WJ, Lawnick MM, Keast SL, Bain LW Jr, et al. The major trauma outcome study: establishing national norms for trauma care. J Trauma. 1990;30:1356–65.
8. Chesnut RM, Marshall LF, Klauber MR, Blunt BA, Baldwin N, Eisenberg HM, et al. The role of secondary brain injury in determining outcome from severe head injury. J Trauma. 1993;34:216–22.
9. Chesnut RM, Marshall SB, Piek J, Blunt BA, Klauber MR, Marshall LF. Early and late systemic hypotension as a frequent and fundamental source of cerebral ischemia following severe brain injury in the Traumatic Coma Data Bank. Acta Neurochir Suppl (Wien). 1993;59:121–5.
10. Manley G, Knudson MM, Morabito D, Damron S, Erickson V, Pitts L. Hypotension, hypoxia, and head injury: frequency, duration, and consequences. Arch Surg. 2001;136:1118–23.
11. Kauvar DS, Lefering R, Wade CE. Impact of hemorrhage on trauma outcome: an overview of epidemiology, clinical presentations, and therapeutic considerations. J Trauma. 2006;60(6 Suppl):S3–11.
12. Butcher I, Maas AI, Lu J, Marmarou A, Murray GD, Mushkudiani NA, et al. Prognostic value of admission blood pressure in traumatic brain injury: results from the IMPACT study. J Neurotrauma. 2007;24:294–302.
13. Zafar SN, Millham FH, Chang Y, Fikry K, Alam HB, King DR, et al. Presenting blood pressure in traumatic brain injury: a bimodal distribution of death. J Trauma. 2011;71:1179–84.
14. Halpern CH, Reilly PM, Turtz AR, Stein SC. Traumatic coagulopathy: the effect of brain injury. J Neurotrauma. 2008;25:997–1001.
15. Talving P, Benfield R, Hadjizacharia P, Inaba K, Chan LS, Demetriades D. Coagulopathy in severe traumatic brain injury: a prospective study. J Trauma. 2009;66:55–62.
16. Maegele M. Coagulopathy after traumatic brain injury: incidence, pathogenesis, and treatment options. Transfusion. 2013;53(Suppl 1):28S–37S.
17. Genét GF, Johansson PI, Meyer MA, Sølbeck S, Sørensen AM, Larsen CF, et al. Trauma-induced coagulopathy: standard coagulation tests, biomarkers of coagulopathy, and endothelial damage in patients with traumatic brain injury. J Neurotrauma. 2013;30:301–6.
18. Galvagno SM Jr, Fox EE, Appana SN, Baraniuk S, Bosarge PL, Bulger EM, et al. Outcomes after concomitant traumatic brain injury and hemorrhagic shock: a secondary analysis from the pragmatic, randomized optimal platelets and plasma ratios trial. J Trauma Acute Care Surg. 2017;83:668–74.
19. Kirkpatrick AW, Vis C, Dubé M, Biesbroek S, Ball CG Laberge J, Shultz J, et al. The evolution of a purpose designed hybrid trauma operating room from the trauma service perspective: the RAPTOR (resuscitation with angiography percutaneous treatments and operative resuscitations). Injury. 2014;45:1413–21.

Permissions

All chapters in this book were first published in WJES, by BioMed Central; hereby published with permission under the Creative Commons Attribution License or equivalent. Every chapter published in this book has been scrutinized by our experts. Their significance has been extensively debated. The topics covered herein carry significant findings which will fuel the growth of the discipline. They may even be implemented as practical applications or may be referred to as a beginning point for another development.

The contributors of this book come from diverse backgrounds, making this book a truly international effort. This book will bring forth new frontiers with its revolutionizing research information and detailed analysis of the nascent developments around the world.

We would like to thank all the contributing authors for lending their expertise to make the book truly unique. They have played a crucial role in the development of this book. Without their invaluable contributions this book wouldn't have been possible. They have made vital efforts to compile up to date information on the varied aspects of this subject to make this book a valuable addition to the collection of many professionals and students.

This book was conceptualized with the vision of imparting up-to-date information and advanced data in this field. To ensure the same, a matchless editorial board was set up. Every individual on the board went through rigorous rounds of assessment to prove their worth. After which they invested a large part of their time researching and compiling the most relevant data for our readers.

The editorial board has been involved in producing this book since its inception. They have spent rigorous hours researching and exploring the diverse topics which have resulted in the successful publishing of this book. They have passed on their knowledge of decades through this book. To expedite this challenging task, the publisher supported the team at every step. A small team of assistant editors was also appointed to further simplify the editing procedure and attain best results for the readers.

Apart from the editorial board, the designing team has also invested a significant amount of their time in understanding the subject and creating the most relevant covers. They scrutinized every image to scout for the most suitable representation of the subject and create an appropriate cover for the book.

The publishing team has been an ardent support to the editorial, designing and production team. Their endless efforts to recruit the best for this project, has resulted in the accomplishment of this book. They are a veteran in the field of academics and their pool of knowledge is as vast as their experience in printing. Their expertise and guidance has proved useful at every step. Their uncompromising quality standards have made this book an exceptional effort. Their encouragement from time to time has been an inspiration for everyone.

The publisher and the editorial board hope that this book will prove to be a valuable piece of knowledge for researchers, students, practitioners and scholars across the globe.

List of Contributors

Jacopo Andreuccetti, Cecilia Ceribelli, Ottavia Manto, Massimo Chiaretti, Paolo Negro and Domenico Tuscano
Department of General Surgery and Organ Transplantation, "Sapienza" Università di Roma, Umberto I Policlinico di Roma, Rome, Italy

Hakan Guven, Bora Koc, Fazil Saglam and Gokhan Adas
Department of Surgery, Okmeydanı Training and Research Hospital, İstanbul, Turkey

Irem Akin Bayram
Faculty of Medicine, Department of Radiology, İstanbul University, İstanbul, Turkey

Bora Koc
Department of Surgery, Başkent University, Oymacı sokak No: 7 Altunizade, İstanbul, Turkey

Naoto Fukuda, Joji Wada and Michio Niki
Department of Surgery, Kawasaki Kyodo Hospital, Kawasaki 210-0833, Japan

Yasuyuki Sugiyama and Hiroyuki Mushiake
Department of Surgery, Teikyo University School of Medicine, University Hospital, Mizonokuchi, Kawasaki 213-8507, Japan

I Michael Leitman, Kei Suzuki, Aaron J Wengrofsky, Eyal Menashe, Michal Poplawski, Charles M Geller, David Lucido, Thomas Bernik and Byron Patton
Departments of Surgery, Albert Einstein College of Medicine-Beth Israel Medical Center, 10 Union Square East, Suite 2M, New York, NY 10003, USA

Kar-Mun Woo
Emergency Medicine, Albert Einstein College of Medicine-Beth Israel Medical Center, New York, NY, USA

Barbara A Zeifer
Radiology, Albert Einstein College of Medicine-Beth Israel Medical Center, New York, NY, USA

Laura Godat, Leslie Kobayashi, Todd Costantini and Raul Coimbra
Division of Trauma, Surgical Critical Care, and Burns, University of California, San Diego, 200 West Arbor Dr., #8896, San Diego CA 92103-8896, United States of America

Katsutoshi Sato, Yoshiharu Hamanaka, Norimasa Mitsui, Shinji Hirai and Naru Chatani
Department of Thoracic Surgery, Hiroshima Prefectural Hospital, Hiroshima, Japan, Ujinakanda 1-5-54, Minami-ku, Hiroshima, 734-8530, Japan

Takashi Nishisaka
Department of Pathology, Hiroshima Prefectural Hospital, Hiroshima, Japan, Ujinakanda 1-5-54, Minami-ku, Hiroshima, 734-8530, Japan

Kazumasa Orihashi
Department of Cardiovascular Surgery, Hiroshima University Hospital, Hiroshima, Japan, Kasumi 1-2-3, Minami-ku, Hiroshima, 734-8551, Japan

Richard C Turner
Department of Surgery, Hobart Clinical School, University of Tasmania, Hobart, Australia

Christina M Steffen and Peter Boyd
Department of Surgery, Cairns Base Hospital, Cairns & Hinterland Health Service District, Cairns, Australia

Fatih Altintoprak and Orhan Veli Ozkan
Department of General Surgery, Faculty of Medicine, Sakarya University, Sakarya, Turkey

Yusuf Arslan, Omer Yalkin and Yener Uzunoglu
Department of General Surgery, Research and Educational Hospital, Sakarya University, Sakarya, Turkey

Ali I Yahya, Hussen E Shwereif, Mustafa A Ekheil, Ahmed S Thoboot, Kalid A Algader, Fatma O Gyaed and Abdsalem S Aldarat
General surgery department, Zliten Teaching Hospital and Edwaw District Hospital, Zliten, Libya

Federico Coccolini, Paolo Bertoli, Michela Giulii Capponi, Marco Lotti, Roberto Manfredi, Michele Pisano, Elia Poiasina, Eugenio Poletti and Luca Ansaloni
General and Emergency Surgery Department, Ospedali Riuniti, Bergamo, Italy

Ferdinando Agresta
General Surgery Department, Adria Hospital, Rovigo, Italy

Andrea Bassi and Feliciano Crovella
General Surgery Department, Cotugno Hospital-CTO, Naples, Italy

Fausto Catena
General and Emergency Surgery Department, Ospedale Maggiore, Parma, Italy

Roberto Ferrara
General Surgery Department, Ospedale Centrale, Bolzano, Italy

Paolo Negro and Francesco Gossetti
General Surgery Department, La Sapienza Univesity Hospital, Rome, Italy

Micaela Piccoli, Gianluigi Melotti and Domenico Marchi
General Surgery Department, New Sant'Agostino Hospital, Modena, Italy

Michele Schiano di Visconte and Gabriele Munegato
General Surgery Department, Conegliano Hospital, Treviso, Italy

Massimo Sartelli
General Surgery Department, Macerata Hospital, Macerata, Italy

Mario Testini
Endocrine, Digestive and Emergency Surgery Department, Aldo Moro University Hospital, Bari, Italy

Andrea M Pakula and Ruby A Skinner
Department of Surgery, Division of Trauma and Surgical Critical Care, Kern Medical Center, Bakersfield, California

Wendy Phillips
Department of Nutrition and Dietary Services, Kern Medical Center, Bakersfield, California

Ram Venkatesh Anantha and Muriel Brackstone
Division of General Surgery, Department of Surgery, Schulich School of Medicine and Dentistry, Western University, London, Ontario, Canada

Neil Parry
Division of Critical Care, Department of Medicine, Schulich School of Medicine and Dentistry, Western University, London, Ontario, Canada
Trauma Program, London Health Sciences Centre, London, Ontario, Canada

Ken Leslie
London Health Sciences Centre, Victoria Hospital, Room E2-217, 800 sCommissioners Road East, London, Ontario N6A 5 W9, Canada

Phillipe Abreu-Reis and Guilherme Czelusniak Oliveira
Federal University of Parana, Curitiba, Brazil
Hospital do Trabalhador, State Health Department, Parana, Brazil

Adonis Nasr and Flávio Daniel Saavedra Tomasich
Department of Surgery, Federal University of Parana, Curitiba, Brazil

Arthur Curtarelli de Oliveira
University Positivo, Curitiba, Brazil
Hospital do Trabalhador, State Health Department, Parana, Brazil

Hammad Sadique
University of Birmingham, UK

Mark Malota and Reinhard Kopps
Krankenhaus München Harlaching, Departement of Surgery, Munich, Germany

Markus C Kowarik
Klinikum Rechts der Isar, Munich, Germany

Barbara Bechtold
Krankenhaus München Harlaching, Departement of Anaesthesiology, Munich, Germany

Shamsi EL-Hasani
Minimal access and bariatric unit, King's College Hospital NHS Foundation Trust, Princess Royal University Hospital, Orpington, London BR6 8ND, UK

Abdulzahra Hussain
Honorary Senior Lecturer at King's College Medical School, London, UK

Muhammad R Khan and Sameer ur Rehman
Department of Surgery and Medical College, Aga Khan University & Hospital, Stadium Road, Karachi, 74800, Pakistan

Frederico Teixeira, Eduardo Hiroshi Akaishi, Adriano Zuardi Ushinohama, Tiago Cypriano Dutra, Sérgio Dias do Couto Netto, Edivaldo Massazo Utiyama, Celso Oliveira Bernini and Samir Rasslan
Division of Clinical Surgery III, Department of Surgery, São Paulo University School of Medicine, São Paulo, Brazil

Ayman El-Menyar
Clinical Research, Trauma Surgery Section, Hamad General Hospital, Doha, Qatar

Ahammed Mekkodathil
Clinical Medicine, Weill Cornell Medical School, Doha, Qatar

Rafael Consunji
Hamad Injury Prevention Program, Trauma Surgery Section, Hamad General Hospital, Doha, Qatar

Hassan Al-Thani and Gaby Jabbour
Trauma Surgery Section, Hamad General Hospital, Doha, Qatar

Khalid A. Alyafei
Department of Pediatrics, Division of Pediatric Emergency Medicine, Hamadc Medical Corporation, Doha, Qatar

Kai Liu, Jiaxiang Meng, Shuofei Yang and Baochen Liu
Medical School of Nanjing University, Nanjing 210002, Jiangsu Province, P. R. China

Weiwei Ding, Xingjiang Wu and Jieshou Li
Research Institute of General Surgery, Jinling Hospital, 305 East Zhongshan Road, 210002 Nanjing, Jiangsu, China

Nan-Ping Yang
Department of Surgery & Orthopedics, Keelung Hospital, Ministry of Health & Welfare, Keelung, Taiwan

Dachen Chu
Faculty of Medicine, School of Medicine, National Yang-Ming University, Taipei, Taiwan
Institute of Public Health and Community Medicine Research Center, National Yang-Ming University, Taipei, Taiwan
Department of Neurosurgery, Taipei City Hospital, Taipei, Taiwan
Department of Health Care Management, National Taipei University of Nursing and Health Sciences, Taipei, Taiwan

Dinh-Van Phan, Ren-Hao Pan and Chien-Lung Chan
Department of Information Management, Yuan Ze University, Taoyuan, Taiwan
Innovation Center for Big Data and Digital Convergence, Yuan Ze University, Taoyuan, Taiwan

Nien-Tzu Chang
Department of Nursing, School of Nursing, College of Medicine, Chang-Gang University, Taoyuan, Taiwan
School of Nursing, College of Medicine, National Taiwan University, Taipei, Taiwan

Jin-Chyr Hsu
Department of Medicine, Taipei Hospital, Ministry of Health & Welfare, Taipei, Taiwan

Arianna Birindelli
Department of Surgery, University of Bologna, Bologna, Italy

Massimo Sartelli
Department of Surgery, Macerata Hospital, Macerata, Italy

Salomone Di Saverio
Department of Surgery, Maggiore Hospital, Bologna, Italy

Yoram Kluger
Division of General Surgery, Rambam Health Care Campus, Haifa, Israel

Gustavo P. Fraga
Division of Trauma Surgery, Hospital de Clinicas, School of Medical Sciences, University of Campinas,Campinas, Brazil

Carlos A. Ordonez
Department of Surgery, Universidad del Valle, Fundacion Valle del Lili, Cali, Colombia

Michael Sugrue
Letterkenny Hospital, Donegal, Ireland

Osvaldo Chiara
Niguarda Hospital, Milan, Italy

Luigi Bonavina, Yuri Macchitella and Emanuele Astis
Department of Surgery, IRCCS Policlinico San Donato, University of Milan Medical School, Piazza Malan 1, 20097 San Donato Milanese (Milano), Italy

Mircea Chirica
Department of Digestive Surgery, Saint-Louis Hospital, Paris, France

Ognjan Skrobic, Aleksander Simic and Predrag Pesko
Department of Surgery, University of Belgrade, Belgrade, Serbia

Yoram Kluger
Department of General Surgery, Rambam Health Care Campus, Haifa, Israel

Nelson A. Andreollo and Gustavo P. Fraga
Department of Surgery, University of Campinas, Campinas, Brasil

Sandro Contini
University of Parma, Parma, Italy

Luca Ansaloni and Federico Coccolini
General Surgery I, Papa Giovanni XXIII Hospital, Bergamo, Italy

Fausto Catena
Emergency Surgery Department, Maggiore Parma Hospital, Parma, Italy

Carlo Locatelli
Institute of Toxicology, University of Pavia, Pavia, Italy

Osvaldo Chiara
Emergency Department, Niguarda Hospital, Milan, Italy

Jeffry Kashuk
Department of Surgery, University of Jerusalem, Jerusalem, Rehovot, Israel

Massimiliano Mutignani
Department of Endoscopy, Niguarda Hospital, Milan, Italy

Cesare Cutrone
Department of Otolaryngology, Azienda Ospedaliera, Padova, Italy

Marco Dei Poli
Intensive Care Unit, IRCCS Policlinico San Donato, San Donato Milanese, Italy

Tino Valetti
Department of Anesthesiology, Papa Giovanni XXIII Hospital, Bergamo, Italy

Michael Kelly
Department of Surgery, Wagga Wagga Hospital, Wagga Wagga, Australia

Michele Pisano
General Surgery Papa Giovanni XXII Hospital Bergamo, Bergamo, Italy

Luigi Zorcolo
Colorectal Unit, Department of Surgery, University of Cagliari, Cagliari, Italy

Cecilia Merli
Unit of Emergency Medicine Ospedale Bufalini Cesena, AUSL Romagna, Romagna, Italy

Fikri M. Abu-Zidan
Department of Surgery, College of Medicine and Health Sciences, UAE University, Al-Ain, United Arab Emirates

Itamar Ashkenazi
Hillel Yaffe Medical Center Hadera, Hadera, Israel

Miklosh Bala
Trauma and Acute Care Surgery Unit Hadassah, Hebrew University Medical Center, Jerusalem, Israel

Gustavo P. Fraga
Division of Trauma Surgery, Department of Surgery, School of Medical Sciences, University of Campinas (Unicamp), Campinas, SP, Brazil

Ioran Kluger
Department of General Surgery, Division of Surgery, Rambam Health Care Campus, Haifa, Israel

Patrick B. Murphy, Richard Hilsden and Jennifer Koichopolos
Division of General Surgery, Department of Surgery, Schulich School of Medicine and Dentistry, Western University, London, Canada

Dave Paskar
Divisions of General Surgery Trauma & Critical Care Medicine, University of Toronto, Toronto, Canada

Tina S. Mele
Divisions of Critical Care, Department of Surgery, Schulich School of Medicine and Dentistry, Western University, London, Canada

Chip-Jin Ng, Shih-Hao You, Yi-Ming Weng, Chung-Hsien Chaou and Chen-June Seak
Department of Emergency Medicine, Chang Gung Memorial Hospital and Chang Gung University, Linko, Taiwan

I-Lin Wu
Department of Emergency, Taoyuan Armed Forces General Hospital, Taoyuan, Taiwan

Yi-Ming Weng
Department of Emergency Medicine, Prehospital Care Division, Taoyuan General Hospital, Ministry of Health and Welfare, No. 1492 Zhongshan Rd., Taoyuan Dist, Taoyuan City 330, Taiwan
Faculty of Medicine, National Yang-Ming University School of Medicine, Taipei, Taiwan

Cheng-Yu Chien
Department of Emergency Medicine, Ton-Yen General Hospital, Zhubei, Hsinchu County, Taiwan

G. Sganga
Istituto Clinica Chirurgica, Divisione Chirurgia Generale e Trapianti d'Organo, Università Cattolica del Sacro Cuore, Fondazione Policlinico Universitario Agostino Gemelli, Rome, Italy

C. Tascini
U.O. Malattie Infettive, Azienda Ospedaliera Universitaria Pisana, Pisa, Italy

E. Sozio
U.O. Medicina d'Urgenza Universitaria, Azienda Ospedaliera Universitaria Pisana, Pisa, Italy

M. Carlini
Chirurgia generale Ospedale Sant'Eugenio di Roma, Rome, Italy

P. Chirletti
Dipartimento di Chirurgia Università La Sapienza, Policlinico Umberto I, Rome, Italy

F. Cortese
UOC Chirurgia di Urgenza Ospedale San Filippo Neri, Rome, Italy

R. Gattuso
Dipartimento di Chirurgia Generale e Trapianti d'Organo, UOC Chirurgia Vascolare, Università La Sapienza, Policlinico Umberto I, Rome, Italy

P. Granone
Istituto Patologia Chirurgia, Unità Operativa Complessa Chirurgia Toracica, Università Cattolica del Sacro Cuore, Fondazione Policlinico Universitario Agostino Gemelli, Rome, Italy

C. Pempinello
Ortopedia e Traumatologia dell'Ospedale S. Gennaro ASL Napoli 1 Centro, Naples, Italy

M. Sartelli
U.O Chirurgia Generale Ospedale di Macerata, Macerata, Italy

S. Colizza
Master Sepsi in Chirurgia, Università Cattolica, Rome, Italy

A. E. Sharrock, V. J. Gokani, R. L. Harries, L. Pearce, S. R. Smith, O. Ali, H. Chu, A. Dubois, H. Ferguson, G. Humm, M. Marsden, D. Nepogodiev, M. Venn, S. Singh and C. Swain
Association of Surgeons in Training (ASiT), Royal College of Surgeons England, 35 - 43 Lincoln's Inn Fields, London WC2A 3P3, UK

J. Kirkby-Bott and A. E. Sharrock
Department of Emergency Surgery, Southampton General Hospital, Tremona Road, Southampton, Hampshire SO16 6YD, UK

Takahiro Kinoshita, Kazuma Yamakawa, Jumpei Yoshimura, Atsushi Watanabe and Satoshi Fujimi
Division of Trauma and Surgical Critical Care, Osaka General Medical Center, 3-1-56 Bandai-Higashi, Sumiyoshi-ku, Osaka 558-8558, Japan

Yosuke Matsumura
Department of Emergency and Critical Care Medicine, Chiba University Graduate School of Medicine, 1-8-1 Inohana, Chuo-ku, Chiba 260-0856, Japan

Kaori Ito
Department of Emergency Medicine, Division of Acute Care Surgery, Teikyo University School of Medicine, 2-11-1 Kaga, Itabashi-ku, Tokyo 173-8606, Japan

Hiroyuki Ohbe and Shigeki Kushimoto
Division of Emergency and Critical Care Medicine, Tohoku University Graduate School of Medicine, 1-1 Seiryo-cho, Aoba-ku, Sendai 980-8574, Japan

Kei Hayashida
Department of Emergency and Critical Care Medicine, School of Medicine, Keio University, 35 Shinanomachi, Shinjuku-ku, Tokyo 160-8582, Japan

Junichi Matsumoto
Department of Emergency and Critical Care Medicine, St. Marianna University School of Medicine, 2-16-1 Sugao, Miyamae-ku, Kawasaki 216-8511, Japan

Index

R

S

T

U

V

www.ingramcontent.com/pod-product-compliance
Lightning Source LLC
LaVergne TN
LVHW080702210926
848485LV00003B/407
9781639274888